Medicinal Plants
of the
Heartland

Connie Kaye

and

Neil Billington

Library of Congress Catalogue Card Number 96-086527
ISBN Number 0-9627422-8-7

1st Edition

Authors:
Connie Kaye
Neil Billington

Publisher:
Cache River Press
2850 Oak Grove Rd.
Vienna, IL 62995

Printed in the U.S.A.

To
Aristotel Pappelis
and
my mothers, Betty and Lola Mae,
who gave me the knowledge
and courage to be all that I can be.

Connie Kaye

To
Gordon (Daddy) Knight
who introduced me to biology
and
Patrick Fair and Paul Hebert
who helped fine-tune my
development.

Neil Billington

The Authors

Connie Kaye, Ph.D.

Connie obtained a Bachelor of Science in Zoology in 1968 from Southern Illinois University at Carbondale, SIU-C. Her interest in medicine was jump-started when she supported herself working as a nurses aide in the early 1960s. After receiving her degree, Connie worked as a bacteriologist in Peoria, Illinois, before returning to Carbondale to begin a family. She returned to SIU-C, earning a Master of Science degree in 1983, and a Doctor of Philosophy in 1989, both in botany. She specialized in botanical cytology, concentrating her research on the effect of plant growth regulators on ribosomal cistron regulation in the nucleoli of epidermal onion cells.

Connie's paternal great-grandmothers were both part Cherokee Indian. Being a botanist has given her the opportunity to research the native plants of the Heartland and their medicinal uses by her ancestors. Connie has also worked for the United States Department of Agriculture Forest Service located at Harrisburg, Illinois, collecting, pressing, drying and mounting herbarium specimens. Connie is currently teaching adult education courses on the medicinal plants of Southern Illinois at local junior colleges.

Neil Billington, Ph.D.

Neil Billington obtained a Bachelor of Science (Honors) in Animal and Plant Ecology in 1978 from Loughborough University in England. He earned his Doctor of Philosophy in 1985, also from Loughborough University, on the ecology of phytoplankton. Neil's interest in medicinal plants began when he worked in a wholefood cooperative in Loughborough, England. He also grew herbs for both culinary and medicinal use in his garden in Shepshed, England.

Neil moved to North America in 1983, working in Canada for eight years at the University of Windsor and the University of Guelph. He spent his summers in the Canadian Arctic studying the ecology of tundra ponds. While there, he maintained an interest in the food and medicinal plants used by the Canadian Indians and Inuit. He is currently an Assistant Professor of Zoology at Southern Illinois University at Carbondale, specializing in fish genetics in the Cooperative Fisheries Research Laboratory.

The Cover

T he drawing on the cover emphasizes the impact Native Americans have had on the development and growth of medicine throughout the Heartland. The circle represents the "dream catcher" because it was through visions (dreams) that the Medicine man or Shaman received his knowledge of where and how to use certain herbs.

The four plants on the shield are important medicinal plants used by the American Indians long before European settlers arrived in the Heartland. The plants are: coneflower, one of the most widely used medicinal plants of the Plains Indians; trumpet honeysuckle, used for numerous medicinal remedies and in basket weaving; horsemint, used by many Northeastern Indians as a panacea, especially for respiratory ailments; and evening primrose, a very popular medicinal herb of the American Indians, later called the "King's Cure-All" when introduced to European herbalists by returning settlers.

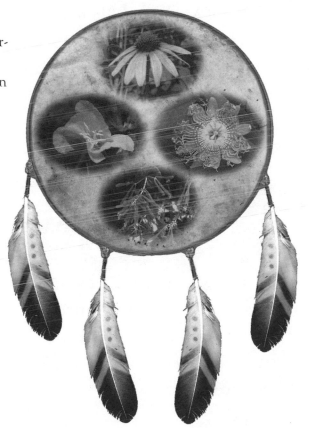

Contents

Foreword

What began as a spiritual quest to write a book about the medicinal plants found in Southern Illinois, eventually grew to encompass the area we identified as the Heartland: eastern Michigan south to western Florida, and eastern Texas north to eastern North Dakota. Of the one thousand plant species that are used directly or yield some by-product used by the pharmaceutical industry, approximately five hundred grow as native, naturalized or cultivated plants in the United States. This book describes two hundred fifty of the plants most commonly found in the Heartland. Each description includes the historical medicinal uses, the active components, the present recommended medicinal uses, and current research that confirms the medicinal usage.

The authors extend special thanks to the following people: to Marjorie Russell for her invaluable editing skills; to Karen Fiorino for the beautiful cover design; to Eric Ulaszek for his editing skills and for providing many of the plates in the color section; to the Plant Biology Department at Southern Illinois University at Carbondale for allowing us to use the slides from the Welch Collection; to Don Ugent, curator of the Welch Collection, who provided plates that are also included in the color section and allowed us the use of his copy of Millspaugh's three volume edition of *American Medicinal Plants*; to Mike Loizides for providing several line drawings and the cover design concept; to Lonnie Russell for his guidance and direction in the production of this book; and to Vickie Heide for reviewing the historical chapter on medicinal plants.

Beth and Jodi Shimp not only provided editorial assistance, but also moral support; and Aristotel Pappelis contributed invaluable advice and assistance to every stage of the book from planning and organizing to production.

This book is intended primarily as a reference book. It is NOT intended to take the place of the advice of a physician, nor is it meant to be a practical guide to self medication. ALWAYS consult a qualified medical or herbal practitioner before using any herbal medications. The authors and publisher shall have neither liability nor responsibility to any person or entity with respect to any loss, damage or injury caused, or alleged to be caused, directly or indirectly, by the information contained in this book.

Introduction

Many people may think that herbs are primarily used for adding flavors to our favorite food dishes. According to Thorndike-Barnhart, an herb is defined as "a plant whose leaves or stems are used for food, medicine, seasoning or perfume." Given the immense range of modern herbs and their current uses, this definition needs to be expanded to include the plant's flowers and roots. Perhaps the definition should read: An herb is a plant that is used for medicine or its health-giving properties, as an ingredient in food for flavor or for its preservative properties, that has cosmetic or cleansing actions, and/or can be used as a dye for food and materials.

Throughout history, the major role of herbs has been to provide mankind with food, medicines and cosmetics. The same herbs that have nourished us and cured our illnesses have also, sometimes, been used to kill.

The first herbs known to mankind were spices such as nutmeg, cinnamon, cloves, pepper, used to preserve meats and fish long before the spices were appreciated for their flavor. Excavations of tombs, temples and cities have shown the importance of spices in religious ceremonies, embalming of the dead, in medicine and folklore, in the preservation and cooking of food, in skin and hair care, cosmetics and as dyes for food and fibers. The legends of the ancient world abound with accounts of the magical powers of herbs. At one time, aromatic plants (spice plants) were such a highly-prized commodity (at times more precious than gold), that their place of origin was the best-kept trade secret of antiquity. Man sailed the world, many lives were lost and new lands were discovered in the search for these places of origin, and for new, exotic spices.

Each civilization had its written authority on the lavish uses of spices. The Greeks had Hippocrates, the "Father of Medicine," who wrote about the importance of spices in medicine and cooking. The historian Herodotus, believed that cassia (senna) grew in swamps protected by ferocious bat-like animals. The Roman writer Pliny, author of several natural history books, was perhaps the first to realize that the tales of spices growing in darkest African swamps and jungles were nothing but hoaxes meant to drive the market prices of spices beyond the reach of most people. The rich indulged themselves by bathing lavishly in aromatic baths and using many after-bath perfumes, ointments and creams. The cost was immaterial. It is said that the Roman emperor Nero burned a whole years supply of Rome's cinnamon at the funeral of his wife.

The use of spices was not confined to aromatic baths. The motto for Roman kitchens must have been "spices, and more spices with everything." All meat and fish dishes were heavily overpowered by spices, particularly for flavoring, but also for masking the odor of decay. The conquering Roman armies carried spices everywhere they went. Their gift to Britain consisted of some four hundred aromatic plants; mustard seeds have even been found at a Roman site in Silchester.

The knowledge and use of these plants was brought to the New World, the Americas, by the Europeans in their search of exotic spices and new lands to conquer. To their amazement, they found a new land rich in plants that were being used by the natives for numerous medicinal purposes, as well as for preserving food for the long, cold winters. The settlers and Indians traded their knowledge of plants and their medicinal remedies. Medicinal plants became a part of their daily lives. However, with the advancement of technology, the use of synthetic drugs became increasingly more prevalent.

A new age is at hand. People are returning to the herbal remedies used by their grandmothers and great-grandmothers because the cost of buying synthetic drugs is rapidly becoming prohibitive. They are realizing that many plants provide the raw materials for the preparation of medicines and that many of those raw materials can be found in plants growing in their backyards. Such raw materials include those extracted from garlic, various mints, onions, oregano and those pesky dandelions. Many well-known kitchen herbs like caraway, coriander, fennel, garlic and pepper, also have medicinal uses as flavoring for drugs and as treatments for many aches, pains and other ailments. Furthermore, many medicinal plants are still being used in the preparations of tobacco, beer and wine, perfume and cosmetics.

The same plants that have provided herbal medicines for centuries are still being used around the world because they provide the vitamins and minerals the human body needs to function as a "well-oiled machine." They also provide a complex combination of active components that act synergistically to give the desired medicinal affect without side effects or long term resistance. Presently researchers are studying the chemical and physiochemical actions of the active components of known plants and new plant species throughout the world, thus providing a scientific basis for comparing herbal and synthetic remedies. However, the destruction of natural plant habitats, in particular the tropical rain forests, may also destroy species that might otherwise be shown to be valuable in treating such devastating viruses as HIV.

Many plants used for healing by the settlers and North American Indians have been found to contain active components with medicinal properties. For example, bloodroot, containing the antiseptic alkaloid sanquinarine, is used as an anti-plaque agent in dentistry. Coneflower, regarded as a panacea by many Plains Indian tribes, contains the antibacterial agent echinacin B, which promotes tissue granulation, and a penlodecadiene which possesses anti-tumor activity. Lobelia, containing the alkaloid lobeline, is used in certain over-the-counter "quit-smoking" remedies and as an expectorant in the treatment of asthma, although it has been mainly replaced by synthetics. Mayapple is the source of legal drugs used in the treatment of cancer of the testicles and venereal warts. Wild black cherries contain benzaldelyde, an anti-cancer, antispasmodic, antiseptic, anesthetic and narcotic agent. Willow, containing salicin in the bark, is the main ingredient in aspirin for treating rheumatism, headaches and toothaches. Chewing on a willow twig to release the "Indian aspirin" is excellent for relieving toothaches.

This book is intended as an educational and reference manual of the medicinal plants found throughout the Heartland, an area encompassing eastern Michigan south to western Florida, and eastern Texas north to eastern North Dakota. It is not intended to be a field or medical guide. This book includes a brief historical perspective on the uses of medicinal plants, the known active components that give plants medicinal qualities, how to collect, dry, prepare and store medicinal herbs, and a description of approximately two hundred-fifty of the most common medicinal plants found in the Heartland, including ferns, grasses, cacti, trees, shrubs, vines, wild flowering plants and cultivated garden plants.

Special reference will be made to the medicinal remedies of the Cherokee, Choctaw, Illinois-Miami, Lakota-Dakota, Kickapoo, Osage, Potawatomi and Winnebago Indian tribes, the first occupants of the Heartland. Although herbal remedies still have beneficial actions and play a very important role in medicine, they are not the panaceas they were once claimed to be. Many are harmless in small doses, but can be poisonous if taken in excess or over a prolonged period of time. They may react adversely with other medicines, foods, and/or aggravate a pre-existing condition. Pregnant women, especially those in the first trimester of pregnancy, should not use any herbal preparation internally, except perhaps for the mildest of herbal teas. Several grasses, trees, weeds and fungi may cause allergic reactions, asthma, hay fever or dermatitis in many people. Follow this basic rule: *always consult a qualified medical or herbal practitioner before self treatment with any medicinal herb*.

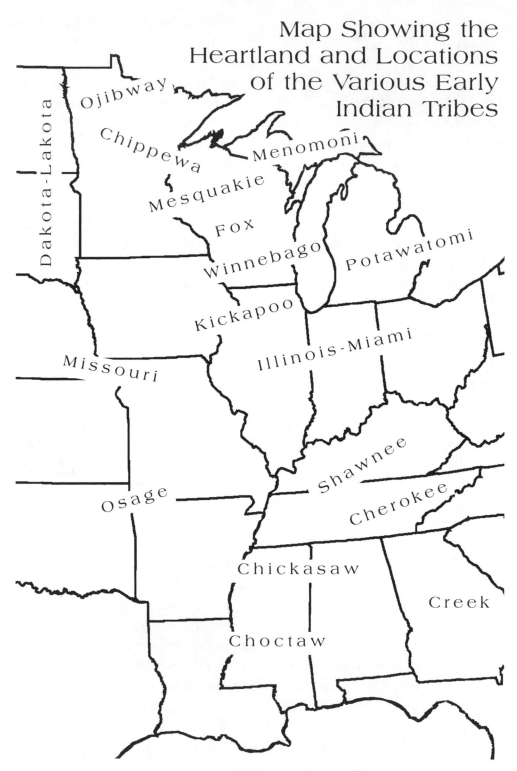

Map Showing the
Heartland and Locations
of the Various Early
Indian Tribes

Ojibway

Dakota-Lakota

Chippewa

Menomoni

Mesquakie

Fox

Winnebago

Potawatomi

Kickapoo

Illinois-Miami

Missouri

Osage

Shawnee

Cherokee

Chickasaw

Creek

Choctaw

An Historical Perspective

Since the earliest days of mankind, plants have been used to heal. Modern medicine is based on man's historic knowledge of plants and trees. Nature has provided the plants (pharmacy) and man has provided the chemical-pharmaceutical translation of the healing properties. The prehistoric herders of tribal communal flocks, with plenty of free time to observe the effects of various plants on their animal charges, became the first sages and medicine men. With time, they evolved into the herbalists of ancient Persia and the philosophers of antiquity. The history of medicinal plants is a history of economic botany, the plants used by man in pharmaceutical, food, cosmetic and perfumery industries. The oldest known systems of healing were those of China, India and ancient Egypt, followed closely by those developed by the ancient Greeks and Romans.

From the third century B.C. to the seventh century A.D., Chinese medicine was influenced by the philosophy and example of Taoist sages who believed in the prevention of disease through moderation, acupuncture, plants, massage, diet and gentle exercise to correct imbalances within the body. The Indian system of yoga, known as Ayurveda ("science of life"), worked to maintain health and prevent disease through a balance of diet, exercise, thought and environment to help the sick person develop positive emotions and qualities. Ancient Egyptian medicine united magic, prayers, spells and sacrifices with empirical treatments and some surgery. The use and need for exotic herbs and the use of the aromatic spices anise, cumin, marjoram, cassia and cinnamon, in their embalming methods, stimulated world trade.

Hippocrates (460-366 B.C.) introduced to Western medicine the theory of the "healing crisis," which has also been called the holistic approach. According to this theory, during a healing crisis the body goes back through the development of the illness, one stage at a time. One after another, various symptoms of the disease disappear as toxins are eliminated from the body. The crisis is identified as a period of regression, meaning a process of reforming the body back to health as the original condition. In general, sickness came first and the crisis followed the treatment. Hippocrates' "advice" was to let the crisis, or nature, take its course.

Hippocrates described health primarily as that state in which the body fluids ("blood, phlegm, yellow bile and black bile") and "humors" (earth, air, fire and water) are in correct proportion to each other. The humors interact with each other, with a person's diet, activities and environment. Hippocrates noted a correlation between changes in the seasons and shifts in the balance of the humors. Annual cycles of humoral imbalance were corrected naturally with the advent of a new year. These observations led Hippocrates to formulate a general theory of healing which advised patients to treat disease by the principle of opposition to the cause. Accordingly, Hippocrates used foods and herbs as a way of affecting an exchange between the four humors and the four seasons. In addition, he employed the four qualities hot, cold, dry and wet. Hippocrates believed that in winter, when it was very cold and wet, a person should eat foods that were dry and warming. On hot, summer days, a person should eat foods that were light, cooling and with many fluids in order to counteract the heat and dryness. To maintain a healthy body, Hippocrates recommended sound nutrition, purgatives, and if needed, botanical "drugs." He described the medicinal properties of three hundred to four hundred species including burdock, mint, peony, rosemary, thyme and violet.

The philosopher Aristotle (384-322 B.C.) also wrote about medicinal plants. His pupil Theophrastus (372-287 B.C.), the Father of Botany, wrote detailed descriptions of the plants found growing in the botanical gardens of Athens. He also wrote the first complete description of opium and its affects.

Two great figures in Roman medicine were two Greek physicians, Galen (130-200 A.D.) and Dioscorides (first century A.D.). Galen, physician to Marcus Aurelius, wrote a "recipe book" of one hundred thirty antidotes and medicines. Dioscorides wrote the first true herbal, *De Materia Medica*, which described the appearance and medicinal properties of about five hundred plants, and how to prepare some one thousand simple drugs. *De Materia Medica* became the prototype for future pharmacopoeias, books which describe medicines and their preparations. The earliest surviving pharmacopoeia was a Byzantine manuscript prepared around 512 A.D., called the *Codex Vindobonaensis*. It featured four hundred full-page natural paintings of plants which were attributed to the greatest botanical illustrator of ancient times, Krateuas. Krateuas was the physician who poisoned the tyrannical king, Mithradates VI Eupator.

When Christians made their way to the British Isles in 597 A.D. with some plants and a limited medicinal knowledge taken from their Greek and Roman masters, they found an extensive Druid herbal and medicinal tradition existing in Wales which dated back at least a hundred years. An Anglo-Saxon medical tradition began to develop combining the herbal traditions of the Druids with Greco-Roman traditions.

In the seventh and eighth centuries, Arabic physicians translated the Greek and Roman herbals. They also added their traditional herbal medicines and those acquired along the spice trade routes to the Far East. The famous Arabic physician, Avicenna wrote the *Canon on Medicine* which included a description of medicinal plants, diseases and treatment. When Alexandria was conquered by the Moslems in 641 A.D., they found that alchemists had invented the Alembic, a crude distillation apparatus used for extracting the aromatic oils that were used in perfumes.

During the Dark Ages, a period dated from 641 A.D. when Alexandria fell, to 1096 A.D. when the first Christian Crusades took place, Anglo-Saxon medicine was dominated by the monasteries and the "herb lady." The monasteries perpetuated the healing doctrines and herbal knowledge of Galen and Dioscorides, while the general populatio's folk healers, usually women, stirred a pot mixed with ancient herbal lore, pragmatic healing and pagan sorcery.

Knowledge of herbs and their cultivation was proclaimed pagan by the Church during the Dark Ages because of the many mystical and magical rites connected with their use. However, the Church did adopt versions of primitive superstitions such as the tying of herb bundles to doors to keep out witches, or the wearing of amulets of dried herbs to ward off disease. In the Dark Ages, many herbal manuscripts were destroyed by those who were not interested in science or culture. In the seclusion and security of their monasteries, monks kept the knowledge of herbs and their properties alive. They studied, translated and meticulously copied for posterity the few remaining herbals. In the tenth century, the first Anglo-Saxon herbal, *The Leech Book of Bald*, written by a monk in the common tongue, emphasized a combination of ritual and magical medicine.

In the Middle Ages, monks and nuns revived the cultivation of herbs. They became physicians and nurses as well as healers of the soul. The herb garden, called the "Physick Garden," (Physick meant pertaining to things natural) became an important part of every cloister and monastery. Alembic laboratories, also called distilling plants, predecessors of our modern pharmaceutical industry, were set up in monasteries and hospitals to process medical potions and liqueurs. Although many of the herbal concoctions eventually became obsolete, we still use many as spices and condiments in food, medicinal teas, infusions and liqueurs such as Benedictine, Peres Chartreuse and Trappistine.

The Crusaders, upon returning from their missions, introduced the material goods of the Middle East and Orient to Europeans. Arabian herbal traditions took root throughout Europe. Sweet, exotic spices became popular healing agents. Men took to the high seas to find new trade routes for spices such as black pepper, cinnamon, cardamon, sandalwood, nutmeg, cloves and mace. With the discovery of a whole new world by the Spaniards and Portuguese came new plants such as the love apple (tomato), Jesuit bark (the bark of the cinchona tree from which came quinine), and tobacco.

Throughout Europe, the study of native plants was frowned upon. The old folk herbalist was gradually ostracized, legally and socially, by the so-called "proper" schools of medicine. Their folk remedies became an increasing threat to the medical academies. However, herbals were continually being written in the native languages and folk medicine endured. Probably the most famous of the herbals was written by the alchemist Paracelsus (1493-1541 A.D.).

Paracelsus changed the course of Western medicine with his belief that all medicinal substances, plant or otherwise, contained an essential principle that was pure and entirely beneficial. He conducted extensive research to develop a treatise of common herbs and minerals. He was the first to recommend the use of mercury for treating syphilis. He also believed that God placed plants on Earth for human use, and that God provided signs embodied in the plants to indicate their potential uses. This idea became known as the "Doctrine of Signatures."

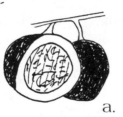
a.

Doctrine of Signatures

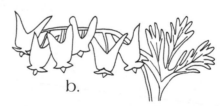
b.

The Doctrine of Signatures was received with wide acclaim because people saw the need to attach religious significance to plants for healing. An excellent example is the passion flower. When it was first introduced into Europe by the Spanish, Catholics saw it as a symbolic representation of the Passion of Christ. The corona was the crown of thorns, the five sepals and five petals symbolized the ten Apostles (absent are the traitor Judas and Peter who betrayed Christ three times),

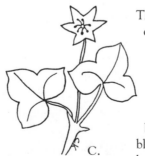
c.

The Doctrine of Signatures encompassed the concept that the walnut (a) which looks like the human brain could be used to cure madness and migraine headaches; Dutchman's breeches (b), clearly a man's plant because of the flower's resemblance to a man's breeches, could be used to cure venereal disease; and, hepatica (c) with its lobed leaves, could be used to cure liver diseases.

and the other parts of the flower represented the nails and the wounds. They also believed that disease was a manifestation of evil and that there must be an outward sign to describe the particular healing qualities of a plant.

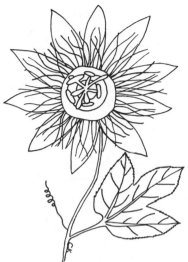

The English herbals were as florid and spicy to read as were the lives of their authors. John Gerard (1545-1612), a physician and gardener, was the best known and most controversial, except for perhaps Culpeper. Generally, Gerard was a reliable witness, listing wild flower locations around London. However, in his publication *Herball or Generall Historie of Plantes* (1597), he claimed to have seen barnacles hatching out of geese, a popular belief of the time.

Passion Flower

Nicolas Culpeper (1616-1654), a Puritan apothecary rather than a physician of the established medical community, translated *The London Pharmacopoeia* from Latin to English, publishing it as the *Physicall Directory*. His writings and practices were not at all accepted by the physicians of the day. He subscribed to the Doctrine of Signatures as did the physicians, but also to astrological botany as prescribed by Arabic physicians. Astrological botany allied plants to the planets according to color and shape, and then connected the astrological influence of the planet with the plant. Culpeper used the combination of astrology and signatures in his book, *The Complete Herbal*.

When the Europeans came to the Americas, they found that the Native Americans had already identified and established a vast pharmacopoeia of indigenous medicinal plants. Some of the more common ones were birch, blackberry, butternut, corn, coneflower, ginseng, goldenseal, horsetail, oak, slippery elm, sumac, sweet flag, water hemlock, wild ginger and willow.

The Native American herbalist relied on cultural and personal knowledge. Cultural knowledge was handed down from one generation to the next. Personal knowledge developed because of the Indians' nomadic lifestyle and geographic migrations. The Indians believed that the basic cause of an illness originated in the spirit world. Health and healing were part of a way of relating to the entire world. The Native American tradition of "Good Medicine" meant living in harmony with nature. Nature's harmony itself was Good Medicine. The Shaman, or medicine man, sought the knowledge of Good Medicine by communicating through visions with the Great Spirit. Various rites were performed to persuade the spirits to intervene in the fate of a sick person. The goal of the healing ceremony was for the sick person to attain complete harmony with nature and the universe, in itself of great psycho-therapeutic value. The Navaho used sweat baths, baths in a distillate of the yucca root and/or sandpaintings in their healing ceremonies.

The Native American healer classified herbs and medicines according to the four directions and the two powers, the Great Spirit (Grandfather Earth) and Creation (Grandmother Earth).

The healer viewed plants as a chemical combination that helped the human body become part of the whole of Creation. An Indian medicine man said of plants: "They were, and are, infused with the same spirit, power, and life forces that animate and flow through all the universe." Believing this, the healers called plants "medicine people." Plants represented a complete system for analyzing the physical, psychological and spiritual needs of individuals, with an emphasis on direct experiences and a relationship with nature as the healing force.

European settlers brought with them their knowledge of medicine, much of which was based on the Doctrine of Signatures and an underlying belief in magic and witchcraft. The knowledge of European herbal medicine, plus Indian knowledge, provided a situation where cross-borrowing took place quickly and extensively. The settlers adopted the medicinal remedies of bloodroot, wild cherry, mayapple, catnip, blackberry, licorice and red cedar from the Indian herbalist. In turn, the Indians adopted alfalfa, comfrey, dock and plantain.

In 1822, Dr. Samuel Thomson of New Hampshire, a self-taught physician, wrote an eight hundred-page manual of Indian and colonial herb practices. With his accumulated knowledge of herbal medicine, he realized that certain plant compounds were valuable diagnostically. He patented the formulas because his prescriptions, widely-accepted by the common people but not the medical professionals, were quickly copied. This was the beginning of the popularity of patented medicines. Over the years, many of his "cures" were proven to be correct, with at least fifty prescribed species still valued by herbalists. R.V. Pierce, a physician in the early 1800s, developed several patented "scientific" medicines. His "Golden Medical Discovery," probably his most famous medicine, was a nutritional tonic preparation that combined the remedial properties of the best-known herbal alterations known at that time. It included gentian root (*Gentiana lutea*), sacred bark (*Rhamus purshiana*), Oregon grape root (*Berberis aquifolium*), bloodroot (*Sanguinera canadensis*), wild cherry bark (*Prunus virginia*), queen's root (*Stillingia sylvatica*) and stone root (*Collinsonia canadensis*). Golden Medical Discovery was intended to produce gradual changes, "arousing the excretory glands to remove morbid materials, and at the same time toning secretory organs." Dr. Pierce's 'Favorite Prescription' was formulated especially for women to help relieve the discomfort of functional menstrual disturbances (including delayed menstruation, cramping and menopausal discomfort) and associated nervousness. Dr. Pierce's "Favorite Prescription," contained the best-known herbal emmenagogues known at that time, valerian root (*Valerian offinale*), black haw (*Viburnum prunifolium*), blue cohosh root (*Caulophyllum thalictroides*), unicorn root (*Nodicias dioca*), black cohosh root (*Cimicifuga racemosa*) and Oregon grape root (*Berberis aquifolium*).

The Shakers (Church of the United Society of Believers), prime friends of the Indians, were the first to extensively cultivate medicinal plants in mass quantities. They specialized in growing and merchandising a wide variety of healing plants that were used by Dr. Thomson and others. They became America's first reputable pharmaceutical manufacturers. Immediately prior to the Civil War, three hundred fifty-four kinds of herbs were available from the gardens of the Shakers. These included catnip, chicory, elderberries, horseradish, mullein, pennyroyal, sage, sarsaparilla, tansy and wintergreen.

Many physicians prescribed medicines containing medicinal plants into the early twentieth century. Research and technological advances have made it possible to synthetically manufacture many of the active components found in plants. Unfortunately, along with these advances came soaring production costs. People are gradually looking for alternatives through herbal medicine. People are listening to the Indian belief that man must co-exist with nature.

> "The Great Spirit is our father, but the earth is our mother. She nourishes us; that which we put into the ground, she returns to us, and healing plants she gives us likewise."
>
> Big Thunder, a North American Indian

They also realize that the anecdote, "much ado about nothing" no longer applies to preventive health care. Perhaps this book will help those who are searching for answers in their quest to learn more about medicinal plants and how to apply that knowledge to their daily lives.

Active Components
of Medicinal Plants

T hroughout the ages, man has used medicinal plants without knowing the source of their effective medicinal properties. The rapid development of organic chemistry and pharmacology beginning in the nineteenth century has given man the tools to determine which active component or group of components are responsible for a given therapeutic effect.

The plants used in herbal remedies contain chemical substances (principle constituents or 'active' components), which may have a healing effect on the human body. They affect the condition and function of the human body, clear residual symptoms or destroy the cause of the disease by increasing the body's resistance to disease, inhibit the natural aging process or stimulate the adaptation of the organism to certain conditions. The power to heal is within each individual, but there are times when the body needs a boost. The active components of medicinal plants provide that boost.

Medicinally active components usually occur in groups of closely related compounds that complement the healing effects of each other. This synergistic action is considered by herbalists to be advantageous in treatments with medicinal plants. The physiological effect of each separate alkaloid (quite different from that of a combined group) has a specific characteristic and different pharmacological effect in the body.

The active components of plants effective in the nutritional and healing mechanisms within the human body, are the products of the plant's primary or secondary metabolism. Primary metabolism, a process that occurs during photosynthesis, produces sugars, amino acids and fatty oils. Products of secondary metabolism serve as defense mechanisms for the plant against attacks by insects and other invertebrates. These products, including essential oils, glycosides, tannins and bitter principles, are also effective in bolstering nutritional and healing mechanisms within the human body. The active components of plants which belong to several chemical groups such as alkaloids, glycosides, saponins, bitter compounds, tannins, essential oils, terpenes, resins, fatty oils, mucilages, pectins, proteins, and vitamins, will be described briefly.

Alkaloids

Alkaloids are the most efficient and therapeutic plant substances. Alkaloids are a diverse group of organic aromatic, nitrogenous compounds (usually crystalline compounds insoluble in water) with a marked physiological effect on the nervous and circulatory systems. They generally have a bitter flavor, are poisonous to varying degrees, and may act as analgesics, local anesthetics, tranquilizers, antispasmodics, heart constrictors and/or hallucinatory agents. The most common are atropine (jimsonweed, *Datura stramonium*), caffeine (coffee beans and tea leaves), colchicine (saffron, *Crocus sativus*), lobeline (Indian tobacco, *Lobelia inflata*), nicotine (tobacco, *Nicotiana tabacum*) and protopine (bloodroot, *Sanguinava canadensis*). Isolated alkaloids may have a more potent action than the plant material from which they were extracted. Many isolated alkaloids have therapeutic value, but due to their toxicity they must be used only by qualified medical personnel. In folk medicine, plants containing alkaloids were used only for external applications.

Bitter Compounds

Bitter compounds are terpenoid or glycosidic substances that commonly have a strong, bitter taste irritating to the taste buds. Herbalists use bitter compounds in tea mixtures as appetizers to stimulate the appetite and the flow of digestive juices. Some bitter compounds such as choleretics and cholagogues activate the secretion and flow of bile, while others such as diuretics increase urine flow. Bitter compounds are found in many members of the daisy and gentian families such as American wormwood and blessed thistle.

Carotenoids

Carotenoids are yellow or red pigments found in photosynthetic plants. There are two types, carotenes and zanthophylls. Carotenes, hydrocarbons (tetraterpenes), and yellow pigments are converted to vitamin A in the human body. The common carrot is probably the most widely-used vegetable containing carotene. Zanthophylls are oxygenated derivatives of carotenes. There are two types of zanthophylls, lutein, the predominant zanthophyll found in most leaves, and lycopene which gives the reddish color to tomatoes.

Essential (volatile) Oils

Essential oils are lipid components of plant cells that vaporize when heated. Their principal constituents are complex mixtures of terpenoid substances including terpenes and sesquiterpenes. Essential oils accumulate in certain tissues, in specialized cells or in intercellular spaces. They may occur in only one part of a plant, such as in rose petals, or in morphologically related parts like flowers and fruits. Many plants containing essential oils are well known for their fragrance and are commonly used in the food and perfumery industries. Essential oils can be used in an infusion, decoction, poultice, or by themselves. They are preferably extracted from fresh or dried herbs by steam or water distillation, or by distillation in alcohol. Some of the isolated components of essential oils such as menthol, camphor and thymol, also have important medicinal properties and are included in proprietary medicines.

Essential oils have varied physiological effects. Aromatic spices such as anise and fennel, and flavoring agents may also act as digestive tonics as does caraway. Others have antiseptic (bloodroot, garlic, self-heal), carminative (chamomile, fennel, pennyroyal, tansy), expectorant (elderberry, Indian tobacco, thyme), rubefacient (horseradish, mustard, mugwort, wintergreen), anti-rheumatic (arrowhead, boneset, evening primrose and lavender), anthelmintic (alumroot, mayapple, tansy), and anti-inflammatory (black cohosh, hops, pot marigold) properties. Essential oils and the plant parts containing them must always be stored in the dark in airtight containers.

Fatty (fixed) Oils
Fatty oils of plant origin are mixtures of triglycerides, glycerol and fatty acids that are insoluble in water but dissolve in organic solvents. Examples of fatty oils with medicinal application are maize oil, soybean oil and castor oil. Fatty oils are used in medical preparations and industrial, food and cosmetic products. Many vegetable oils also contain substantial amounts of unsaturated fatty oils.

Glycosides
Glycosides, products of secondary metabolism in plants, are complex organic substances which separate into a sugar component and a non-sugar component when hydrolyzed (split by the action of water, acids or enzymes). Glycosides include some of the most potent plant drugs and some of the plants containing these drugs are among the most toxic known. Because of their toxicity, these plants must never be self-administered. Cardiac, mustard, cyanogenic and phenolic glycosides are classified according to their chemical composition.

Cardiac glycosides contain various sugars attached to hydroxyl groups or the hydroxyl group is connected to a fatty acid. Cardiac glycosides found in foxglove and lily-of-the-valley, affect contractions of the heart muscles and are used to correct arrhythmia in the heartbeat.

Mustard glycosides contain bonded sulfur and are characteristic of mustards and other members of the mustard family such as horseradish. They are also associated with the enzyme myrosinase. Activation of myrosinase breaks down the mustard glycoside into the sugar and non-sugar (allyl isothiocyanates, also called mustard oils) components. Mustard oils have antiseptic properties due to the activity of the bonded sulfur compound.

Cyanogenic glycosides contain a non-sugar compound, a cyanahydrin that is bonded to a sugar. Hydrolysis by enzymes release poisonous hydrogen cyanide (prussic acid). Cyanogenic glycosides have antispasmodic, purgative and sedative actions of varying potency. They may be found in some plants of the rose, legume, honeysuckle and flax families.

Phenolic glycosides have a wide range of chemical structures that are divided into four main groups:

A) Simple phenolic glycosides contain phenol, a simple aromatic. These include salicylic derivatives found in willow and balm of Gilead, methylarbutin found in barberry, and arbutin, which on hydrolysis releases the mild diuretic hydroquinone.

B) Coumarin or phenylpropane derivatives have a characteristic sweet smell like newly-cut hay. Some coumarins have the ability to strengthen capillary walls or to adsorb ultraviolet radiation, an ability valuable in sunscreens. Others are poisonous or are phototoxic, that is, they heighten sunburn during exposure to ultraviolet light. Coumarin glycosides are found in angelica, melilot and Queen Anne's lace.

C) Anthraquinones are generally aromatic pigmented phenolic compounds which break down to lose their sugar component, and when ingested, exert a laxative action within six to eight hours (senna)

D) Flavonoids are aromatic phenolic compounds formed from flavones which are yellow plant pigments. Flavonoid glycosides are classified as anthocyanins or bioflavonoids. Anthocyanins (from the Greek words *anthos* meaning flower and *kyanos* meaning dark blue) are largely responsible for the red, purple and blue color of flowers such as hollyhock, mallow, cornflower, peony and sweet violet. The bioflavonoid rutin, found in ground ivy, hawthorns and hops, affects the strength and permeability of capillary walls and is used to treat hypertension and various disorders. The bioflavonoids silybin, silydramine and silychistin, found in milk thistle, are used to treat liver disorders.

Mucilages and Pectins

Plant mucilages and pectins are amorphous mixtures of polysaccharides that form viscous colloidal systems in water. Pectins from blackberry and Queen Anne's lace are used in the treatment of diarrhea and in the preparation and preservation of fruits. Mucilages (dandelion, peppermint-spearmint) are therapeutically helpful because they reduce mechanical and chemical actions. They form protective barriers over the mucous membranes and prevent irritants from reaching inflamed surfaces. They are used in treating infections of the chest, throat and intestinal tracts. In small doses, they have an anti-diarrheal effect; in large doses, they are purgative. Applied in poultices, mucilages alleviate the pain of bruised tissues and soften the skin.

Resins

Resins, found in trees and shrubs such as birch and willow, are often associated with essential oils. Resins, produced by special plant cells, are secreted into intracellular spaces or resin ducts. Some are phenol derivatives, while others are terpenoid derivatives. They occur as solids when cooled and melt when heated. Some resins are mixed with essential oils to form balsams.

Saponins

Saponins characteristically have the ability to reduce the surface tension of water, producing a soapy foam in water. Saponins (derived from the Latin word *sapo*, meaning soap) are excellent emulsifiers and destroy the membranes of red blood corpuscles, a process called hemolysis. Saponins are often associated with cardiac glycosides and consist of a triterpene non-sugar portion, such as sapongenin, and a sugar portion, such as glucose or galactose. The chemical composition of some saponins like those found in fenugreek, are similar to that of sex hormones. The saponin-containing plants sarsaparilla and wild yam are the source of the substances used in the manufacture of contraceptive pills. Plants in which large quantities of saponins occur are highly toxic and should not be taken internally. However, plants in which small quantities occur are safe to use. Saponins also have an irritating effect on mucous membranes of the respiratory and digestive tract. They are used medicinally as expectorants, cathartics, diuretics and antiseptics, especially for the urinary tract. Since saponins aid the absorption of various substances, they are effective constituents of tea mixtures.

Tannins

Tannins are complex, colorless polyphenolic compounds and have the characteristic ability to coagulate proteins, heavy metals and alkaloids when they dissolve readily in water. Tannins have astringent and antiseptic properties that hasten the healing of wounds and inflamed mucous membranes. The action of tannin also induces sensitivity and relieves pain. Medicinally, tannin-containing plants are used for diarrhea, bronchitis, slow-healing wounds, mouth infections and hemorrhoids. Large doses or prolonged use of tannins may be harmful. Tannins are found in the rose, willow and birch families.

Collecting, Drying and Storing Medicinal Plants

Medicinal plants can be found growing in the wild, or they may be cultivated and obtained through commercial growers and suppliers. There are those who believe it is best, whenever possible, to obtain medicinal plants from a qualified herbalist or reputable supplier. That recommendation is based on several factors: cultivation aids in proper identification of the plant; it assures perpetuation of the species; organically grown herbs are free of pesticides; plants are usually collected at their peak of medicinal value; and are more likely to be properly dried and stored to ensure preservation of the medicinal properties. In addition, the herbs are ready for immediate use.

If possible, it is best to purchase herbs from a reputable local herbalist, rather than from nutrition or "health" stores that may be selling packaged herbs from unknown sources. There is no guarantee that over-the-counter packaged herbs are labeled accurately. There is also the possibility that the fancy packaged herbs, although packaged in the United States, actually came from overseas. Many herbs are grown in eastern Europe, Asia and South America. To save time, picking and processing has often been automated. And often the entire herb has been collected when perhaps only the leaves or flowers are used in preparing the desired medicinal herbal. Chamomile is an excellent example of this. Even though only the flowerheads are used in medicinal teas, the entire stem and leaves may also be harvested. Furthermore, some countries allow the use of pesticides that have been banned in the United States.

Many of the common, wild medicinal herbs found in the Heartland can also be grown in a private garden, or even indoors in containers. Each plant part needs to be collected, dried and stored in a manner that will ensure the optimum quality and quantity of the active components.

Proper Collection of Medicinal Plants

It is important to collect the medicinal part of the plant at its optimum growth point. For leaves, this is just before flowering. Collect flowers just before full bloom. Collect roots and rhizomes when the aerial parts of the plant begin to wither and die. Collect the bark in the spring or autumn when it is damp and easy to peel off. Always remove any damaged parts and check for insect infestation.

There are certain procedures to follow when collecting the various parts of either wild or cultivated plants in order to guarantee the best quality and quantity of the active components.

Aerial Parts (flowering stems)
Cut off the aerial parts of the plant, harvest only the upper three-fourths of the plant, leave enough of th stem and leaves to assure the maintenance of photosynthesis. This way, new foliage will grow that can be harvested later. Only the top growth should be gathered from tall plants such as mullein. Prostrate, creeping plants should be gently washed in water to remove soil particles.

Breaking or tearing the stems damages the plant tissues and initiates the plant's defensive metabolic processes. Use sharp gardening shears when cutting the stem in order to minimize this effect. Whenever possible, collect only plants that are young and fresh.

Transport all aerial parts such as the leaves, flowers or fruits in a basket, rather than in a plastic bag, in order to prevent condensation.

Flowers
Collect undamaged flowers by hand at midday in dry weather when they are first fully open. Be careful not to touch or bruise the petals. To prevent condensation from forming, transport the flowers in a basket rather than a plastic bag.

Fruits and Seeds
Collect seeds when they are fully ripe and ripe fruits before they get too soft. Catch the seeds by hanging the flowerhead by its stalk over a tray. Berries can be forked off their stalks when partially dried.

Leaves
Collect fresh leaves that are free of disease or insects before they flower, when they contain the maximum amount of active components. Be careful not to crush or bruise the leaves when collecting them.

Roots, Rhizomes and Bark

Collect roots and rhizomes in the fall or spring during the dormant period when they contain the greatest amount of active components. Annuals may be collected in the autumn of the first year of growth and perennials can be collected in the second or third year of growth. Be careful not to bruise or cut the root or rhizome while removing it from the soil. While removing loose soil, do not scrub with a brush as this may cause the loss of essential oils. Washing under a strong jet of water is preferred.

Collect bark from young trunks or branches (or felled ones) in damp weather when it is easier to remove. A basket, plastic or paper bags may be used when collecting roots, rhizomes or bark. Wash under a strong jet of water to remove any soil and unwanted pests.

In addition, there are nine rules to follow when collecting wild medicinal plants:

Rule 1. Correct identification. It is imperative to know beyond question that the correct specie is being collected. This book is intended to aid in the identification of herbs by giving a brief description of each species, accompanied by an illustration (selected photographs may also aid in the identification). However, it cannot be emphasized enough that **mistaken identification may be fatal.** Many poisonous and non-poisonous plants look very similar, especially before flowering. Examples of these Jekyll/Hyde look-alikes are sweet cicely and water hemlock, comfrey and foxglove or milkweed and dogbane. If in doubt, always seek professional advice.

Rule 2. Always obtain permission from the landowner before collecting wild medicinal plants, and always leave several plants of each species to ensure their continued survival. Too many species are presently endangered by over harvesting and because of the encroachment of man on their environment. Black cohosh (*Cimicifuga racemosa*), American ginseng (*Panax quinquefolium*) and coneflower (*Echinacea* sp.), once important medicinal plants prized by the American Indians, early settlers and herbalists, are currently being over-harvested in some areas of the Heartland. However, they are being cultivated commercially in the United States and Europe and are available in all health stores. In many states, the collection of ginseng requires special permission from state agencies.

Rule 3. When collecting medicinal plants always wear gloves as some plants such as stinging nettle may cause contact dermatitis. Also, use proper tools such as knives, special digging implements, and cutting shears. Proper tools make collecting easier and make it easier to obtain better quality, crude active components.

Rule 4. Use a proper receptacle for collecting. Use a basket for collecting flowers and delicate leaves. Roots, rhizomes, stems and most leaves may be placed loosely in a carry-all such as a back pack, plastic bag, or an oblong cylinder called a vasculum.

Rule 5. Collect hearty, undamaged plants. Do not collect diseased or pest-infested parts.

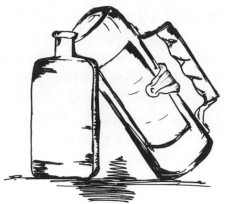

Rule 6. Label each plant. Write the name or description of each plant with a pencil (ink from a ballpoint pen may run) on an index card or small piece of paper. Include a description of the collection area for future reference.

Tincture Bottle and Vasculum

Rule 7. Do not collect plants along roadsides, railroads or farmlands where weed killers and pesticides have been used. They may contain undesirable concentrations of heavy metals or poisonous chemicals that may be metabolized by the plant and become incorporated in some of the active components.

Rule 8. Collect in dry, sunny weather between 10 a.m. and 5 p.m. Wet, damp plants quickly spoil from overheating and moisture condensation. The resulting fermentation and biochemical processes in the wilting plant or various plant parts changes their appearance and active components by breaking down, or decreasing, the concentration of the active components.

Rule 9. Dry the collected plant or plant parts as quickly as possible after harvesting.

Proper Drying of the Medicinal Plant

The removal of a leaf, flower, or other plant part is followed by metabolic changes in the plant part removed. The cells begin to die as soon as their supply of water and nutrients cease. If they are not immediately laid in a thin layer to dry, the excised part may begin to spoil from overheating and moisture condensation. As decomposition proceeds, the chemical composition also changes. Incorrect drying increases this effect and the possibility of loss of the medicinal properties. Plants may lose up to one-third of their potency and their natural coloration if dried in direct sunlight.

Plants can be dried by artificial heat in a good quality drying oven or dehydrator. Drying removes water and should be done gradually. Drying time is dependent on the species and part of the plant being dried. To ensure that the essential oils do not evaporate, the top of plants that have essential oils should not be damaged before, during or after drying. Dry flowers and leaves in thin layers so they do not need to be turned frequently. Dry at a temperature of approximately 90° to 100°F for the first twenty-four hours; then, if required, reduce the temperature to 70° F. Dry leaves, stems and flowers until they are brittle and all parts break easily. Correctly dried flowers retain their coloration. However, over time, they may begin to turn brown or lose their scent. Replace old flowers throughout the growing season with a fresh supply. Drying too long depletes the essential oils.

When drying large quantities, spread the plant parts in wooden, slatted trays that can be easily stacked and placed where it is easy to turn the plant material to allow proper access of air. Plants can also be dried, tied in small bunches, stem up, on lines strung across a drying room. The drying room should be dark and have plenty of circulating air in order to prevent mildew, spoilage and/or loss of color. Properly dried herbs should smell and look much like the fresh plant. The color should be only slightly muted and the smell as strong or stronger than that of a fresh plant.

All green parts should be removed from the roots and rhizomes before drying. Thick roots and rhizomes can be cut into small pieces to allow proper drying. Thick roots, rhizomes and bark may need a higher initial temperature (up to 120° F), that is gradually lowered to 70° F, if dried in a dehydrator.

For large roots and thick pieces of bark, a simple dryer can be made by replacing the shelves of an old utility cart with one or two strong metal screens spaced twelve to eighteen inches apart. Hang a seventy-five to one hundred watt light bulb from the underside of the top shelf. Use cardboard or newspaper to cover the sides.

Proper Storage of Medicinal Plants

Proper storage is as equally important as the collection and drying processes to preserve the medicinal components. Always store the herbs under dry, cool, dark, dust-free conditions. Glass containers "breathe" easier than do plastic or tin. Plants containing essential oils may be stored loosely in brown glass jars. Bags or boxes may be used temporarily to protect dried herbs from light and moisture.

Storage containers should be clearly labeled with the name and part of the herb, the date collected and the date stored. Containers with poisonous active components must always be clearly marked with either the skull and cross-bones or the word **POISON** in large red letters in order to insure that here won't be any danger of mistaken identification resulting in possible accidental poisoning.

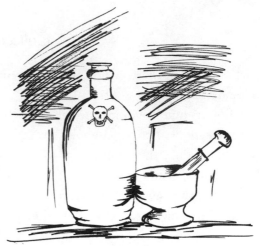

Plants that are hygroscopic (absorb moisture from the air) should not be stored for too long. Storing for a prolonged period may cause chemical changes to occur due to reactivation of enzymes. Heartland plants in which this can occur include mullein, angelica and parsley root.

Long-term storage of medicinal plants will result in the gradual break-down of the medicinal potential. Do not use herbs or plant parts that are over two years old. Preferably, replace aerial herbs yearly.

Culinary herbs can be frozen, in water, either in ice trays or in plastic bags. Freezing is the preferred method of long-term storage and is more convenient than drying. Freezing is unsuitable for medicinal herbs.

Preparation of Medicinal Plants

In order of their common usage, home remedies, or herbals, are administered in the form of teas, infusions, decoctions, syrups, tinctures, oils, poultices, compresses, ointments or herbal baths made with dried or fresh material. Dried herbs usually have a higher concentration of essential oils than fresh herbs due to the loss of water. A general rule of thumb is, if using fresh material, double the recommended amount of dried material. Use glass, ceramic, pottery or an unchipped enameled container for making herbals. If possible, use fresh spring water or distilled water. Always use a muslin strainer or unbleached coffee filter to strain teas, infusions, decoctions or tinctures. Avoid using metal containers or utensils. The metals may leech into the tea, infusion, decoction or tincture and bind with the active components, rendering them useless.

Compresses

Compresses are pads of muslin or gauze dipped in a cold or hot medicinal solution, such as an infusion or decoction, and applied to the skin. They are usually covered and bandaged in place. Keep the compress on the area being treated for up to thirty minutes, depending on the condition and herb being used. Remove the compress when the treated area becomes uniformly flushed or if a tingling sensation or feeling of relief develops. Remove the compress if the area becomes red or feels uncomfortable.

Clean, bruised fresh leaves or roots, held in place by a bandage, make the simplest compresses. The herbs used for compresses can be warm and stimulating as in the case of cayenne or ginger which increase circulation and energize areas of body that are congested or debilitated.

Decoctions

Decoctions are a method for extracting the active components from hard plant parts such as the bark, stems, roots, hard fruits (nuts) and some seeds by boiling them in water. This method is not suitable for plants containing essential oils, mucilage, enzymes or glycosides which may be affected by heat.

To prepare a decoction, pour one cup of water over one to three teaspoons of dried herb in a nonmetallic container. Slowly bring to a boil and simmer gently for fifteen to twenty minutes. Woody parts may need to be boiled for as long as an hour. Strain the decoction while hot. Drink immediately or store up to seven days.

Herbal Baths

There is probably nothing that is more soothing and relaxing than an herbal bath. Baths involve the total immersion of the body or the immersion of just the limbs, hands or feet in water. The best method is to add a strong infusion or decoction to bath water. For a relaxing, soothing bath, add two pints of the herbal solution to the bath water. Another method is to put the herb(s) in cheesecloth or a muslin bag and hang under the running, hot water. With this method, however, the full, soothing effect of the herbs may not be realized.

Infusions

Infusions are used for extracting the active constituents from an herb by steeping it in hot water. It is a good method for aromatic herbs containing essential oils which would lose up to sixty percent of their effectiveness if boiled.

The infusion is prepared by pouring a cup of boiling water onto one to three teaspoons of dried, or two to six teaspoons of fresh, herb. Cover the container with a tight-fitting lid to prevent the volatile oils from escaping. The aroma of the steeping infusion indicates that the herb's essential oils are escaping and that the container's lid needs to be tightened. Steep the infusion ten to fifteen minutes, strain and drink when warm.

For those who do not like using measuring utensils, fill a pint jar half full with the dried herb or completely full if using fresh material. Pour the boiling water into the container, cover and steep ten to fifteen minutes, shaking occasionally. The mixture is then strained and usually taken immediately. Most infusions can be stored in the refrigerator for five to seven days.

Another method is to put the herbs in a glass container with room-temperature water, and allow it to stand for a few hours in a warm place in a manner similar to making sun tea.

Oils and Ointments

The extraction of essential oils from aromatic herbs by steam distillation concentrates the active components into a few drops of oil which may be harsh and irritating. To make a safe, less concentrated oil at home, macerate two ounces of dried herb, or four ounces of fresh, and mix with one pint of virgin olive, safflower or pure vegetable oil in a clear glass jar. Cover and place the container in a warm place, out of direct sunlight, for three to five days. Shake the jar vigorously at least once a day. Strain the oil into a clean bottle.

Another method is to combine the herbs and oil or one cup of herbal tincture and oil in a medium or large pot. Heat the uncovered mixture gently for one hour (DO NOT BOIL as boiling may destroy the volatile oils). Strain and bottle the oil when cool.

Herbal creams or ointments can be made by adding one to one and one-half ounces of melted beeswax to the prepared oil. Comfrey makes an excellent first aid cream.

Poultices

A poultice is made from macerated fresh or dried, powdered herbs, an herb tea, infusion or decoction mixed with hot water. Oatmeal can be added to the mixture to make a paste (use two ounces herb with twenty ounces oatmeal). The resulting paste is applied directly on the skin. Cover the poultice with a warm towel, gauze or bandage to hold it in place. Remove the covering when cool (the covering can sometimes be reheated a few times). Poultices are effective for drawing out an infection or foreign bodies such as a splinter, and relieving muscle spasms and pain. Burdock, comfrey or slippery elm are safe, traditional poultice herbs. Apply mustard, cayenne or other irritating herbs in a plaster, between cheesecloth or muslin layers.

Syrups

Honey-based herbal syrups are a simple and effective way to preserve the healing qualities of some herbs. Syrups are used to soothe sore throats and provide temporary relief from coughs and colds. To make an herbal syrup, combine two ounces of the dried herb or four ounces of fresh, with one quart water in large pot. Boil the mixture down until it is reduced by half, then add one to two tablespoons of honey. Syrups may be stored up to one month. Wild black cherry makes an excellent syrup for sore throats and coughs.

Teas

Medicinal teas are not pleasant tasting, and are much more potent than packaged herb beverages. Teas are made by steeping one ounce (about two handfuls) of dried flowers, leaves or stems per two cups of hot water for five to ten minutes. Strain in a muslin strainer before use. Avoid contact with metals, if possible.

Tinctures

Tinctures are excellent for preserving and concentrating the healing qualities of herbs. They are effective in very small quantities because they are so concentrated. Use caution when using tinctures because of their potency. The dosage, dependent on the tincture and the ailment, ranges from several drops to one tablespoon of tincture taken directly or in a cup of hot "tea."

A tincture is prepared by prolonged steeping of a fresh or dried herb in alcohol to draw out the active constituents. Tinctures are usually made from unprocessed plant material but may also be prepared from dried extracts. Quantities vary according to the herb, but generally the preparation is one part crushed plant material to five parts or four ounces powdered or finely cut herb with one pint of sixty percent alcohol or spirits such as brandy or vodka. **DO NOT** *use rubbing (isopropyl) or wood (methyl) alcohol. Both are poisonous and may cause blindness, brain damage or even death.* Mix the preparation in a glass container, cap and allow to stand in a cool, dry place for three to seven days, depending on the herb used. Stir or shake once or twice a day. The liquid is then poured off and pressed out of the soaked herb. Add enough alcohol or sixty percent alcohol solution to bring 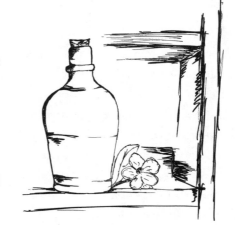 the tincture to the required volume. The tincture is then left to stand, undisturbed, until clear. It should then be filtered before being stored. Tinctures may be stored for three to six months.

If a tea without alcohol is preferred, add one teaspoon or one tablespoon of tincture to one cup of simmering water and allow it to sit uncovered ten to fifteen minutes, or until cool enough to drink. Another method to prepare an alcohol-free tea is to substitute cider vinegar for the alcohol.

Medicinal Actions of Plants

Just as the active component of a plant determines its effect on the human body, a medicinal herb can be characterized by its therapeutic effect or medicinal remedy. Some of the most common therapeutic effects are listed below.

Alterative - A substance capable of favorably altering or changing unhealthy conditions of the body and tending to restore normal bodily function.

Amenorrhea - A medical term for the absence or abnormal cessation of menstruation.

Analgesic - A substance that allays pain without causing loss of consciousness.

Anodyne - An analgesic substance that relieves pain.

Anti-coagulant - A substance that prevents the formation of a blood clot.

Anthelmintic - A substance used to eliminate or destroy parasitic intestinal worms. Also called vermifuges.

Anti-inflammatory - A substance that counteracts inflammation.

Anti-scorbutic - A remedy for scurvy, usually a substance that supplies vitamin C.

Antispasmodic - A substance used to prevent or ease muscle spasms or convulsions.

Aromatic - A plant or medicine with a fragrant, spicy smell and often a pleasant pungent taste, used to mask less pleasant drugs.

Astringent - A substance that causes contraction of the tissues and stops bleeding.

Bitter tonic - A substance with a bitter taste which stimulates the flow of saliva and gastric juices. Such tonics are taken to increase the appetite and aid the digestive process.

Carminative - A substance which checks the formation of gas and helps to expel whatever gas has already formed. Used to relieve colic or flatulence.

Catarrh - An inflammation of a mucous membrane, usually the nasal and air passages, characterized by congestion and the secretion of mucus.

Cathartic - An agent such as a laxative or purgative, used to encourage the evacuation of the bowel. A laxative is a gentle cathartic, while a purgative is more forceful and is used for severe constipation.

Cholagogue - A substance that promotes the discharge of bile from the gall bladder and bile ducts into the duodenum.

Choleretic - A substance that stimulates the production of bile in the liver.

Demulcent - A medicinal liquid of a bland nature taken internally to soothe inflamed mucous surfaces and to protect them from irritation.

Diaphoretic - A substance taken internally to promote sweating.

Diarrhea - An abnormal increase in the frequency of intestinal evacuations characterized by a fluid consistency.

Diuretic - A substance that increases the volume and flow of urine, thereby cleansing the excretory system.

Dysmenorrhea - Painful menstruation.

Emetic - A substance used to induce vomiting.

Emmenagogue - A substance that promotes or stimulates menstrual flow. Once a euphemism for an abortifacient, a substance that induces abortion.

Emollient - A substance applied externally to soothe, soften or protect the skin.

Expectorant - A substance that stimulates the formation and expulsion of mucus from the respiratory tract.

Febrifuge - An antipyretic substance that reduces or prevents fever.

Galactagogue - A substance that promotes or increases the secretion of milk.

Laxative - A substance that loosens the bowels and eases constipation.

Leucorrhea - A yellowish discharge from the vagina.

Purgative - A substance that causes fast, vigorous evacuation of severely constipated bowels more quickly and forcefully than a laxative. Sometimes synonymous with cathartic.

Rubefacient - A substance which, when rubbed into the skin, reddens the skin by attracting blood to the area.

Sedative - A substance that tends to calm, relieve anxiety and tension. It may cause drowsiness.

Stimulant - A substance which increases or quickens the various functional actions of the body, such as quickening digestion, raising body temperature and other effects.

Stomachic - A substance which gives strength and tone to the stomach or stimulates the appetite by promoting digestive secretions.

Tonic - A substance that stimulates and invigorates the body or an organ.

Vulnerary - A substance that counteracts inflammation and promotes the healing of wounds.

See the Appendix for a complete glossary of medical terms and a list of plants by medicinal remedy.

Anatomy of
Medicinal Plants

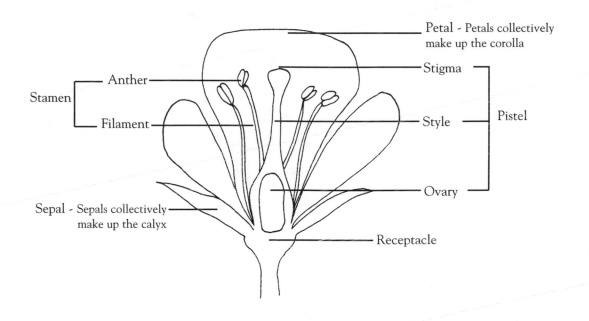

Petal - Petals collectively make up the corolla

Stigma

Style

Ovary

Pistel

Stamen

Anther

Filament

Sepal - Sepals collectively make up the calyx

Receptacle

Flower Forms

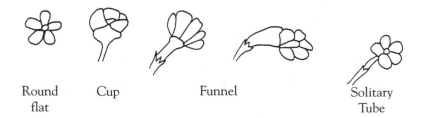

Round
flat

Cup

Funnel

Solitary
Tube

Flower Arrangements

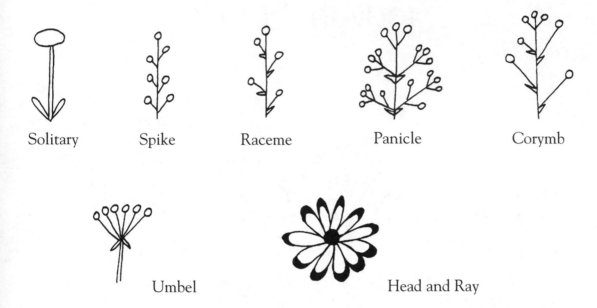

Solitary   Spike   Raceme   Panicle   Corymb

Umbel   Head and Ray

Flowerhead in the sunflower family (Asteraceae)

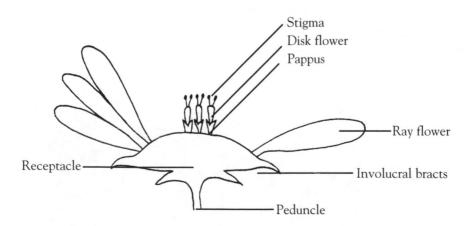

Stigma
Disk flower
Pappus

Ray flower

Receptacle

Involucral bracts

Peduncle

Leaves

Leaf Parts

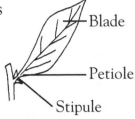
Blade
Petiole
Stipule

Sessile leaf
(no petiole)

Leaf Arrangements

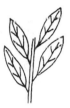
Alternate

Opposite

Whorled

Basal

Simple Leaves

Entire

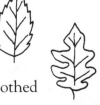
Toothed

Pinnately
lobed

Palmately
lobed

Once-Compound Leaves

Pinnate

Palmate

Leaf Shapes

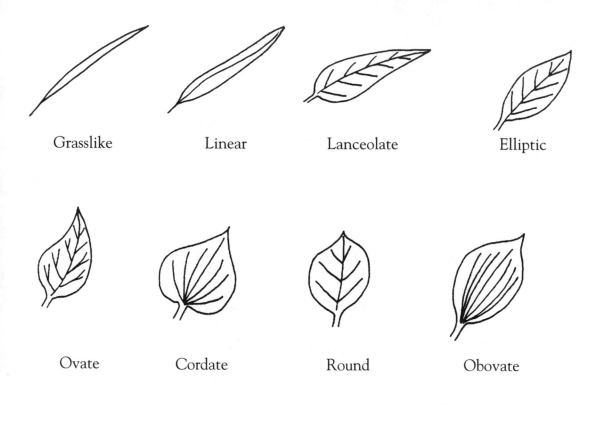

Grasslike   Linear   Lanceolate   Elliptic

Ovate   Cordate   Round   Obovate

Venation

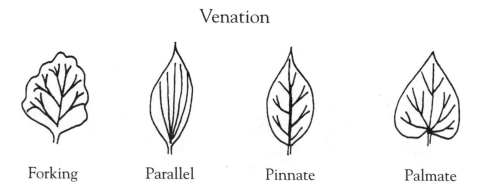

Forking   Parallel   Pinnate   Palmate

34

Root Types

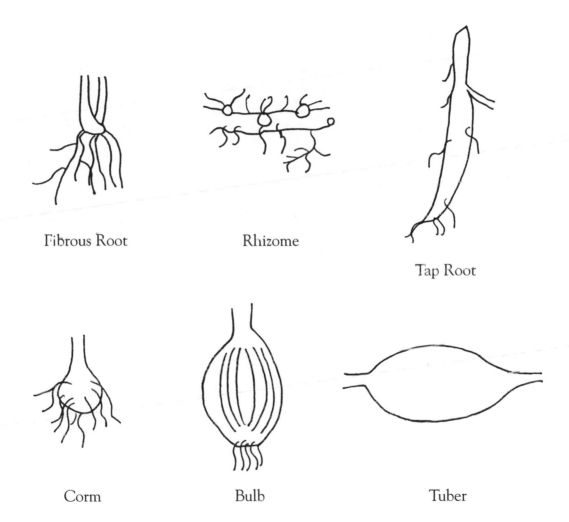

Fibrous Root

Rhizome

Tap Root

Corm

Bulb

Tuber

Medicinal Plants

Ferns, Grasses and Cacti

Bracken Fern

Pteridium aquilinum L.

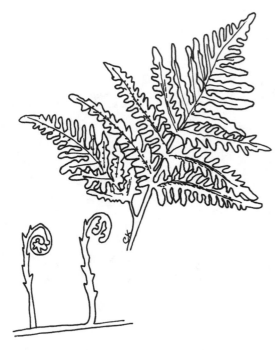

Common names
Brake fern, hogbrake, pasture brake.

Habitat
Open thickets, dry woods and fields throughout the Heartland, but mostly absent from the Great Plains.

Description
Bracken fern is a member of the Polypodiaceae (fern) family.

Bracken fern has a long, prolific root which extends horizontally. The rugged, stiff, dark green fronds (leaves) stand one to four feet tall with three branches containing rows of feathered, blunt-tipped leaflets which are reddish at the bases. Brown fruiting bodies called nectarines, located on the under surface, contain the spores, called sori. The shoot, or fiddlehead, resembling an eagle's claw, is covered with woolly, silver-gray hair.

Medicinal Uses
The fiddleheads of bracken fern have been a gourmet delicacy for centuries. According to legend, if you gather the sori on St. John's Eve, June 23, and hold them in your hand, you'll become invisible at the moment of St. John's birth.

The rhizomes, boiled into a strong tea, were used by several Indian tribes as an anthelmintic and diuretic for treating diarrhea, flatulence, mastitis and to expel intestinal parasites. Many Indians inhaled the smoke from the dried fronds to help ease headaches. The Cherokee used the roots of bracken ferns to soothe upset stomachs, as a blood purifier and as an antiseptic for treating wounds and scratches. The Ojibwa used a root decoction for nursing mothers and to curb stomach cramps.

Bracken fern contains the active component tannin. Herbalists recommend using the fiddleheads, collected before the fronds uncurl, in an infusion as an anti-carcinogenic, antiseptic, anti-viral and astringent. Boiled with water and sugar, the fiddleheads can be eaten, and the water which is rich in tannins, can be saved for later use to relieve various lung and liver ailments, or as an excellent dye for cotton fabrics. Boiling destroys the enzyme thiminase which depletes the body of vitamin B_1.

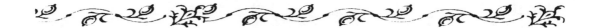

Studies have shown that bracken fern contains three carcinogens which may cause stomach cancer if ingested in large quantities over an extended period of time.

Long-term usage of bracken fern may cause constipation and interfere with calcium absorption which can cause extensive kidney damage. The concentration of the enzyme thiminase is very high and potentially very dangerous in mature, bitter fronds. Mature bracken ferns should not be used internally unless under the strict supervision of a qualified medical or herbal practitioner.

Cattail
Typha latifolia L.

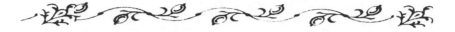

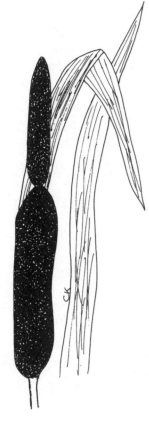

Common names
Black cap, cat-o-nine tails, marsh pestle, water torch.

Habitat
Rich wet soils, marshes, swamps, wet ditches and stream edges throughout the Heartland.

Description
Cattail is a member of the Typhaceae (cattail) family.

Cattail is a perennial with long, tapering, pointed, sword-like, alternate green leaves. The stiff, erect flowering stalk is topped with two flowering spikes, one above the other. The upper stalk bears the yellow, pollen-laden male flowers, and the lower stalk bears the hot dog-shaped brown female flowerhead.

Medicinal Uses
The peeled, young shoots of cattails less than eighteen inches long can be eaten raw or cooked as a potato substitute. Just before blooming, when enclosed in a husk, the top spike steamed or boiled, can be eaten like corn-on-the-cob. Pollen sections next to the base of the leaves and the rhizomes can be ground into a flour for making bread.

Many American Indian tribes used cattails for numerous medicinal remedies. They used the downy insides of the seedhead to soothe and relieve the pain of burns, wounds, carbuncles, external inflammations and boils. They applied the chopped root directly onto minor wounds and burns. They also used the chopped roots in an infusion to treat diarrhea, gonorrhea and intestinal parasites. The Dakota, Fox, Omaha, Pawnee, and Winnebago Indians applied the down of cattails to scalds and burns, in a manner similar to using baby powder. The Delaware regarded the root infusion as a cure for kidney stones. The Houma used a stem decoction for treating whooping cough. The Washone ate the young flowerheads to treat diarrhea. The Ojibwa, Potawatomi, Chippewa and Algonquin used a crushed root poultice to treat boils, carbuncles and sores.

Horsetail
Equisetum arvense L.

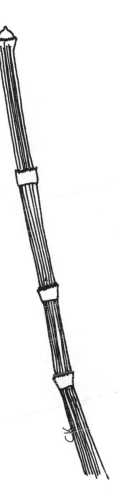

Common names
Scouring rush, bottle bush, mare's tail.

Habitat
Light sandy soils in fields, roadsides and waste grounds throughout the Heartland.

Description
Horsetail is a member of the Equisetaceae (horsetail) family. The generic name, *Equisetum*, is from two Latin words *equus* (horse) and *seta* (bristle).

Horsetail is a perennial, non-flowering herb with black rhizomes and two types of hollow stems with six to nineteen grooves. Horsetail appears in the spring; the fertile stems are joined, lack chlorophyll and have a compact terminal cone of sporangia. The sterile summer stems are green with grooved toothed sheaths at the joints with solid branches in whorls.

Medicinal Uses
Horsetail, a fern-like plant, is a relic of a dominant group of land plants of the mid-Paleozoic age which were once quite tall and tree-like, growing up to ninety feet tall and one foot in diameter. Horsetail, containing large quantities of silica, is used to clean metal and other hard surfaces. The Paiute Indians used dried horsetail ashes to treat sore mouths and canker sores. Nevada Indians made whistles from horsetail and drank a decoction to cleanse the urinary tract. The Cherokee and Ojibwa Indians made a decoction for treating constipation, bladder and kidney ailments.

Horsetail contains the active components silicic acid, aconite acid, the saponin equisetonin, minerals, tannin, traces of the alkaloids nicotine, palustrine, palustrin and equisitine. Herbalists recommend using the green stems in a tea mixture as an anti-diaphoretic and diuretic for anemia, kidney and bladder disorders including cystitis and urinary stones, enlarged or inflamed prostate, tuberculosis, calcium deficiencies, arteriosclerosis and hemorrhages. Studies have shown that silica aids in the absorption of calcium.

Externally, the tea mixture is used in compresses or bath preparations for stubborn wounds, skin rashes and skin ulcers.

Prickly Pear

Opuntia compressa (Salisb.) Macbr

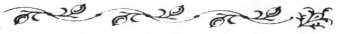

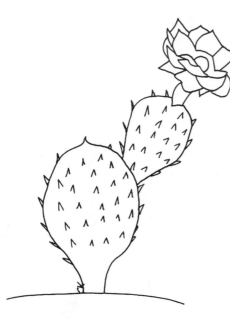

Common names
Beaver tail, Devil's tongue, Indian fig, prickly cactus, slipper thorn.

Habitat
Open fields throughout the Heartland.

Description
Prickly pear is a member of the Cactaceae (cactus) family.

Prickly pear has flat-jointed stems with very sharp spines instead of leaves. Lush red and golden flowers grow on a pod-like joint. It has pale oval seeds.

Medicinal Uses
Indians, plainsmen, mountain men, prospectors, trappers and settlers used compresses containing the acrid, sticky juice from the carefully peeled stems to heal abrasions and wounds. They also boiled the stems in water to provide a wash for sore eyes and a decoction for headaches, rheumatism and even insomnia. Poultices were prepared from mashed pulp and applied to various sores, such as saddle sores, on man and on animals, especially horses, mules and burros. Young joints, harvested before the spines had time to grow, roasted or boiled, were used as compresses for arthritis. Western frontiersman simmered well-washed roots in milk for treating dysentery. Black slaves also used the same remedy for treating severe diarrhea and to restore mucus to the intestinal tract.

Prickly pear is an excellent source of the active components potassium, beta carotene, vitamin C, calcium and phosphorous. Herbalists recommend using the fruits as an excellent gentle diuretic for expelling kidney stones and soothing ulcers. Don't be frightened if urine turns a bright crimson color after eating the fruit.

Use extreme caution when handling and collecting prickly pear and always wear gloves because the spines have been known to penetrate even leather gloves.

Quack Grass
Agropyron repens L.

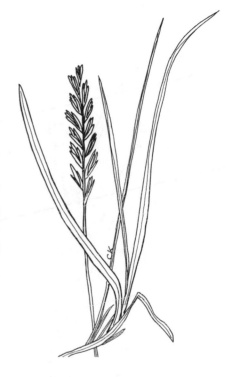

Common names
Couchgrass, wheat grass.

Habitat
Fields and waste grounds throughout the Heartland.

Description
Quack grass is a member of the Poaceae (grass) family. The generic name, *Agropyron*, comes from the Greek words *agros* (field) and *pyros* (wheat).

Quack grass is a long perennial grass with creeping rhizomes, that bears both sterile and fertile hollow, jointed stems, called culms. Linear leaves and sheaths encircle the culms. The flowers in flat spikelets are in long, stiff, loose terminal spikes and bloom in June and July. The fruit has one seed.

Medicinal Uses
American Indians used quack grass as a diuretic for treating kidney stones, urinary incontinence and to expel intestinal worms. The Cherokee used an infusion for treating urinary tract gravel and incontinence. They also used the infusion in a bath to reduce swollen arthritic joints. The Iroquois used the rhizomes with alder twigs in an infusion for treating urinary disorders.

The roasted herb has a pleasant aroma and sweet taste, and was once used as a substitute for coffee and as a raw material for making beer and spirits.

Quack grass contains the active components potassium, silica, saponins, sugars, the phenolic glycosides avenein and vanillin, mucilage, vitamins A and B, iron, a volatile oil with agropyrone, and a fixed oil with triticin, inositol and mannitol. Herbalists recommend using the dried rhizomes in a tea mixture as an antibiotic and diuretic for disorders of the kidney, bladder and urinary tract and for gout and rheumatism.

Recent studies have shown that the broad antibiotic properties of agropyrone is useful in the treatment of inflammatory disorders.

Sweet Flag

Acorus calamus L.

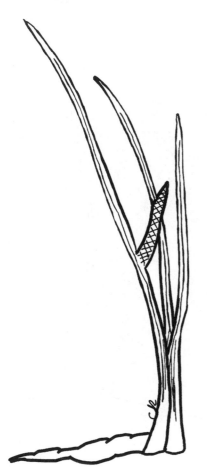

Common names
Calamus, pineroot, sweet cane, sweet root, sweet sedge.

Habitat
Marshes and other low areas throughout the Heartland.

Description
Sweet flag is a member of the Araceae (arum or calla) family. The generic name, *Acorus*, is derived from the Greek word *kore* (pupil of the eye) or from the Latin word for aromatic plant, referring to the usage by Dioscordis to cure eye troubles. The species name, *calamus*, is from the Greek word *kalamos* (reed), referring to the ancient custom of throwing sweet flag on dirt floors instead of rushes.

Sweet flag is an aromatic, grass-like perennial herb growing three to four feet tall. It has a long, branching, aromatic rootstock with coarse secondary roots. The flowering stems are three-angled with erect, thick, sword-shaped leaves. Tiny light brown or greenish brown flowers are in dense cylindrical spikes and bloom from May through August. Small, gelatinous, berry-like fruits contain three to five seeds.

Medicinal Uses
Sweet flag has been traded commercially in the Near East for four thousand years. Sweet flag was used as a common remedy two thousand years ago in India and by the early Greeks. In the Old Testament, Moses was commanded by God to use calamus (sweet flag) in an ointment he was to prepare for use in the tabernacle (Exodus 30). Sweet flag has also been used by many European herbalists as a folk remedy for a variety of uses. The roots, coated with sugar, were eaten as candy and as a breath sweetener. Distilled from the leaves and roots, the yellow, aromatic oil of sweet flag was used in hair powders, perfume, and as a flavoring in liqueurs, beer, gin, vinegar and snuff.

The Dakota, Omaha-Ponca, Pawnee and Winnebago Indians held sweet flag in very high esteem. They used it in a decoction for fevers and chewed the roots as a cough remedy and to relieve painful toothaches. The Meskwaki used a root tea for treating tuberculosis, coughs and stomachaches. The Potawatomi used the dried, macerated roots to stop

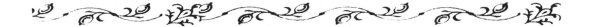

hemorrhages and in a snuff to cure catarrh. The roots were prepared in various folk remedies for treating inflammations of the liver, spleen and stomach, testicle tumors, ulcers, colds, coughs, dyspepsia, hysteria, insomnia, malaria, melancholy, headaches, gout, rickets, rheumatism and scrofula. The root stalk was considered to have tranquilizing effects, and when chewed raw, it temporarily sedated a throbbing toothache.

American Indians and early pioneers used a decoction made from the roots of sweet flag to treat colic, dyspepsia, stomach cramps, typhoid fever, coughs and constipation. In Appalachia, the freshly cut, spicy leaves were used as an insecticide. Sachets were hung or laid with clothing to keep moths away and the leaves were spread on cabin floors to ward off insects. It was also thought that sweet flag excited sexual desire because of its spicy aroma and pleasing taste.

Sweet flag contains the active components sesquiterpenes, tannin, resin, mucilage, an essential oil, the bitter principle acorin, a phenolic ether, a volatile oil with aserone, calamene, linalool, eugenol, azulene, pinene, cineole and camphor. Herbalists recommend using the fresh or dried roots as an aromatic bitter, anti-spasmodic, anti-convulsant and central nervous system depressant. The fresh root can be chewed for relieving the discomfort of flatulence and heartburn. In a tea, the dried roots can be used for indigestion, fevers, colds and coughs.

The Chinese recommend using sweet flag to treat dizziness, deafness, epilepsy and toothaches. They also used sweet flag, with its mild sedative effects, to break habitual tobacco usage.

Sweet flag was once considered carcinogenic. However, further tests have shown that only the variety native to India contains the carcinogen beta-asarone which also acts to sterilize female insects by preventing ovary development.

The beta-asarone-free oil from American sweet flag has been found to be an effective, safe antihistamine.

Trees, Shrubs
and Vines

Balm of Gilead

Populus canadicans L.

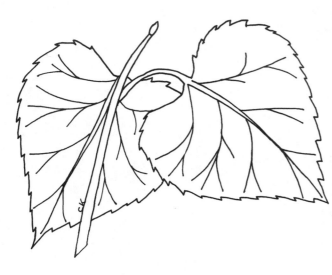

Common names
Poplar, cottonwood.

Habitat
Moist forests and occasionally culti-vated. Found primarily in Wisconsin, Minnesota and Iowa.

Description
Balm of Gilead is a member of the Salicaceae (willow) family.

Balm of Gilead is a small tree with a fissured, black trunk with broad, flat ridges. The broad-ovate leaves are finely toothed. The fruits are in a catkin.

Medicinal Uses
The Colonists introduced the practice of steeping fresh blossoms in cold water, straining, and drinking the resulting tea to purify the blood. Mashed leaves were made into compress-es to alleviate headaches. The juice was used as eardrops for relieving painful earaches. The roots, raw or boiled, were used in a warm poultice to relieve the swelling, pain and inflammation of sprains, bruises and rheumatic areas. Dissolved or held in suspension by alcohol, the chopped bark was highly recommended by settlers for treating inflammations of the kidneys, chest and digestive system. Tinctures were also used for treating scurvy, arthritis and gout. Steeped in Jamaican rum, the buds were considered an excellent remedy for treating cuts and bruises. Resin from the buds, extracted by alcohol before the buds burst into leaves, was used in salves and ointments to treat burns, scalds, scratches, inflamed wounds, coughs, colds, flu and pneumonia. An antiseptic gargle was used to treat sore throats. In an aromatic tea, the resin was believed to be even more soothing and stimulat-ing than Oriental tea.

Balm of Gilead contains the active components salicin, phenolic acid, a resin with palicin and populin, a volatile oil with cineole, bisabolene, bisabolol and humulene. Herbalists rec-ommend using the bark in a decoction as an anti-bacterial and expectorant for lung infec-tions. The decoction is also used as a gargle for sore throats, and mixed in an ointment to ease the pain and inflammation of rheumatism.

Studies have shown that bisabolol has anti-microbial and anti-inflammatory properties. Salicin has sedative properties.

Barberry
Berberis vulgaris L.

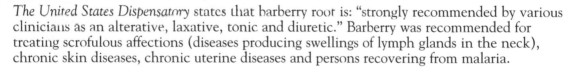

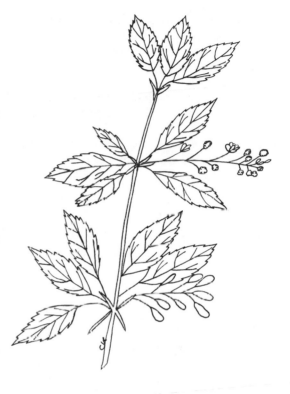

Common name
Yellow root, dragon grape, sow berry.

Habitat
Pastures, thickets, fence rows and occasionally cultivated. Found in Michigan, Ohio, Indiana, Illinois, Missouri and Minnesota.

Description
Barberry is a member of the Berberidaceae (barberry) family.

Barberry is a perennial, deciduous shrub. The obovate, small, serrated leaves are green above and gray below. The small yellow flowers, in drooping racemes, bloom in May and June. It has a scarlet to purple, oblong berry.

Medicinal Uses
According to Culpeper, "the inner rind of the barberry tree, boiled in white wine and a quarter of a pint drunk every morning, is an excellent remedy to cleanse the body of choleric humors, and free it from such diseases as choleric causeth, such as scabs, itchy tetters, ringworms, yellow jaundice and biles."

The United States Dispensatory states that barberry root is: "strongly recommended by various clinicians as an alterative, laxative, tonic and diuretic." Barberry was recommended for treating scrofulous affections (diseases producing swellings of lymph glands in the neck), chronic skin diseases, chronic uterine diseases and persons recovering from malaria.

Barberry contains the active components tannin, the triterpene myricadial, the flavonoid glycoside myricitrin, resin, the alkaloids berberine, berbamine, columbamine, palmatine and oxyacanthine. Herbalists recommend using small doses of the bark in a decoction (large doses may cause stupor) as an antiseptic, choleretic, diuretic, laxative and stomachic. The decoction is used for kidney, liver and gallbladder disorders, inflammation of the gastrointestinal tract, post-partum hemorrhage, excessive menstruation, vomiting, diarrhea and respiratory failure. The decoction is also used as a douche for treating leucorrhea, and in a compress for healing cuts and ulcers. The root bark steeped in beer is used as an astringent for diarrhea, dysentery, hemorrhages and jaundice.

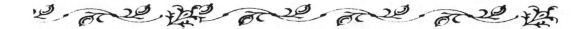

The non-toxic berries, rich in vitamin C, sugars and pectin, are used as an astringent and anti-scorbutic. A refreshing herbal tea is used by herbalist to relieve sore throats and upset stomachs. The berries are used as a flavoring in many teas to treat fevers, especially typhus, and to treat certain vitamin deficiencies such as scurvy.

Studies have shown that myricitrin is an antibacterial agent and encourages bile flow. Myricadriol may cause salt retention and potassium excretion.

Barberry bark, containing berberine, is very toxic and should be used only under the strict supervision of a qualified medical or herbal practitioner.

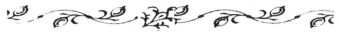

Bearberry
Arctostaphlos uva-ursi (L.) Spreng.

Common names
Bear's grape, hog cranberry, Uva-ursi.

Habitat
Sandy, rocky soils in Minnesota, Wisconsin, Michigan, northern Illinois and northern Indiana.

Description
Bearberry is a member of the Ericaceae (heath) family. The generic name, *Arctostaphlos*, is derived from two Greek words, *arktos* (a bear) and *staphyle* (grapes).

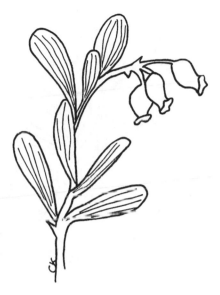

Bearberry is a low, evergreen shrub with long, rooting branches. Small, oval, leathery leaves are dark green on the upper surface with a pale, distinct net-veined under surface. It has small white or pink-tipped flowers in short dense raceme s and produces a shiny red, globose drupe with five seeds. The flowers bloom in May and June.

Medicinal Uses
The Indians and settlers smoked bearberry leaves as a tobacco substitute or drank a leaf tea to increase urine flow. Pioneers mixed a small amount of dry powdered leaves from whole leaves previously soaked in an alcoholic beverage, in a cup of hot water to make a tea for treating chronic inflammation of the kidneys or bladder.

According to Millspaugh "Uva ursi is an ancient astringent... in late years it has been called attention to as uterine excitant, very useful in prolonged parturition from debility... I could hardly point to a drug more adapted to diseases of the kidneys, bladder and urethra than arbutin, which is changed in the renal tract to hydrokinone, a source of phenol, which is in itself a germicide, the arbutin being more or less innocuous and at same time a diuretic; it has however, caused an eruption in the skin."

Bearberry contains the active components allantoin, the glycosides arbutin and methylarbutin, tannins, the crystalline principle ursone, gallic and phenolic acid. Herbalists recommend using the powdered leaves in an infusion as an antiseptic, astringent, diuretic and tonic for urinary disorders, hemorrhage, bronchitis, cystitis, nephritis, kidney and gall stones, gonorrhea, diarrhea and uterine contractions.

Bearberry should be taken internally only under the supervision of a qualified medical or herbal practitioner. Used for long periods of time, bearberry may cause skin eruptions, constipation, nausea or more serious side effects. Arbutin hydrolyzes to the toxic urinary antiseptic hydroquinine which is poisonous in large doses. Normal medicinal usage is perfectly safe.

Birch

Betula sp.

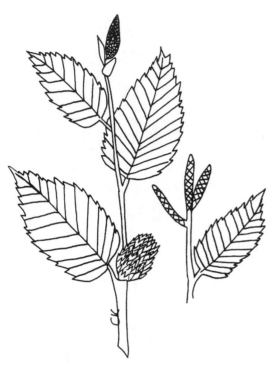

Common name
River birch, white birch, yellow birch.

Habitat
Rich, moist woodlands along rivers and streams throughout the Heartland.

Description
Birch is a member of the Betulaceae (birch) family.

Birch (*Betula alba, B. allegheniensis, B. nigra*) are tall, deciduous trees with pendulous brown branches that have resinous wart-like structures, called lenticels, on the surface. Pointed, oval, alternate, leaves are doubly-serrated. Monoecious, purple-brown male flowers are in drooping catkins; female flowers are smaller, green catkins. The fruit is a winged achene.

Medicinal Uses

American Indians and settlers used the fresh leaves of black birch in an unboiled tea steeped in hot water until cool. One to two cups drank daily was used as a mild sedative that produced no drug-like hangover, to encourage quiet, peaceful sleep and to relieve headaches. A similar medicinal tea from the leaves and dried bark was used for treating fevers, kidney stones and abdominal gas pain. A bark poultice was applied to heal burns, wounds and bruises. Catawba Indians simmered the buds to make a syrup, to which sulfur was added, to make a salve for treating ringworms, sores, wounds and dermatitis.

Birch species contain the active components methyl salicylate, betulinol, a camphor-like betulin saponin, resin, tannins, sesquiterpenes, betuloventic acid and vitamin C. Herbalists recommend using the bark, buds and young leaves of the various birch species as an anodyne, astringent and diuretic. A leaf infusion is used by herbalists as a diuretic to treat fluid retention due to heart or kidney malfunction. To obtain the best results, add a pinch of baking soda to the infusion to promote the extraction of the diuretic hyperoside. The infusion is powerful enough to dissolve kidney and bladder stones, to lower blood cholesterol levels, to stimulate bile flow and as an antibiotic agent against harmful bacteria. The infusion is also an excellent gargle for sore mouths and canker sores.

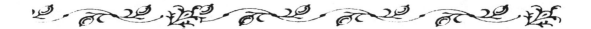

Commercial birch oil, known as oil of wintergreen, is used in antiseptic ointments for skin diseases, musculoskeletal pain of osteoarthritis, low back pain, and as a counterirritant for sore, stiff muscles and joints. Some herbalists mix this oil with other aromatic oils as an insect repellent.

Studies have shown that methyl salicylate is an anti-inflammatory and excellent analgesic that relieves pain and reduces the risk of heart disease. Recent research has shown that betulinic acid has promising results against melanoma, a skin cancer that strikes one in fifteen people. Betulinic acid may reduce the possibility of developing melanoma as well as reduce the size of existing tumors.

Bittersweet
Celastrus scandens L.

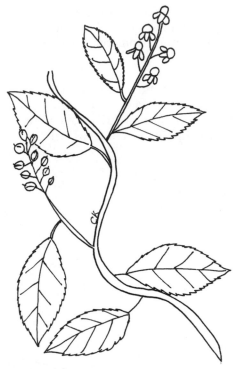

Common names
Fever twig, staff tree.

Habitat
Dense, moist thickets, fence rows, waste grounds and roadsides throughout the Heartland.

Description
Bittersweet is a member of the Celastraceae (staff tree) family. The genus name, *Celastrus,* is from the Greek for a kind of evergreen plant; and the species name, *scandens,* is from Latin meaning "climbing," referring to the plant's general growth habit.

Bittersweet is a perennial vine with twining woody stems and has broad, oval, alternate leaves with uneven margins. It has tiny inconspicuous flowers in loose terminal clusters with five green-white oblong petals. It blooms in June and produces brilliant orange, round, finely wrinkled, pea-sized berries.

Medicinal Uses
The Chippewa Indians used a stem decoction of bittersweet as a physic and as a wash for skin eruptions. A root-bark decoction was used to induce menstruation and perspiration. Both Indians and settlers used bittersweet bark as an astringent, diaphoretic, emetic and diuretic for the treatment of fevers, tuberculosis, venereal diseases, diarrhea, dysentery and leucorrhea. They also mixed powdered bark with animal fat as a salve for treating rheumatism, skin cancers, tumors, burns and swellings. An extract of the roots and stems provided an excellent insecticide. Millspaugh in his book *American Medicinal Plants,* described bittersweet as a excellent blood purifier for the removal of liver obstructions.

Herbalists recommend using a root-bark decoction as a diaphoretic, diuretic and emetic for chronic liver and skin ailments, rheumatism and suppressed menses. Externally, it can be used in an ointment for burns and skin eruptions and in a douche for leucorrhea.

Bittersweet Nightshade
Solanum dulcamara L.

Common names
Woody nightshade, scarlet berry.

Habitat
Waste areas, thickets, open fields and boggy areas throughout the Heartland.

Description
Bittersweet nightshade is a member of the Solanaceae (nightshade) family.

Bittersweet nightshade is a perennial, woody at its base, with long climbing or trailing stems. Alternate, ovate leaves are serrated or deeply lobed at base and pointed toward the tip. Violet flowers with five spreading, recurved petals and yellow anthers are in long stalked terminal cymes located in the upper leaf axils. It blooms from June through October and has scarlet red, ovoid berries.

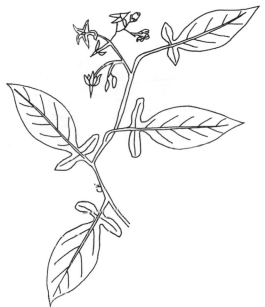

Medicinal Uses
Galen in A.D. 150 recommended using bittersweet nightshade as a treatment for tumors, cancer and warts. Dr. O.P. Brown in 1875 said that "The Complete Herbalist regard this plant as important as any in the Herbal Kingdom, and too little justice is done to it by those under whose care the sick are intrusted."

Many Indian tribes of northeastern America used bittersweet nightshade as a medicinal herb. The Nootka Indians used a decoction as an analgesic for colic. The Delaware used a salve for treating dermatological problems. The Malachite used a root infusion for nausea.

Bittersweet nightshade contains the active components tannins, saponins, the steroidal glycosidic alkaloids soladulcine, solanine and dulcamarine. Herbalists recommend using an infusion of the green shoot tips as an antiseptic, expectorant, mild diuretic and stimulant for chronic bronchitis, asthma, rheumatism and chronic skin disorders.

Large doses of the alkaloid solanine paralyzes the central nervous system without affecting peripheral nerves or voluntary muscles. It also slows the heart and respiration, lowers body temperature, causes vertigo, deliriums and convulsions, with the end result possibly being death.

All parts of bittersweet nightshade are poisonous and should never be collected and used for self medication without supervision from a qualified medical or herbal practitioner.

Blackberry - Raspberry

Rubus sp.

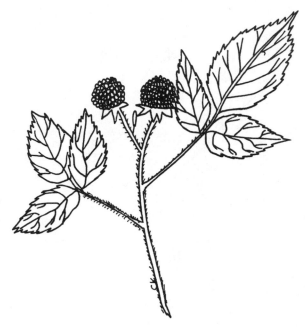

Common names
Blackberry, cultivated raspberry, black raspberry, raspberry.

Habitat
Roadsides, open fields and cultivated throughout the Heartland.

Description
Rubus species are members of the Rosaceae (rose) family.

Rubus species (*Rubus allegheniensis, R. idaeus, R. occidentalis, R. pennsylvanicus*) are perennial shrubs, wild or domesticated, tall or short, with erect, thorny or thornless, woody stems. Odd-pinnate leaves with three to seven serrated, ovate leaflets that are glossy above and white-felted below. The white flowers are in dense terminal, axially drooping racemes and bloom from June through August. The black, red or yellow juicy fruit is a compound drupe.

Medicinal Uses
Since ancient Greek times *Rubus* species have been used interchangeably for a multitude of medicinal remedies. A leaf tea has been used by pregnant women to prevent miscarriage, to ease labor pains and to increase the milk supply of nursing mothers. An infusion has been used to treat stomach disorders, enteritis, diarrhea, flu and colds. A fresh berry tea was used as a gargle for sore throats, as a mouth wash, and as a base for summer drinks, candies, syrups, pies, brandy and wines. Bath preparations were excellent for treating skin rashes, wounds and fungal infections.

The Cherokee, Chippewa, Omaha, Potawatomi and Rappahannock Indians used a root bark decoction for treating dysentery, diarrhea (especially in children), parturition, dyspepsia, rheumatism, measles, and as an eye wash. The Cherokee chewed the roots and berries for treating coughs, diarrhea, fevers, scurvy, sore throats and toothaches.

At one time, American physicians officially recognized using a decoction of the dried bark of roots and rhizomes as an astringent, blood purifier and spring tonic in a manner similar

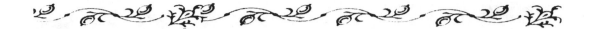

to uses by the Indians. Many a colonist deemed his medicine chest incomplete without blackberry brandy as a rapid remedy for diarrhea; eating large quantities of the ripe berries was also an effective remedy for diarrhea.

Rubus species contain the active component tannin, pectin, sugar, vitamins A, B and C, fragarine, citric and malic acid, iron, calcium and phosphorous. Herbalists recommend using the leaves and berries in an infusion or herbal mixture as an anti-fungal, antiseptic, astringent, cholagogue, diuretic, emmenagogue, expectorant and tonic. The infusion or herbal mixture is used for lung, stomach, intestinal and female disorders, especially menstrual pains.

Studies have shown that flagarin, and other unidentified substances found in the leaves and berries, have oxytocic properties, serving to relax the uterine muscles and relieve menstrual pains.

Butternut
Juglans cinerea L.

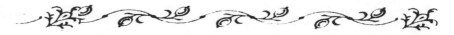

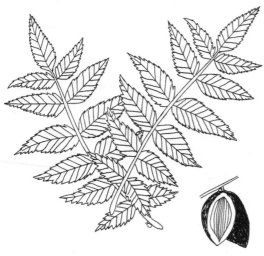

Common names
Lemon nut, oil nut, white walnut.

Habitat:
Rich woodlands from Michigan to Georgia, Arkansas to North Dakota.

Description
Butternut is a member of the Juglandaceae (walnut) family. The generic name, *Juglans*, means "regal nut of Jupiter."

Butternut, a native of North America and a close relative of the black walnut (*J. nigra*), is a tall tree forty to sixty feet high, with light gray bark and broad, furrowed ridges. It has odd-pinnate compound leaves, with eleven to seventeen opposite, serrated leaflets. It produces small, green-yellow elliptical nuts with the sticky husk covered with hairs in a thick, deeply furrowed shell.

Medicinal Uses
The American Indians obtained the oil from the ripe nuts by boiling them in water and skimming off the oil which rose to the surface. The tasty nuts were dried and eaten later. The oil was used for treating fungal infections and to expel tapeworms. Indians used a warm bark compress on wounds to stop bleeding and to promote healing.

As far back as the Revolutionary War, butternut was used to treat dysentery and constipation without causing cramps. During the Civil War, a strong decoction of bark and leaves was used as an external wash for ulcers, open sores and other skin troubles. The decoction was also an effective gargle and mouth wash for sore throats, canker sores and other mouth irritations such as those caused by the rubbing of artificial teeth, like Washington's wooden set. The nut kernels were a favorite prescription for mental patients.

Butternut contains the active components juglone, phosphorous, magnesium, silicon and calcium. Herbalists recommend using the inner bark of the roots and nut kernels in a decoction as an emetic, stimulant and tonic for stimulating the flow of bile in liver disorders, to purify the blood and stabilize the brain. The nuts have the lowest carbohydrate content of all nuts and are ideal for people on a low carbohydrate diet.

Studies have shown that juglone has antiseptic and anti-tumor activity. Juglone is also an excellent herbicide.

58

Cramp Bark
Viburnum prunifolium L., *V. opulus* L.

Common names
Black haw, red elder.

Habitat
Dry, rocky hillsides, fence rows, roadsides, thickets and low woods from Michigan to Florida, Texas to Iowa.

Description
Cramp bark is a member of the Caprifoliaceae (honeysuckle) family. Both *Viburnum prunifolium* and *V. opulus* have been called cramp bark; however, *V. prunifolium* is is preferably called black haw by most botanists, and *V. opulus* is called cramp bark.

Cramp bark is a large shrub to small tree. It has bright green leaves that are elliptic to broadly ovate and finely toothed. Small white flowers in flat clusters bloom from March through May. It also has black oval drupes.

Medicinal Uses
A root or stem bark tea made from cramp bark was used by the American Indians for relieving painful menses, to prevent miscarriage and to relieve spasms after childbirth.

The root or stem bark of cramp bark contains the active components resins, valeric acid, the coumarin scopoletin, the bitter glycoside viburnin, triterpenoid saponins, salicosides, tannins and arbutin. Herbalists recommend using a decoction as an antispasmodic, astringent, nervine, uterine sedative and tonic. The decoction is used as an excellent muscle and nervous relaxant particularly good for easing painful periods and birthing pains, to prevent excessive menstrual flow at menopause, and for uterine infections and septic poisoning during childbirth. A decoction of twigs is used for diarrhea, uterine pains and general spasms. Collect bark and twigs in the spring to make a tincture because the dried bark loses strength with time.

Cramp bark was listed in *The United States Pharmacopeia*. It is now listed in *The National Formulary* as a nerve sedative and antispasmodic for treating asthma and hysteria. At one time, selling cramp bark was a small business in the United States. Dried or powdered, it

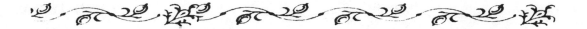

was sold in local pharmacies for treating painful menstruation, cramps, amenorrhea, threatened abortion, bleeding and pregnancy. A tea was also used for treating asthma, charley horses, epilepsy and convulsions.

Studies have shown that scopoletin is a muscle relaxant, and that viburnin is a mild sedative of the nervous system. *V. prunifolium* contains three times the amount of viburnin. As a muscle relaxant and mild sedative, cramp bark is an excellent remedy for reducing spasms and painful cramps. In Europe a cramp bark tea is used to relieve all types of spasms, including menstrual cramps.

The berries contain the active components chlorogenic acid, beta sitoslerol, urosolic acid and vitamin C. Herbalists recommend using the berries as an anti-scorbutic to prevent and treat scurvy. The berries, tasting like dates and with a texture like prunes, were traditionally used in "Pioneer Jam" for treating scurvy. In China, the berries and fruit are used as an emetic, laxative and anti-scorbutic. *However, the berries are potentially poisonous when unripe and may cause nausea.*

Dogwood
Cornus florida L.

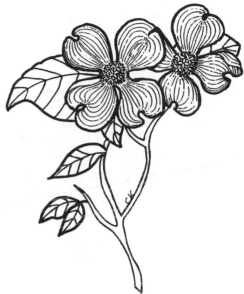

Common name
Dog tree, flowering dogwood.

Habitat
Rocky woods, wooded slopes and low slopes throughout the Heartland.

Description
Dogwood is a member of the Apiaceae (carrot) family.

Dogwood is a beautiful American tree ten to thirty feet tall. Oval, opposite leaves are dark green above and lighter below. Flowers, occurring in a small bunch surrounded by four large white, involucral bracts, bloom in May. The dogwood produces red, berry-like fruits.

Medicinal Uses
All Northeastern Indians used a red dye from the roots to color the porcupine quills and eagle feathers used to trim their clothing. They steeped the inner bark of the stems and root to make a fever remedy for malaria. The bark was used in a poultice for treating sores, and in rubbing ointments for relieving leg pains. The Delaware, Alabama and Houma Indians used the inner bark in a tea for treating fevers and diarrhea. The Cherokee used the tea for treating backache, chickenpox, colic and measles.

The Indians introduced the medicinal uses of dogwood tea to the white settlers. The settlers also used the tea for treating cholera, sore mouths, and jaundice, to expel worms and as a bitter, spring tonic to cleanse and rejuvenate the body after a long, cold winter.

According to Millspaugh: "Dogwood bark has properties calculated to invigorate the vital forces, and the organic nervous energy." During the Civil War dogwood was used a substitute for quinine and to treat chronic diarrhea. Peeled twigs were used by Creole Blacks of Virginia as toothpicks to clean, preserve and whiten their teeth. The juice preserves and hardens the gums.

Dogwood trees contain the active components tannic and gallic acids, resin, lignin, minerals and the glucoside cornin. Herbalists recommend using the bark in a decoction as an astringent, cholagogue, diaphoretic, stimulant and tonic for cancer, colic, dyspepsia, fever, hepatitis, hysteria, jaundice, malaria and typhus.

Elderberry

Sambucus canadensis L.

Common names
Black elder, elder, pipe tree.

Habitat
Rich, moist soil of woodlands and roadsides throughout the Heartland.

Description
Elderberry is a member of the Caprifoliaceae (honeysuckle) family.

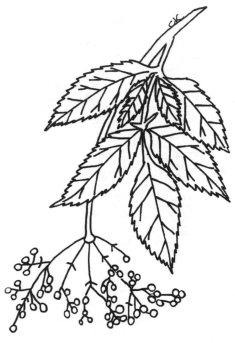

Elderberry is a small deciduous tree or climbing shrub with a corky bark and arched, gray-brown, deeply furrowed branches. It has odd-pinnate, opposite leaves with five or seven oval to lanceolate, serrated leaflets, with or without very small stipules. Small fragrant creamy-white flowers with yellow anthers are arranged in flat-topped terminal umbel-like cymes and bloom in June and July. Small, dark purple edible drupes are borne on red stalks.

Medicinal Uses
Elderberry has been found in Stone Age sites. It was perhaps one of the original Grecian formulas for dyeing hair black, and was considered the home of the goddess Freya. According to an ancient recipe, washing the face with elderberry flower water in the morning and at night, and leaving it there to dry, would remove freckles and harden the skin. During the Middle Ages, it was believed that elderberry sprigs gathered on the last day of April would ward off witches if put on the windows and doors of houses, and that fairies and elves would appear if you sat underneath an elderberry tree on a midsummers night.

American Indians used the leaves and flowers in an antiseptic wash for skin diseases. They used the berries to dye their hair black and the strands of grass were used in their basket designs. Some old Indian herbalists listed the flower and bark as a diuretic, purgative and emetic, depending on dosage. According to J. L. Lighthall, an Indian herbalist: "a tea of flowers had diaphoretic effect when taken hot, a diuretic effect when taken cold, and a tea of the bark, taken in tablespoon doses 3 - 4 times daily was a mild purgative, while doses of 3 - 4 swallows every 5 minutes would produce an emetic effect." The Illinois-Miami Indians used a root and bark decoction for fainting spells. The Iroquois used the inner bark in a decoction to ease toothaches. The Meskwaki used the root bark decoction to free lung phlegm and in extremely difficult cases of parturition when the baby was dead.

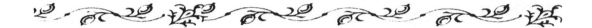

Elderberry wines (a safe hypnotic) and cordials have been made for centuries. Elderflower fritters can be made from either fresh or dried flowers. A delightful tea made from the dried blossoms was used for colds and to promote sleep. The flowers contain an oil that is used in perfume and cosmetics.

Elderberry contains the active components anthocyanin pigments, triterpenes, the flavonoid glycosides rutin and quercitrin, sugar, vitamin A, very high amounts of vitamin C, thiamine, niacin, calcium, the cyanogenic glycosides valerianic, palmitic, linoleic and linolenic acids. Herbalists recommend using the flowers and/or fruits in an infusion as an alterative, astringent, diaphoretic, diuretic, expectorant, mild gentle laxative and mild sedative. The flower infusion is used for colds, respiratory infections and mild nervous disorders. The flowers in bath water, soften the skin, soothe sore muscles and serve as an excellent remedy for irritable nerves. The berries eaten raw are said to help arthritis and gout The berry infusion is used for treating colds, insomnia, migraine headaches, to soothe children's upset stomachs, to relieve gas, and for weight loss as a diuretic and detoxifying agent. The berry juice mixed with honey makes an excellent cough syrup.

Elderberry leaves contain cyanogenic glycosides (substances that release cyanide and an unidentified cathartic) and should not be used internally because of their strong purgative and potentially poisonous properties. Used externally, however, the bruised leaves rubbed on skin will keep flies away.

Hawthorn
Crataegus sp.

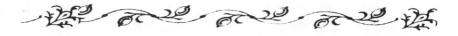

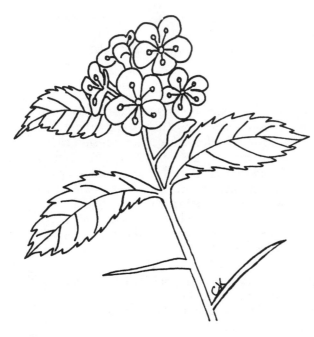

Common names
May blossom, whitethorn.

Habitat
Moist woodlands throughout the Heartland.

Description
Hawthorn is a member of the Rosaceae (rose) family. The generic name, *Crataegus*, is from the Greek word *kratos*, meaning hardness of the wood.

Hawthorn is a deciduous thorny shrub with dark green, wedge-shaped, deeply lobed leaves. White flowers, mostly in dense corymbs, have five petals and a five-parted, bell-shaped-tube calyx. They bloom in spring and early summer. The berries have one to five seeds.

Medicinal Uses
The fruits and flowers of hawthorn are famous in American, Indian, Chinese and European herbal folk medicine as a heart tonic. In China and France, the berries were used for treating diarrhea and dyspepsia, and to aid digestion. An infusion or tea mixture was used in both herbal medicine and proprietary medicine to treat various heart and circulatory disorders, migraines, menopausal conditions and insomnia.

Hawthorn contains the active ingredients saponins, tannin, procyanidin, organic acids, trimethylamine, flavonoid glycosides, pectin, vitamin C and B-complex. Herbalists recommend using an infusion of the flowers, leaves and/or fruits as an astringent, cardiac, diuretic, sedative and tonic for sore throats, diarrhea, abdominal distention, heart and circulatory ailments.

Recent studies confirm that the flavonoids are useful in relieving hypertension and arteriosclerosis by reducing blood pressure and dilating the coronary vessels. Procyanidin also acts to slow the heart beat. British research has shown that the berries reduce high blood pressure caused by hardening of the arteries and kidney disease, and that the flowers improve the health of patients suffering from "aging heart" and heart-valve disease.

Hercules' Club
Aralia spinosa L.

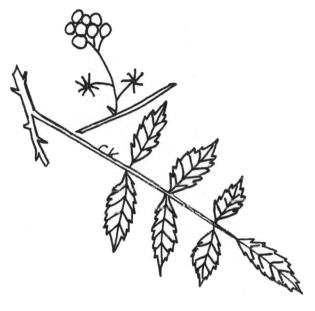

Common names
Angelica tree, Devil's walking stick, prickly elder.

Habitat
Rich woods and thickets through the Heartland.

Description
Hercules' club is a member of the Araliaceae (ivy) family.

Hercules' club is a perennial with many sharp spines on the woody stems and leaf stalks. The huge, oval, toothed leaves are twice-divided with numerous leaflets. Tiny white flowers in umbels bloom from July through September. It produces a bluish colored fruit.

Medicinal Uses
The Cherokee Indians used a root decoction as a "blood purifier," carminative, diaphoretic, emetic and tonic for treating colic, paralysis, rheumatism, fever and venereal diseases. The Chippewa used the decoction as a gargle for sore throat and toothaches. The Mississippi valley Indians and Rappahannock poulticed the roots onto boils and other sores.

Black slaves used the fresh root to draw out the venom from snakebites, and applied the dried, powdered root to the bite to prevent infection. The water used to store the fresh roots was used to treat irritated eyes.

Hercules' club contains active components the saponin aralien, a volatile oil and an acrid resin. Herbalists recommend using a bark decoction as an alterative, diaphoretic, purgative and strong emetic for fevers, colic, rheumatism and chronic constipation. A tincture of the berries is used for toothaches and rheumatic pain.

Handle Hercules' club with care as the roots may cause dermatitis. Large amounts of the berries can be poisonous.

Honeysuckle

Lonicera japonica Thunb. and *L. sempervirens* L.

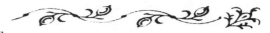

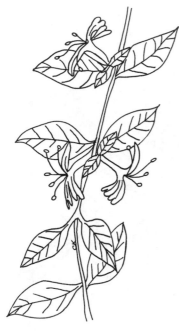

Common names
Japanese honeysuckle, trumpet honeysuckle.

Habitat
Woods, thickets and along roads throughout the Heartland.

Description
Honeysuckle is a member of the Caprifoliaceae (honeysuckle) family.

Honeysuckle is a perennial woody vine with opposite, oval leaves with smooth margins and the tip rounded or pointed. The lower leaves have short petioles, but upper ones may be perforate (joined around the stem). Red, white, creamy or yellow flowers are a distinctive trumpet shape. Outer flared petals, may be equal but usually have unequal, upper and lower lips and bloom from April through August. It produces red berries, often in pairs.

Medicinal Uses

Early settlers used honeysuckle as a cathartic, diuretic and emetic in an infusion for treating nausea, constipation and urinary retention. The Indians chewed the leaves and applied the maceration on bee stings. They used the leaves in an infusion as a wash for sores and used the roots in a poultice to reduce swellings. The berries were eaten raw to expel worms from pregnant women, and in an infusion to cure lung ailments and fevers. A root tea was used as a diuretic for treating urinary ailments. Many tribes wove the vines into baskets.

Honeysuckle contains the active component salicylic acid, mucilage and invertin. Herbalists recommend using an infusion as an anti-bacterial, astringent, diaphoretic, diuretic, emetic, expectorant and laxative for bacterial dysentery, enteritis, laryngitis, fever and flu. A syrup is used for respiratory disorders, fevers, constipation, edema and asthma. The leaves, infused in oil, are excellent for relieving cramps and nervousness. A decoction of the bark is used as a gargle for sore throats or in a lotion for itchy skin and skin eruptions. The sweet-scented flowers are used in perfumes. Externally, the flowers are used in a wash for treating rheumatism, infected wounds, tumors and scabies.

Recent studies have shown that the flowers lower cholesterol and have anti-viral and anti-bacterial properties.

Hops
Humulus lupulus L.

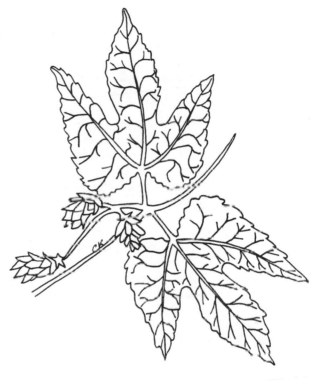

Common names
Hop vine, northern vine, European hop.

Habitat
Ditches, wetlands, wet areas and cultivated throughout the Heartland.

Description
Hops is a member of the Cannibaceae
(hemp) family.

Hops is a perennial, climbing herb with
long, leafy angled stems and branched
rhizomes. Opposite, palmate, coarsely-
serrated leaves have three to five lobes.
It has dioecious green flowers; male
flowers are in druping axillary panicles,
tiny female flowers are clustered in
ovoid, cone-like spikes (hops) with persistent overlapping bracts. It blooms
from July through September. The fruit
is an achene enclosed in the perianth.
All parts of the plant are roughly hairy.

Medicinal Uses
Hops has been used in brewing since Roman times. However, there was widespread resistance to its use in Europe, particularly in England, until the seventeenth century. During
the reign of Henry VIII, petitions against hops as "a wicked weed that would spoil the taste
of the drink and endanger the people" were presented to the Parliament. After hops was
accepted in the brewing business, brews flavored the old way with rosemary or ground ivy
were known as ale, while those brewed with hops were given the German name "bier." The
bitter substitute obtained from the granular hairs of the strobili, which when dried have a
spicy aroma and bitter taste, is used by brewers for giving aroma and flavor to beer.

King George III slept on a hops-stuffed pillow to alleviate some symptoms of his porphyr-
ia. Originally hops were used for their preservative value. Germans add hops to sausages as
a natural preservative. Hops contain a natural substance that prevents the growth of
gram-negative bacteria.

The Delaware, Cherokee, Mohegan and Fox Indians drank a hops tea several times a day to
alleviate nervousness. Hops tea was also drunk in an effort to stop the craving for white

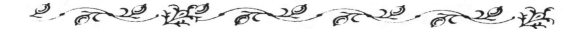

mans' alcohol. The Cherokee used the herb like aspirin to ease pain, to induce sleep, and for treating breast complaints, urinary gravel, inflamed bladder and kidneys and rheumatism. The Delaware applied hot leaves to relieve earaches or toothaches, and drank a flower tea for relieving coughs and flu, and as tranquilizer. A root decoction was used as an antacid and diuretic. They used hops in hot baths for relieving the swelling and pain of arthritis, rheumatism and muscular swellings.

Hops contain the active components a bitter resin compound with valeronic acid and lupulone, the volatile oil with humuline, myrcene, and barnescene, the flavonoid glycosides rutin, linalool, citral, linionene, serolidol, quercitrin, and asparagin, and the oestrogenic substance gamma-linoleic acid (the "wonder drug" GLA found in evening primrose - *Oenthera biennis*). Herbalists recommend using the cones or strobili in an infusion as a mild diuretic, sedative, stomachic and weak antiseptic for digestive disorders, nervous irritability, insomnia, and as an anti-aphrodisiac for men. Hops are used in skin creams and lotions for their skin softening properties. In China alcoholic extracts of hops are used clinically to treat leprosy, pulmonary tuberculosis and acute bacterial dysentery.

An effective way of using hops for insomnia is in a sachet under the pillow. The distilled essential oil is used in perfumes, cereal beverages, mineral waters and tobacco. A decoction of hops with boneset (*Eupatorium perfoliatum*) is used for treating bruises. Hops can be used with other herbs to treat irritable bowel syndrome, Crohn's disease (regional enteritis) and nervous stomachaches. The young shoots and immature leaves make a good addition to salads.

Research shows that hop extracts relax the smooth muscles, especially those of the digestive tract. The components lupulone and humulone, with anti-bacterial activity, play a major role in reducing inflammations of gastric and duodenal ulcers.

GLA is used by the body to produce prostaglandins, which control the physiological responses that lower blood pressure, reduce the risk of thrombosis, stimulate the immune system and regulate brain function.

Women should always wear gloves when handling hops as female hop pickers occasionally suffer disruption or the complete absence of menstruation when the oil of hops containing oestrogenic principles is absorbed through their hands. Pregnant women should never use hops.

Kentucky Coffee Tree
Gymnocladus dioicus (L.) K. Koch.

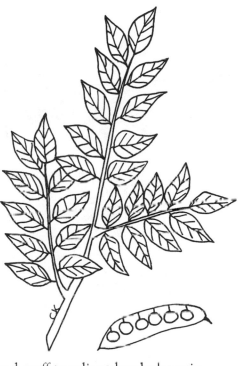

Common name
Coffee tree.

Habitat
Rich, low woods from Ohio to Tennessee,
Oklahoma to South Dakota.

Description
Kentucky coffee tree is a member of the Fabaceae
(pea) family.

The Kentucky coffee tree is a native tree that
grows from forty to one hundred feet tall.
Gigantic, double-compound leaves have seven to
thirteen oval toothed leaflets. A single white
inflorescence has a terminal raceme and blooms in
June. Large brown, flattened, curved seedpods
have six to ten seeds.

Medicinal Uses
The Pawnee were among the Indians who roasted
the seeds and ate them like chestnuts for nutrition
and health reasons. They also used them in a powdered snuff to relieve headache pain.
The Omaha Indians used a root infusion as an enema and hemostat.

Early settlers discovered Kentucky coffee seeds (they somewhat resemble coffee beans) at
about the time the famous frontiersman Daniel Boone was helping to settle Kentucky.
They roasted and ground them as a caffeine-free coffee substitute.

Pioneer women crushed, sweetened and ate the pod with its pulpy filling or made a preserve
which they used as a gentle laxative. A decoction of the leaves and fruit pulp was used to
treat locomotor ataxia, coughs, peritonitis, erysipelas and typhoid. The roots were dried,
pulverized and used in an enema for intestinal disorders such as constipation, diarrhea and
hemorrhoids. A root bark tea was used for relieving coughs, prolonged childbirth, and as a
diuretic and hemostat. The powdered bean was used in a manner similar to smelling salts.

*The poisonous raw seeds contain hydrocyanic acid, the alkaloid cystosine and toxic saponins which
cause severe gastrointestinal irritation and nervous disorders. Kentucky coffee seeds should be used for
self medication only under the supervision of a qualified medical or herbal practitioner.*

Moonseed

Menispernum canadense L.

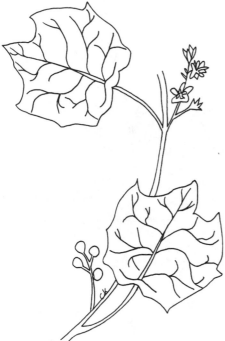

Common name
Yellow sarsaparilla.

Habitat
Moist woodlands and thickets throughout the Heartland.

Description
Moonseed is a member of the Menispermaceae (moonseed) family. The generic name, *Menispernum*, comes from two Greek words, *mene* (moon) and *sperma* (seed).

Moonseed is a perennial, woody climbing vine with a slender stem. Large, broad leaves with three to seven shallow lobes have smooth edges and palmate venation. White or pale-green flowers with a stamen protruding beyond the petals, are in long clusters. They bloom from May through July. The globular, dark blue-black, moon-shaped flattened seed is rough and ridged.

Medicinal Uses
Indians utilized a root tea for treating scrofulous affections, indigestion, arthritis, bowel disorders, female disorders and as a "blood purifier." The Cherokee also used the tea for treating venereal diseases.

The Indians taught the early settlers to use moonseed as an anti-inflammatory, astringent, emmenagogue, stimulant and tonic. They also used the rhizomes and roots in a decoction to treat constipation, syphilis, rheumatism, gout, edema and skin infections. The dried rhizome was officially listed in *The United States Pharmacopeia* from 1882 through 1905. Historically, physicians used a root tincture to treat constipation, edema, indigestion, rheumatism, arthritis and chronic skin infections.

Moonseed contains the active components the alkaloids isoquinoline, berberine and menispine. Herbalists recommend using an infusion of the fruits as an alterative, antibiotic, astringent, diuretic and cathartic for arthritis, syphilis and general debility. Externally, a poultice is used to treat ulcerated sores.

Research has shown that the alkaloids isoquenoline, berberine and menispine have curare-like qualities which paralyze the muscles by blocking nerve impulses.

70

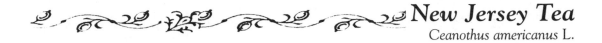

New Jersey Tea
Ceanothus americanus L.

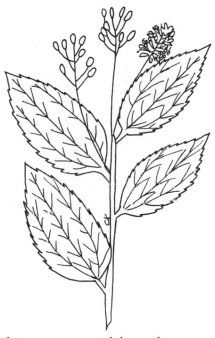

Common names
Mountain tea, red root, wild snowball.

Habitat
Rocky hillsides, roadsides, ravines and open woodlands throughout the Heartland.

Description
New Jersey tea is a member of the Rhamnaceae (buckthorn) family.

New Jersey tea is a shrub. Leaves are oval and toothed with three prominent veins. White flowers are showy, puffy clusters and bloom from April through September. Fruits are triangular seed vessels.

Medicinal Uses
A tea made from New Jersey tea leaves was drank during the American Revolution as a substitute for imported English teas. The tea was also used as an expectorant, mouthwash and gargle for sore throats. A commercial tincture was widely used to increase blood coagulation, particularly after surgery. Early physicians used the root as an astringent, expectorant, stimulant and tonic to treat digestive, ovarian and uterine irregularities.

The American Indians including the Chippewa, Menomoni, Mesquakie and Potawatomi used a root tea for treating colds, fevers, snakebites, stomachs, diarrhea, lung ailments, constipation and as a blood tonic.

New Jersey tea contains the active components tannins, ceanonthin, and the flavonoids afzelin, quercitrin and rutin. Herbalists recommend using an infusion of the leaves and/or roots as an antispasmodic, astringent, expectorant, hemostat, sedative, and stimulant for gonorrhea, dysentery, asthma, sore throats, bronchitis, whooping cough, spleen inflammations, eye diseases in children and to promote blood clotting. The infusion is also used as a douche for treating leucorrhea.

Studies have shown that New Jersey tea lowers blood pressure.

Oak

Quercus sp.

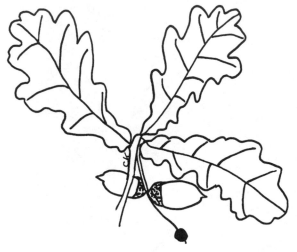

Common names
Black, burr, post, red, Spanish or white oak.

Habitat
Moist bottom land or dry upland woods throughout the Heartland.

Description
Oak is a member of the Fagaceae (beech) family.

Oak trees (*Quercus alba, Q. falcata, Q. macrocarpa, Q. rubra, Q. stellata, Q velutina*) are large, deciduous trees. Leaves are alternate, simple and often lobed. Long, narrow yellow flowers are in drooping catkins and bloom from April through May. The fruit, acorns, are oval thin-shelled nuts, partially surrounded by cups.

Medicinal Uses
Many Indians used oak species interchangeably for numerous medicinal remedies. The Cherokee, Chippewa, Creek, Delaware, Lumbee, Ojibwa, Potawatomi, and Houma Indians used a bark decoction as a panacea. It was used to treat asthma, bronchial and cardiac ailments, chafing, chills, debility, dysentery, dyspepsia, fevers, diarrhea, hysteria, dysmenorrhea, laryngitis, malaria, stomatitis (an inflammation of the mucous membranes of the mouth), sore throat, gynecological disorders and as a wash for sore eyes.

All oak species contain the active component tannins, gallic acid and allagitannin. Herbalists recommend using a decoction of the bark as an astringent and antiseptic for treating chronic diarrhea, dysentery and bleeding from the mouth. The decoction is also used in a douche for leucorrhea, as a gargle for sore throats, a wash for eczema, poison-ivy, rashes, burns, and as a poultice for gangrenous sores.

Experimentally, tannic acid has been shown to have anti-viral, antiseptic, anti-tumor and carcinogenic properties.

The tannic acid in oak species is potentially toxic in large doses or prolonged usage. Therefore, caution should be taken when using for self medication.

72

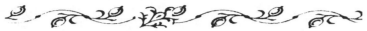

Prickly Ash
Zanthoxylum americanum Mill

Common names
Toothache tree, yellow wood.

Habitat
Open, rocky woodlands, thickets, fence rows and roadsides throughout the Heartland.

Description
Prickly ash is a member of the Rutaceae (yellow wood) family. The generic name, *Zanthoxylum*, may be spelled with an X: *i.e.*, *Xanthoxylum*.

Prickly ash is a small tree with alternate branches, sharp, strong prickles and pinnate leaves. It blooms in April and May. The berries are in clusters at the tip of the branches. The nut has a black-to deep blue shell.

Medicinal Uses
Many Indian tribes used a decoction of prickly ash as a cure for toothaches, hence its common name, toothache tree. The Chippewa used a decoction of the fruit and bark as a gargle for sore throats. The Winnebago used prickly ash to cure gonorrhea. The Meskwaki used prickly ash as an expectorant in cough syrups and as a cure for hemorrhaging and tuberculosis. Illinois-Miami used a poultice to draw off pus.

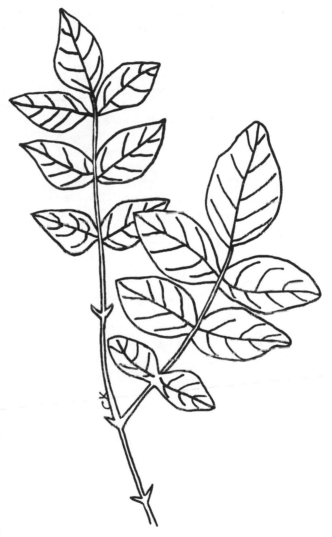

The settlers adopted the medicinal remedies of prickly ash from the Indians. They also used prickly ash as a treatment for diarrhea, fevers and flatulence. Black slaves used the bark to treat toothaches and rheumatism. Millspaugh wrote that prickly ash was used for treating rheumatism and as a powerful stimulant for healing wounds or ulcers. Prickly ash

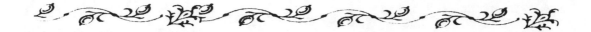

was used by the physicians of Cincinnati for treating the Asiatic cholera outbreak in 1849 and 1850. It was considered superior to other medicines for treating typhus fever, pneumonia and typhoid.

The dried bark was officially listed in *The United States Pharmacopeia* from 1820 to 1926, and in *The National Formulary* from 1926 through 1947. The berries were officially listed in *The National Formulary* from 1916 to 1947 for treating sore throats and tonsillitis.

Prickly ash contains the active ingredients pyrocoumarins, xanthyletin, xanthoxyletin and alkaloids. Herbalists recommend using an infusion of the berries or a decoction of the stem bark and/or root bark as an antispasmodic, astringent, carminative, emmenagogue and stimulant for the ailments listed above. They may also be used as a tonic for stomach disorders and complaints of bad circulation. The powdered bark is used as a poultice on ulcerated sores and wounds, and in an infusion to relieve nervous headaches.

Red Cedar
Juniperus virginianna L.

Common names
Cedar apple, evergreen, savine.

Habitat
Woods, cliffs and fields throughout the Heartland

Description
Red cedar is a member of the Cupressaceae (cypress) family.

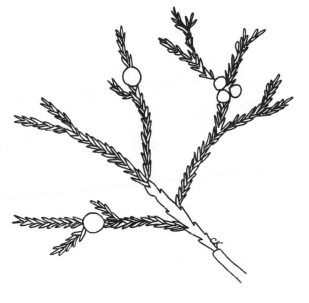

Red cedar is a pyramidal to columnar evergreen tree with reddish brown to gray, fibrous bark splitting into long, flat strips. Opposite leaves are green to blue-green, simple scale-like or needle-like. Male and female cones appear on separate trees in April and May. Male cones are yellowish-brown and papery; dark blue, waxy, berry-like female cones ripen from September to October.

Medicinal Uses
The Cherokee, Dakota, Pawnee, Ojibwa, Omaha and Ponca Indians inhaled the smoke from burned red cedar twigs for head colds, bronchitis and purification rituals. They used the herb and berries in an infusion for treating colds, dysmenorrhea, measles, rheumatism, skin ailments, headaches, swellings, to induce sweating and to expel worms. Red Cloud of the Lakotas used a decoction of the leaves in baths for treating and "curing" Asiatic cholera during an outbreak in 1849 and 1850.

The distilled oil of red cedar has been officially listed in *United States Pharmacopoeia* since 1916 as a diuretic, stimulant, emmenagogue and diuretic.

Red cedar contains the active component cedarwood oil. Herbalists recommend using cedarwood oil as an antiseptic, diaphoretic, diuretic, emmenagogue and rubefacient. Cedarwood oil is used in preparations of insecticides, medicinal liniments and perfumed soaps. The oil was formerly one of the principal ingredients of the popular Extract of White Rose.

Studies have shown that cedarwood oil contains a germicide that is an effective antiseptic.

Sarsaparilla
Smilax sp.

Common names
Catbriar, greenbriar.

Habitat
Dry woods, edges of fields and bluffs throughout the Heartland.

Description
Sarsaparilla is a member of the Liliaceae (lily) family. The common name, sarsaparilla, comes from two Spanish words *sarza* (bramble) and *parilla* (a vine), referring to the thorny stems of the plant.

Sarsaparilla (*Smilax bona-nox, S. glauca, S. rotundifolia*) is a large, perennial vine with tendrils in pairs and alternate, broadly-oval leaves with smooth margins. The female plant has clusters of fifteen to eighty tiny yellow-green flowers. Male flowers are similar, but larger than the female flowers. The plant blooms from July to winter and produces blue-black berries.

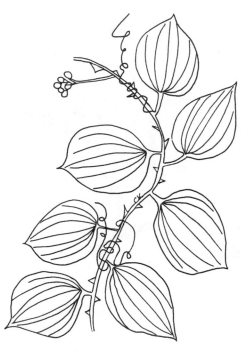

Medicinal Uses
Sarsaparilla has been used in European medicine since the sixteenth century, when it was introduced from Mexico or Peru. It was thought that the juice of the berries given to a new-born made it immune to all poisons. Pirates used sarsaparilla tea as a specific remedy for syphilis and drank large quantities as a tonic. The leaves and berries were used in a tea as an antidote to many deadly poisons.

Native Americans used sarsaparilla roots as an alterative, "blood purifier," pectoral and diaphoretic for treating skin diseases, rheumatism, dyspepsia and gout and expelling the afterbirth. The roots were used in a syrup for coughs and colds. The Natchez rubbed a root decoction on the face to "make one stay young." For local pain, Cherokee and Creek Indians pricked their bodies with sarsaparilla, then rubbed another medicine into the scratch.

Sarsaparilla contains the active components the steroidal saponins sarsapic acid and sarsapogenin which is related to progesterone. These steroidal components are used in the synthesis of progesterone. Research has shown that *Smilax glabra* is highly effective for treating syphilis and mercury poisoning. The roots were once used with wintergreen and sassafras as the major ingredient of root bear; however, this combination of herbs has been replaced by synthetics.

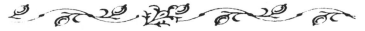

Sassafras
Sassafras albidum (Nutt.) Nees

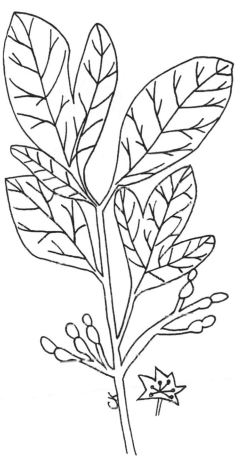

Common name
Ague tree.

Habitat
Dry or moist woodlands, thickets and roadsides from Ohio to Florida, Texas to Kansas.

Description
Sassafras is a member of the Lauraceae (spicebush) family.

Sassafras is a small to medium tree with gray to reddish-brown bark that is roughly furrowed and has a strong aromatic odor and flavor. The leaves are in three shapes: a thumbed mitten, three-fingered glove or a smooth egg-shape. It produces dark blue, pea-sized, one-seeded berries on reddish stalks.

Medicinal Uses
Native to North America, sassafras was used by many American Indian tribes in a root decoction as a diuretic after childbirth, and as a general tonic to heal venereal diseases and rheumatism. It's exportation to Europe exceeded that of tobacco at one time. Grieve stated that: "Oil of sassafras is chiefly used for flavoring purposes, particularly to conceal the flavor of opium when given to children ...it's use has caused abortion in several cases ...prevent and remove the injurious effects of tobacco ...can produce marked narcotic poisoning, and death by causing widespread fatty degeneration of the heart, liver and kidneys, or in a larger dose by great depression of the circulation, followed by a centric paralysis of respiration."

Sassafras contains the active components camphor, resins, albumin, lignin, tannins, sassafrid, a volatile oil with safrole, phellandrene and pinene. Herbalists recommend using a root infusion as an alternate, diaphoretic, diuretic, stimulant and tonic for colds, fever, chronic arthritis, gout, high blood pressure, kidney problems, and stomachaches. Drank regularly, the infusion is a good blood purifier for making a person resistant to colds and throat infections. The infusion can also be used as a wash for inflamed eyes, skin eruptions, rheumatism, gout and arthritis. A compress or salve can be applied to skin rashes such as poison oak or poison ivy.

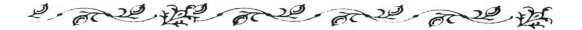

The aromatic oil, distilled from the roots, contains safrole which converts to a carcinogen in rats, but not in humans. It is used to relieve pain of menstrual obstruction and parturition. Sassafras bark is mixed with wintergreen and sarsaparilla to make homemade root beer. Combined with rose hips and capsicum, the bark is used in commercial dental preparations. Sassafras bark, chewed or made into a tea, is an excellent remedy to help one quit tobacco smoking. The peeled twigs are used to disinfect the root canals of infected teeth. Today the dried, powdered leaves are an expensive gourmet item called "gumbo file."

Large doses or prolonged usage of sassafras can cause widespread fatty degeneration of the heart, liver and kidneys and/or a decrease in blood flow which may lead to respiratory paralysis, narcotic poisoning, abortion and possibly death. Always consult a qualified medical or herbal practitioner before using sassafras internally.

Slippery Elm
Ulmus rubra Muhl.

Common names
Indian elm, moose elm, red elm, sweet elm.

Habitat
Moist woods, often disturbed areas from Michigan to Florida, Texas to North Dakota.

Description
Slippery elm is a member of the Ulmaceae (elm) family.

Slippery elm is a slim, wide-branching, flat-topped tree. Dark brown bark is deeply furrowed, rough and scaly. Deep yellowish, olive green rough leaves are lighter underneath. It blooms in March and April and produces winged, round fruit.

Medicinal Uses
The inner, mucilaginous bark of slippery elm has been traditionally used as a diuretic, emollient and demulcent. A decoction has been used as an important, soothing remedy for inflammations, sore throats, bronchitis, upset stomachs, indigestion and stomach ulcers. The decoction is used as a nutritious gruel or food to soothe and heal internal inflammations such as dysentery, diarrhea and urinary disorders. It can also be used as an enema for babies with inflamed bowels, or as a vaginal douche. Ground into a coarse powder, slippery elm bark makes a fine poultice for all externally inflamed surfaces such as ulcers, wounds, bruises, boils and skin diseases.

Due to its strengthening and healing qualities, the bark of slippery elm is considered by herbalists as one of the most valuable remedies for treating sore throats, upset stomachs, stomach ulcers, coughs, pleurisy, diarrhea and dysentery. Research has confirmed the soothing, softening effect of slippery elm on mucous membranes and hardened tissue. Lozenges made from slippery elm are used for coughs and sore throats.

Prepared like oatmeal, the mucilaginous bark is an excellent, nutritional, wholesome food for infants and invalids. To prepare, mix a teaspoon of the powdered bark with cold water to form a thin, smooth paste, then pour in a pint of boiling water, stirring constantly. Flavor with cinnamon, nutmeg or other spices.

Spicebush

Lindera benzoin (L.) Blume

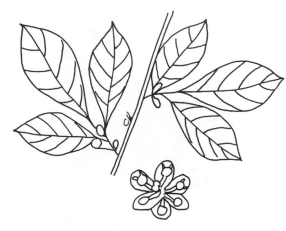

Common names
Feverbush, wild allspice.

Habitat
Moist, rich soils, deep shady woods along streams from Ohio to Florida, Texas to Illinois.

Description
Spicebush is a member of the Lauraceae (laurel) family.

Spicebush is a deciduous shrub and has aromatic, ovate leaves with smooth margins. Tiny, yellow flower in axial clusters bloom in March and April. Its highly aromatic, glossy scarlet berries have one large seed.

Medicinal Uses
American Indians, including the Iroquois, Cherokee, Creek, Rappahannock and Delaware, used spicebush berries in a tea for treating coughs, cramps, delayed menses, dysmenorrhea, hives, croup, measles and as an anodyne. A bark tea was used as a "blood purifier," and to treat colds, rheumatism, fevers and anemia. The oil from the berries was used for treating colic, flatulence and arthritis. The Cherokee steeped the bark with wild cherry (*Prunus serotina*) and dogwood (*Cornus florida*) in corn whiskey to break out measles. The Creek bathed in a tea made of spicebush and willow (*Salix* sp.) to relieve the pain and swelling of rheumatism.

Settlers used spicebush as far back as the Revolutionary War as an allspice substitute, to treat typhoid fever and to expel worms. They called it feverbush because a strong bark decoction caused profuse sweating which activated the immune system and expelled toxins from the body. During the Civil War, Southerners relied on the long leaves, bark and twigs for treating colds, fevers, worms, gas and colic. The young twigs and leaves were also used by the early settlers of Ohio and the Blacks of Alabama as a substitute for tea and allspice.

Spicebush contains the active components borneal, terpinalene, cineole, and phellandrene. Herbalists recommend using the a decoction of the bark, leaves and/or berries as an anthelmintic, anti-periodic, anodyne, diaphoretic, emetic, febrifuge, stimulant and tonic for fevers, respiratory ailments, female problems, anemia and general debility.

 ## Sumac
Rhus sp.

Common names
Dwarf sumac, fragrant sumac, smooth sumac.

Habitat
Woodlands, fields, roadsides, bluffs, and dunes throughout the Heartland.

Description
Sumac is a member of the Anacardiaceae (sumac) family.

Sumacs (*Rhus aromatica, R. copallina, R. glabra*) are shrubs, two to fifteen feet high with straggling branches and pale gray bark. Leaves are one to three feet long with thirty pointed, toothed leaflets (*R. aromatica* has only three leaflets). Green-yellow flowers are in terminal clusters and bloom from May through August. Red, flat, round, hairy berries have a sour, astringent taste.

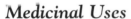

Medicinal Uses
Many Indian tribes used sumac species interchangeably for many medicinal purposes. For peace pipe ceremonies, they used the dried berries or powdered bark mixed with tobacco (some overdosed and hallucinated, believing they were flying through the air). Chippewa, Lumbee, Illinois, Miami, Omaha, Pawnee, and Potawatomi Indians used a flower or root decoction for bladder ailments, stomachache, gonorrhea, labor, diarrhea, dropsy, gingivitis, frostbite and deep arrow wounds. The Cherokee chewed the berries for nausea and drank a bark tea to increase the flow of milk in nursing mothers and to treat sunburn. The Creek used the roots for skin eruptions, sores and venereal diseases, the berries for a mouth wash, and hot steaming foot baths for arthritis, muscular swellings and rheumatism.

Millspaugh wrote about sumac: "Benefit in diabetes ...oil of Rhus ...this waxy oil extracted from the seeds ...can be made into candles, which burn brilliantly, but emit a very annoying pungent smoke. During the summer of 1879, while botanizing ...ate the refreshing berries on three successive nights, following this occurrence I flew (!) over the city of New York with a graceful and delicious motion I would give several years of my life to experience in reality."

Herbalists recommend using an infusion of the berries which are high in vitamin C, leaves, inner bark and root bark as an anti-diuretic, antiseptic, astringent and tonic. The infusion is used for diarrhea, dysentery, asthma, urinary infections, sore throats, chronic gum problems and cold sores.

Caution should be taken when eating the berries in large doses or over an extended period as hallucinogenic effects have been reported.

Walnut

Juglans nigra L.

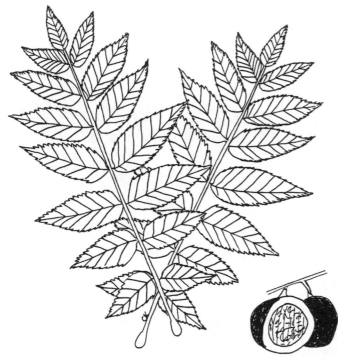

Common names
Black walnut, Jupiter's nuts.

Habitat
Rich, deciduous woods, bottom-lands, floodplains and cultivated throughout the Heartland.

Description
Walnut is a member of the Juglandaceae (walnut) family.

Walnut is a large deciduous tree with a spreading crown. It grows to more than one hundred twenty feet in height. The young trees have ash gray smooth bark and the older trees have a fissured, deep brown bark divided into rough ridges by deep narrow ridges. The odd-pinnate compound leaves have twelve to twenty-three alternate, serrated leaflets. With monoecious flowers, the male flowers are borne in pendulous catkins and the female flowers grow at the ends of twigs in groups of two or three. The green, ovoid fruit (nut) has a thick, fleshy, aromatic husk in a hard, rough deeply-furrowed shell.

Medicinal Uses
In the Middle Ages, walnuts were believed to cure mental disorders because of the resemblance of the nuts to the human brain (in accordance with the Doctrine of Signatures). The juice of the green husks, boiled with honey, was thought to be an excellent gargle for sour mouths and throats. Collected at the end of May, the distilled water of the green leaves was thought to cure running ulcers and sores. It was considered best to bathe the sores in the morning and at night with a wetted cloth.

Walnut contains the active components tannin, juglandin, organic acids, an essential oil, the glycoside hydrojuglone, the bitter compound juglone, beta carotene, iron, linolenic and linoleic acids. Herbalists recommend using an infusion of the outer green layer (pericarp) of the fruit, bark and/or leaflets as an anti-inflammatory, antispasmodic, astringent, mild sedative and vermifuge for treating diarrhea and to check mammary secretions. Externally, the infusion is used as a douche for leucorrhea, or as a mouthwash for sore mouths and tonsils.

82

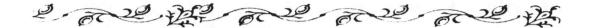

Externally, a thick infusion from the rind of the green fruit is used as a poultice for ringworm, athlete's foot and other fungal skin infections, and hemorrhoids. A decoction of the boiled husks kills parasites and repels fleas.

Rich in oil, high in energy and with almost as much protein as a sirloin steak, the nuts are widely used in the food and confectionery industries. The black walnut is used in soaps, artists paints and to dye the hair and body.

Research has shown that juglone has anti-cancer properties. A spirit distilled from fresh walnuts has been used to calm hysteria and to stop vomiting in pregnant women.

Wild Black Cherry

Prunus serotina Ehrl.

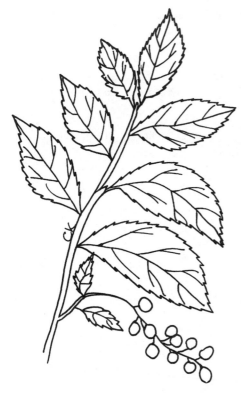

Common names
Choke cherry, Virginian prune, wild cherry.

Habitat
Dry woods throughout the Heartland.

Description
Wild black cherry is a member of the Rosaceae (rose) family.

The wild black cherry is a deciduous tree fifty to eighty feet tall, with black, rough bark. The leaves are toothed. White flowers in erect, long terminal racemes bloom in May. It produces a purplish-black, pea-sized globular drupe.

Medicinal Uses
The Cherokee, Chippewa, Delaware, Illinois-Miami, Lumbee, Mohegan, Ojibwa and Penobscot Indians used a bark and/or root decoction for treating coughs, colds, delayed menstruation, bladder ailments, cholera, ague, worms, hoarseness, fever, parturition, measles, and thrush. A berry wine was drank for difficult pregnancies.

The aromatic, inner bark has traditionally been used in a tea or syrup for treating coughs, fevers, colds, sore throats, diarrhea, lung ailments, dyspepsia and as a "blood tonic."

Wild black cherries contain the active components coumarin, the cyanogenic glycoside prunasin, the enzyme prunase, a volatile oil, tannin, prussic acid and resin. Herbalists recommend using a syrup as an astringent, mild tonic and sedative. The syrup is an important remedy for relieving coughs, bronchitis, heart palpitations and dyspepsia.

Studies have shown that prussic acid increases respiration and then sedates the sensory nerves which promote the cough reflex.

The bark, leaves and pits of wild black cherry are poisonous and contain the cyanide-like glycoside prunasin, that converts to the highly-toxic hydrocyanic acid when ingested. Therefore they should never be used for self medication unless under the strict supervision of a qualified medical or herbal practitioner.

84

Wild Yam
Dioscorea villosa L.

Common names
China root, colic root, devil's bone.

Habitat
Dry or moist woodlands from Michigan to Tennessee, Texas to Minnesota.

Description
Wild yam is a member of the Dioscoreae (wild yam) family. The generic name, *Dioscorea*, is in honor of the ancient Greek physician, Dioscorides; and, the species name, *villosa*, is from the Latin meaning "with hairs."

Wild yam is a perennial with slender twining stems. Its horizontal rhizome has a dry to hard bony texture (Devil's bone). It has alternate, heart-shaped leaves with smooth or slightly wavy margins and pale green, downy undersides. Blooming in June and July, male and female flowers appear separately. Tiny green-yellow male flowers occur in drooping cluster of spikelets and larger female flowers are in a droop spike. They bloom in June and July. The membranous, triangular fruit produces one or two seeds in each compartment.

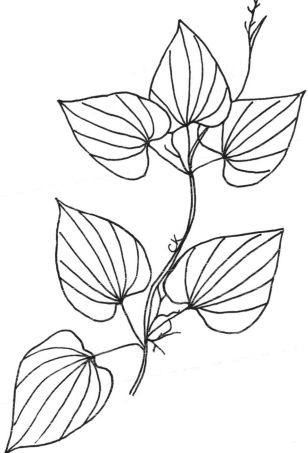

Medicinal Uses
Indians made a wild yam tea to treat nausea in pregnant women and to relieve the discomforts of childbirth. Settlers used wild yam for treating intestinal disorders. Southern slaves used wild yam as a treatment for muscular rheumatism. The dried roots were traditionally used by physicians for treating croup, gastrointestinal ailments, morning sickness, liver ailments, asthma, spasmodic hiccoughs, rheumatism and chronic gastritis of drunkards.

Wild yam contains the active component the steroidal saponin diosgenin (includes dioscin and trillin), phytosterols, the alkaloid dioscorine, tannin and starch. Herbalists recommend using a decoction of the roots as an astringent, cardiac stimulant, emmenagogue and as a

85

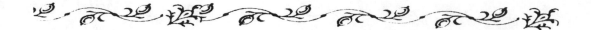

sedative for female disorders, gastro-intestinal disorders, spasmodic hiccoughs and rheumatism.

Diosgenin is used in the manufacture of progesterone and other steroid drugs. Drugs made from diosgenin are used for asthma, arthritis, eczema, dysmenorrhea, premenstrual syndrome, testicular deficiency, impotency, prostate hypertrophy and psycho-sexual problems. They are also used to regulate metabolism, control fertility (contraceptive pills), treat high blood pressure, arterial spasms, and migraine. Diosgenin is an ingredient in widely prescribed cortisone and hydrocortisone medications.

Eating large amounts of fresh wild yam may induce vomiting and other undesirable side affects.

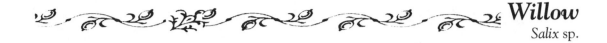

Willow
Salix sp.

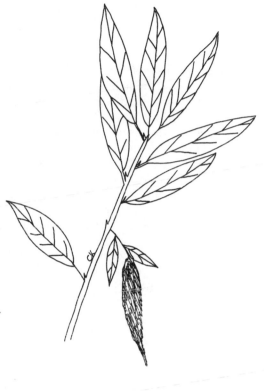

Common names
Black willow, prairie willow, pussy willow, white willow.

Habitat
Prairie willow is found in prairies; black, pussy and white willow along streams, marshes and swamps throughout the Heartland.

Description
Willow is a member of the Saliaceae (willow) family.

Willows (*Salix alba, S. discolor, S. fragilis, S. humilis, S. nigra*) are a deciduous shrub or medium-sized tree with gray fissured bark, ascending branches and flexible yellow-green twigs. Alternate, finely serrate, lanceolate leaves have white, silky hairy on both sides when young and on the underside when mature. The white willow is dioecious with male stallions and female flowers appearing with leaves in erect catkins borne on axils of scaly bracts. It blooms in April and May. The fruit is a capsule containing seeds with long silky hairs.

Medicinal Uses
The ancient Greeks used a bark infusion to treat gout, rheumatism, pain and fevers. The bark has been traditionally used for reducing fevers and relieving pain.

The American Indians used the long, slender willow trees as teepee poles and used the willow species interchangeably for many medicinal remedies. The Cherokee, Chippewa, Cree, Delaware, Fox, Houma and Menomoni Indians used a root and/or bark decoction for treating diarrhea, dysentery, spastic colitis, fever, hoarseness, laryngitis, excessive bleeding, kidney stones and wounds, fainting, stomach trouble, and as a blood tonic for anemia.

Colonists from Europe introduced the practice of steeping the fresh blossoms in cold water, straining and then drinking the liquid to purify the blood. The resin of the often pesky buds was used for treating scurvy, and in spring tonics for purifying the blood. A tea made by steeping one teaspoon of the buds in one cup boiling water was believed to be more soothing and stimulating than Oriental tea.

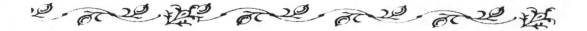

Salacin, a glycoside of salicylic acid, was first isolated from willow bark in 1828 by French and German chemists. Salicin and salicylic acid, are both extremely irritating to the stomach.

In 1898, Felix Hoffman, a chemist at Bayer Company, discovered the acetylated form of salicin, acetylsalicylic acid, which was shown to be considerably less irritating to the stomach. Acetylsalicylic acid was eventually marketed under the name aspirin.

Willow species contain the active components salicin, a close relative of methyl salicylate, a phenolic glycoside, and tannin. Herbalists recommend using a decoction of the bark from two to three year twigs and/or the fragrant, sticky leaf buds as an analgesic, antipyretic, astringent, antiseptic, diaphoretic and tonic for headaches, arthritic-rheumatic inflammation and pain, neuralgia and hay fever. An infusion of the bark and berries of the American black willow (*Salix nigra* or *S. discolor*) is used as an anaphrodisiac, sexual sedative and tonic. Willow has been replaced by synthetics as the source of aspirin (methyl salicylate).

Externally, the bark decoction is used as a hydrating lotion, facial cream, herbal bath or wash to clear the face and skin of pimples, and for treating pus-filled wounds, eczema, burns, arthritic pain, cuts and skin ulcers. A solution of the bark mixed with borax acts as a deodorant wash for offensive smelling perspiration (a few drops of patchouli adds a pleasant scent). The buds were mashed in lard to make a soothing salve for treating sunburns, scalds, scratches and wounds. The salve can also be rubbed on the chest for relieving coughs, colds, flu and pneumonia.

The salicylates found in aspirin are derived from willow, meadowsweet (*Spirea ulmaria*), poplars (*Populus* sp.) and wintergreen (*Gaultheria procumbeus*). Currently aspirin is therapeutically used in maintaining a healthy heart, as well as for the traditional pain-relieving uses of willow bark.

Studies have shown that low doses of aspirin suppress aggregation of blood platelets and suppress prostoglandins. Prostoglandins control the physiological responses that regulate blood pressure, reduce the risk of thrombosis, stimulate the immune system and regulate brain function.

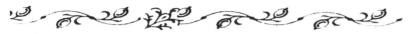

Witch Hazel
Hamamelis virginiana L.

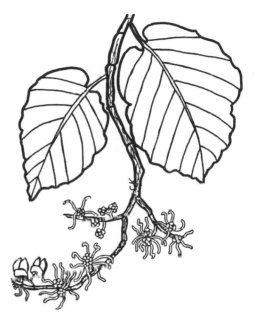

Common names
Pistachio, spotted alder, tobacco wood.

Habitat
Dry to moist woods, rich soils and rocky banks of streams throughout the Heartland.

Description
Witch hazel is a member of the Hamamelidaceae (witch hazel) family. The generic name, *Hamamelis*, is from the Greek referring to its resemblance to an apple tree.

Witch hazel is a shrub. Its slightly lobed leaves with rounded teeth are hairy beneath. Bright yellow flowers with waxy petals bloom from September through November. The fruit is a capsule with two shiny hard seeds.

Medicinal Uses
Indians directly applied witch hazel bark to skin tumors and inflammations. They used the inner bark in a poultice for soothing irritated eyes. They chewed the bark to freshen their breath. A decoction was rubbed on the legs of warriors and athletes to keep them limber and to treat backaches. The Cherokee used a tea for treating colds, fevers, periodic pain, sore throats and tuberculosis. They also used the tea as a wash for sores and wounds. The Menomini used twigs as a charm to "ward-off" bad luck and in sacred ceremonies. The Potawatomi added the twigs in water to heated rocks to create a "sauna" for treating rheumatism and sore muscles.

Witch hazel contains the active components gallic acid, resins, choline, saponin, hamamelin and hamamelidin, an essential oil with the flavonoid glycoside myricetin, iso-quercitrin, acetaldehyde, safrole, sesquiterpene and tannin. Herbalists recommend using witch hazel extract (prepared by aqueous distillation) from the leaves, twigs and/or bark as an alterative, anodyne, antiseptic, astringent, hemostat, refrigerant, sedative and tonic. The extract is used in shaving lotions and to treat bruises and sprains. Witch hazel extract has been used as a folk remedy for treating backache, burns, cancer, diarrhea, dysentery, dysmenorrhea, hemorrhoids, inflammatory menorrhagia, ophthalmia, phlebitis, tumors, ulcers, varicose veins and wounds. Witch hazel extract is also used in an ointment or in suppositories for treating hemorrhoids. Herbalists use a weak decoction as an eyewash to treat conjunctivitis, and in a compress for varicose veins, bruises and to stop bleeding.

Wild Flowering Herbs

Alumroot

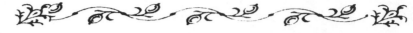

Heuchera americana L.

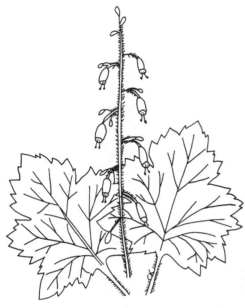

Common names
American sanicle, ground maple, rock geranium.

Habitat
Shady wooded areas and rocky slopes from Michigan to Georgia, Oklahoma to Missouri.

Description
Alumroot is a member of the Saxifragaceae (saxifrage) family. The generic name, *Heuchera*, is in honor of Professor Johann H. Heucher (1677-1747), custodian of the Botanic Garden, Wittenberg, Germany. The common name refers to the alum-like taste of the root.

Alumroot is a perennial with solitary stems. Simple, long-stalked leaves are rounded to kidney-shaped with the upper surface smooth and the lower surface hairy and lobed with prominently toothed margins. Green to green-yellow bell-shaped flowers bloom in June and July. It produces small, dry, oval fruits.

Medicinal Uses
Many American Indian tribes including the Cherokee, Dakotas-Lakotas and Meskwaki, and the early settlers used the fresh or dried leaves and the tuberous root of alumroot in an infusion to treat diarrhea, dysentery, hemorrhoids, hemorrhage, painful menstruation and stomach disorders. The infusion was also used as a gargle for sore throats, and in a poultice on wounds, sores or abrasions. The Indians also chewed the roots for cleansing the teeth of plaque and tartar.

Alumroot was officially listed in *The United States Pharmacopoeia* from 1820 to 1882 as an internal and external astringent. At one time alumroot was the source of tannic acid for commercial preparations. However, alumroot has been replaced by another source.

Alumroot contains the active component tannic acid. Herbalists recommend using a root infusion as an astringent and styptic for diarrhea, dysentery and hemorrhages. The infusion is also used as a gargle for sore throats and in a poultice for wounds, ulcers and abrasions.

Amaranth
Amaranthus sp.

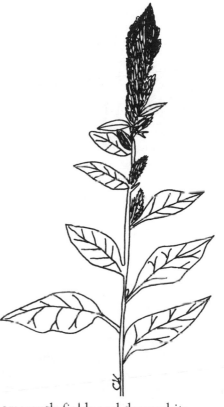

Common names
Amaranthus, smooth pigweed, spiny pigweed, tumbleweed.

Habitat
Open fields, roadsides, waste areas and occasionally cultivated throughout the Heartland.

Description
Amaranth is a member of the Amaranthaceae (amaranth) family.

Amaranth species (*Amaranthus hybridus*, *A. retroflexus*, *A. spinosus*) are erect, branched annuals. Dull green, hairy leaves are ovulate or rhombic. Red or green-tinged small flowers in pyramidal-shaped clusters bloom from July through October.

Medicinal Uses
Amaranth, a major spiritual symbol of the Aztec Indians, was linked to the deities of rain, agriculture and fertility (due to its high yield). The lightly roasted seeds were used in dough mixtures to make a tasty, nutritious bread. Because of its high protein content, amaranth was the principle cultivated crop of the Aztecs, and a key to their survival. Cortez destroyed the amaranth fields and decreed its cultivation punishable by death. This decree alone may have ultimately lead to the complete destruction of this once majestic civilization.

The Zuni Indians of New Mexico believed that the rain gods brought the bright, shiny black seeds from the underworld and dispersed them over their lands. They made a poultice from the entire plant to reduce swellings and to soothe aching teeth. A leaf tea was used to soothe stomachaches, expel intestinal worms and wash arthritic areas of the body.

Archeologists have found seeds of smooth pigweed (*A. hybridus*) in the archeological remains of the Ozark bluff dwellers of northern Arkansas and southern Missouri.

Amaranth species contain more iron and vitamin C than any green vegetable except parsley and spinach. Herbalists recommend using an infusion as a vital anti-scorbutic and astringent for mouth and throat inflammations, sores, wounds, dysentery, intestinal bleeding and diarrhea.

American Ginseng
Panax quinquefolius L.

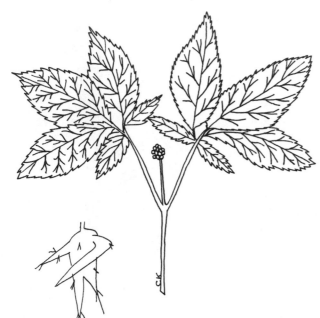

Common Names
Five-finger, manroot, man's health, redberry, tartar root.

Habitat
Rich, moist, hardwood forests from Ohio to Georgia, Oklahoma to Wisconsin.

Description
American ginseng is a member of the Araliaceae (ivy) family. The generic name, *Panax*, comes from the Greek word *panakos* meaning "all remedy," referring to the ancient Chinese belief that the plant was a sovereign remedy for almost all diseases; and *quinquefolius* is from the Latin meaning "five-leafed," referring to the five compound leaflets of the three leaves.

American ginseng is a perennial with a large, forked, pale yellow to tan root and a solitary stem topped with a single whorl of three compound leaves consisting of five leaflets each. Tiny, pale yellow-green flowers can be found in a terminal umbel located where the leaves branch from the main stem. They bloom in July and August. Ruby red, kidney-shaped berries have two to three seeds.

Medicinal Uses
Medicinal usage of Chinese ginseng began more than five thousand years ago in China. The Chinese used ginseng as an aphrodisiac, to restore youth and health and as a panacea for numerous ills. Ginseng (pannag) was mentioned by Judah in the market place of Israel (Ezekiel 27:17). Ginseng was like a golden egg, extremely valuable and difficult to obtain. Many lives have been lost searching the world for ginseng.

American ginseng, native to North America, has medicinal properties similar to those of Chinese ginseng. In the early 1700s the French botanist Father Jarfoux realized that a plant with a similar appearance to the Chinese ginseng was being used for many medicinal remedies by the Indians from the Ozarks and Blue Ridge country.

Each Indian tribe had different methods and/or uses for the American ginseng which had medicinal properties similar to those of Chinese ginseng. With its rejuvenating powers,

94

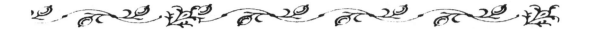

stimulating effect on the gonads, central nervous system and the endocrine glands, American ginseng was used as an aphrodisiac and panacea for treating numerous diseases without any harmful side effects. According to Crow legend, it was revealed in a dream to Gray Bull's wife that chewing American ginseng root would induce childbirth without suffering. The Cherokee used the root for treating colic, dysentery, headache, thrush and weakness of the womb. The Creek used the roots in a poultice to stop bleeding wounds, and in an infusion for treating coughs, hoarseness and dyspepsia. The Delaware, Fox and Mohegan used American ginseng for treating various sexual ailments. The Oklahoma Seminoles used it to stop nosebleeds and to relieve shortness of breath.

Father Jarfous was the first westerner to write a published account of American ginseng. This publication began the great American "Ginseng Rush." Exportation of American ginseng, which had been "cured" as prescribed by the Chinese, began in China and continued via England and France. It is said the Daniel Boone, the great frontiersman of the Heartland, sold a large quantity of ginseng roots in Philadelphia.

Early settlers used American ginseng for treating diarrhea, dizziness, fever, headaches, nervous disorders, sore gums and stomach troubles. Millspaugh recommended using it as an appetite stimulant, cough suppressant and as a tonic to increase overall strength. American ginseng was listed in *The United States Pharmacopoeia* from 1842 to 1882 as a stimulant and stomachic.

American ginseng contains the active components panaquilin, panaxin, panax acid, the volatile oils panacen, sapoginin and ginsenin. Herbalists recommend using a root decoction as a mild tonic and stimulant. In general, American ginseng is used for many of the same ailments and methods utilized in Chinese herbal medicine, that is for treating gastrointestinal, respiratory and urogenital disorders.

Recent research confirms some of the traditional views about ginseng: that panaquilin stimulates intestinal secretion; panaxin stimulates the mid-brain and the heart; panax acid stimulates the heart and general metabolism; panacen and sapoginin stimulate the central nervous system; and ginsenin lowers blood sugar levels. Experiments in Russia have shown that ginseng does improve concentration and endurance.

Currently, harvesting and selling ginseng is regulated and restricted by state agencies, the U.S. Fish and Wildlife Service and the U.S. Department of Agriculture.

Angelica

Angelica atropurpurea L.

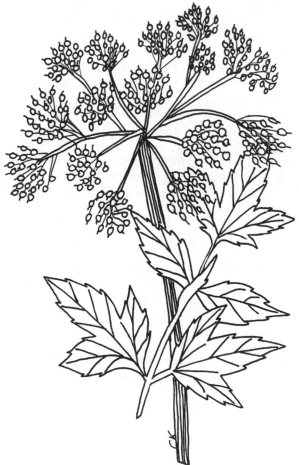

Common names
Alexanders, American angelica, Aunt Jerichos.

Habitat
Rich low grounds, near streams and swamps and occasionally cultivated. Found in Michigan, Ohio, Indiana, Kentucky, Illinois and Wisconsin.

Description
Angelica is a member of the Apiacae (carrot) family. The generic name, *Angelica*, comes from an early legend which tells of an angel revealing the curative powers of this plant to a monk during a plague in Europe during the Middle Ages. The species name, *atropurpurea*, is from Latin (dark purple) referring to the unusual color of the stem.

Angelica is a perennial herb with erect, branching, purple-colored stems. Leaves are divided into three parts with coarsely toothed margins. The tiny, white to green flowers are in umbrella-shaped heads and bloom from May through September. The tiny, rounded fruit has a thin edge or wing resembling a miniature flying saucer.

Medicinal Uses
Indians and settlers used a decoction of angelica as a general tonic for treating anemia, colic, flatulence, gout, indigestion, rheumatism, liver, respiratory and urinary disorders. The decoction was also drank to create an aversion to alcohol. Meskwaki Indians boiled the whole plant to make a tea for treating hay fever. Creek Indians used a tea for treating digestive difficulties and to expel worms.

According to Millspaugh, although the fresh roots are poisonous, the poisonous qualities are lost when dried. He recommended using dried angelica roots as a carminative, diuretic and stimulant to treat urinary disorders, colic and suppressed menstruation.

96

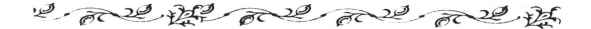

Angelica contains the active components angelic acid, angelicin, a volatile oil with phellandrene, pinene, limonene, caryophyllene and linalool, the coumarins umbelliferone, bergapten and xanthotoxol. Herbalists recommend using an infusion of the dried herb as a diaphoretic, diuretic, emetic, emmenagogue, and expectorant for colds, fever, rheumatism, urinary problems, irregular menstruation, indigestion and respiratory ailments. A poultice of the mashed root can be applied to relieve the pain and inflammation of arthritic joints, wounds and chest discomfort. Scrapings of the root can be smoked to clear head colds. In Appalachia, a root tea is used for colic and lingering illnesses, especially in children.

Studies have shown that pinene is an anti-microbial and expectorant that is effective in the treatment of inflammatory disorders. The coumarin umbelliferone is an effective anti-fungal agent.

Use only the dried herb because the fresh herb is potentially poisonous. The poisonous qualities are lost when the herb is dried. The coumarins bergapten and xanthotoxol can cause photosensitivity; therefore, avoid prolonged usage.

Arrowhead
Sagittaria latifolia Willd.

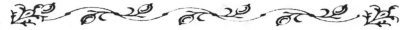

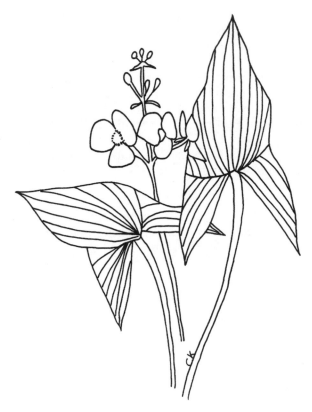

Common names
Arrowleaf, duck potato, swamp potato, wappatoo.

Habitat
Swamps, sloughs, ponds, shorelines and shallow water throughout the Heartland.

Description
Arrowhead is a member of the Alismaceae (water plantain) family. The generic name, *Sagittaria*, comes from Latin for "of an arrow," referring to arrowhead shape of the leaf; and the species name, *latifolia*, from Latin for "wide or broad leaf."

Arrowleaf is a perennial. The above-water, dark green leaves are arrowhead-shaped while the submerged leaves are ribbon-like. The white flowers, in whorls of two to five, have numerous pistils and cluster of yellow stamens. Leaf-like, papery thin bracts in attractive clusters are found below the flowers. It blooms from June through September. Fruits with two wings and round tops contain flat seeds.

Medicinal Uses
Boiled or roasted and with a taste similar to water chestnuts, the large, fleshy, potato-like tubers (starch corms) of arrowhead provided a major food source for many Indian tribes. Lewis and Clark found that the Indians of the Oregon coast considered arrowhead tubers, called wappatoo, so valuable that they would trade their most valued possessions to obtain them. Lewis and Clark named a large island located in the Columbia river, Wappatoo Island, because of the abundance of arrowhead growing there.

The acrid juice of the corms was used by Indians, and later by the settlers, as a diuretic and anti-scorbutic to treat various urinary and kidney ailments. The Cherokee and Chippewa used the tubers in a decoction to treat indigestion, rheumatism, to end lactation in nursing mothers or to wash babies with fever. A poultice was used to treat wounds and sores.

Black Cohosh
Cimicifuga racemosa (L.) Nutt.

Common names
Black snakeroot, bugbane, squawroot.

Habitat
Rich upland woods and hillsides from
Ohio to Georgia, Arkansas to Wisconsin.

Description
Black cohosh is a member of the
Ranuculaceae (buttercup) family.
Cimicifuga, the generic name, is from Latin
meaning to drive away, referring to its use
as an insecticide to drive away insects.

Black cohosh is a perennial with a furrowed stem. It has alternate leaves that are
thrice-divided and sharply toothed. White
flowers in a terminal raceme bloom from
May through September.

Medicinal Uses
Black cohosh was a valuable medicinal
herb to the American Indians who used it
as a general tonic and emmenagogue.
Because it was used to treat all female disorders such as menstrual cramps, delayed
menses, difficult deliveries and others, it
was called squawroot. It was also used to
treat kidney disorders, malaria, sore
throats and rheumatism. The Cherokee
used the roots in a tincture for treating
female disorders, rheumatism, tumors,
backache, respiratory disorders, constipation, fatigue, consumption, hives and
insomnia. The Winnebago and Dakota used the herb for treating snakebites, diarrhea, deep
chest afflictions, spasmodic coughs and menstrual irregularities.

The American settlers learned about the medicinal properties of black cohosh from the
Indians. In addition to the above remedies, they used black cohosh for treating amenorrhea,
bronchitis, chorea (St. Vitus' dance), dropsy, fever, hysteria, lumbago, malaria, nervous
disorders, snakebite and yellow fever.

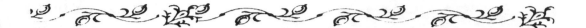

Black cohosh was introduced to the "medical world" in 1831 by Dr. Young as a tonic for treating chorea, bronchitis, rheumatism, neuralgia, dyspepsia, amenorrhea, dysmenorrhea and seminal emission.

King's American Dispensatory (see *The People's Common Sense Medical Advisor, 1918*) says of black cohosh: "This is a very active, powerful and useful remedy, and possesses an undoubted influence over the nervous system ...it is an efficient agent for the restoration of suppressed menses ...in dysmenorrhea (painful periods), it is surpassed by no other drugs, being of greatest utility in irritative and congestive conditions of the uterus and appendages, characterized by intensive, dragging pains ...its action is slow, but its effects are permanent ...black cohosh is a very prompt agent, often relieving in a few hours painful conditions that have existed for a long time."

Black cohosh contains the active components tannin, the triterpene glycosides acetein and cimigoside, the resin cimicifugin, salycilates, isoferulic acid, and ranunculin which yields anemonin. Herbalists recommend using an infusion or tincture of the roots as an antispasmodic, cardiac stimulant (it is safer than digitalis), emmenagogue, expectorant and sedative for bronchitis, cholera, fevers, nervous disorders, lumbago, rheumatism, to ease labor pains and to promote quick delivery.

Research has shown that the resin cimicifugin lowers blood pressure and dilates blood vessels; the salycilates have anti-inflammatory properties; and, ranunculin yields anemonin which depresses the central nervous system. Research has also confirmed the estrogen, hypoglycemic and sedative activities of black cohosh.

Black cohosh should never be used for self medication without supervision of a qualified medical or herbal practitioner. Overdoses may result in intense headaches, dizziness, visual disturbances, slowing of pulse rate, nausea and vomiting. Never use during pregnancy as large doses may cause premature birth.

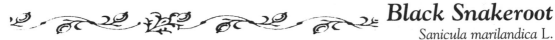

Black Snakeroot
Sanicula marilandica L.

Common names
American sanicle, black sanicle.

Habitat
Rich woods and thickets from Ohio to Georgia, Kansas to North Dakota.

Description
Black snakeroot is a member of the Apiaceae (parsley) family. The generic name, *Sanicula*, is derived from the Latin *sanare*, meaning to heal.

Black snakeroot is a perennial herb with small red furrowed stems. Leaves are palmate and glossy green above, consisting of three to seven leaflets with large teeth. Whitish flowers are in uneven umbels and bloom in June and July.

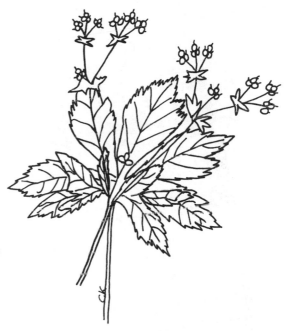

Medicinal Uses
The rhizomes of black snakeroot were used in a tea by the American Indians as an alterative, astringent, expectorant, purgative and vulnerary. It was considered a "cure-all" for treating hemorrhages, intermittent fevers, various skin conditions, menstrual irregularities, pain, kidney ailments, rheumatism, fevers and as an antidote for snakebites.

Black snakeroot contains the active components resin, tannin and a volatile oil. Herbalists recommend using a decoction of the roots as an anti-syphilitic, astringent and tonic. The decoction is an excellent remedy for chronic venereal diseases (including leucorrhea), diarrhea and internal hemorrhaging. With honey, the decoction is an excellent gargle for treating mouth ulcers and sore throats.

Blessed Thistle

Cnicus benedictus L.

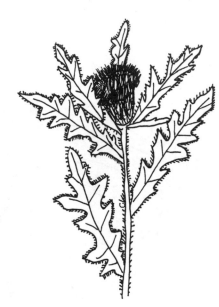

Common names
Bitter thistle, Lady's thistle, St. Benedict's thistle.

Habitat
Roadsides and waste areas throughout the Heartland.

Description
Blessed thistle is a member of the Asteraceae (sunflower) family.

Blessed thistle is an annual herb with branched, spreading stems. Alternate leaves are serrated or pinnately lobed with spiny, prominent wide veins on the underside. Solitary, terminal yellow flowerheads are enveloped by upper leaves and bloom in June and July. It produces ribbed, yellow-brown achene with long yellow pappus. All parts of the plant are hairy.

Medicinal Uses
In 1652, Culpeper said of blessed thistle: "It helps giddiness and swimming of the head ...excellent remedy against yellow jaundice ...it strengths the attractive faculty in man and clarifies the blood ...it cures melancholy and provokes urine."

Indians used an infusion of the flowering tops as a contraceptive. In the 19th century, the flowering tops were used in an infusion to treat internal cancers, hysteria, liver ailments, respiratory inflammations, fevers, diseases of melancholy, urinary retention and to expel intestinal parasites. The juice was used as a hair restorer. The entire herb was boiled in milk to cure dysentery.

Blessed thistle contains the active ingredients tannins, the bitter compound cnicine, essential oils, abundant mucilage and minerals. Herbalists recommend using an infusion of the flowering stems and/or leaves as a anthelmintic, antiseptic, diaphoretic, bitter tonic, choleretic, carminative, emetic, emmenagogue and stimulant. The infusion is used for digestive disorders, migraine headaches, stimulating the appetite, stimulating menstrual flow and to promote the flow of gastric secretions and bile. Blessed thistle is contained in several proprietary medicines and bitter liqueurs. The tender young shoots can be eaten like artichokes, and the leaves are an excellent addition to salads.

Blessed thistle should never be taken during pregnancy. Large doses or prolonged use may irritate the mouth, digestive tract and kidneys. Internal use should be professionally supervised by a qualified medical or herbal practitioner.

Bloodroot
Sanguinaria canadensis L.

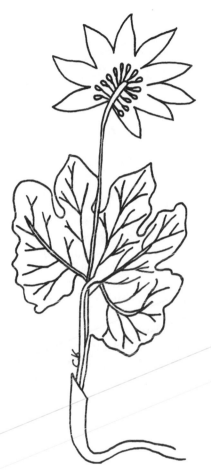

Common names
Sweet slumber, Indian paint, white or red puccoon.

Habitat
Moist, deciduous woods and slopes from Ohio to Florida, Texas to Kansas.

Description
Bloodroot is a member of the Papaveraceae (poppy) family. The generic name, *Sanquinaria*, comes from the Latin word, *sanquinarius* (bleeding) referring to the bright red juice which oozed from a cut or broken root.

Bloodroot is a herbaceous perennial with orange sap flowing throughout the plant. The sap is a deeper, reddish color in the root (thus, the name bloodroot) and has thick, round, fleshy salmon-colored rootstock. Broad, circular, light green palmate leaves with five to nine lobes are paler underneath. White flowers have eight petals with large petals alternating with the smaller ones, and with wax-like golden stamens. It blooms in March and April and produces an oblong, narrow fruit pod.

Medicinal Uses
American Indians were the first to use bloodroot, which they called pocones, as a dye and for medicinal purposes. They used the sap to dye their clothes and paint their bodies to frighten their enemies. An excellent source of tannin, oak bark was added to the dye to set the color making it more permanent. Medicinally, the plant was used to treat hemorrhages, fevers, rheumatism, poor digestion, colds and coughs. Chippewa Indians drank a tea to relieve stomach cramps. The Menomini and Potawatomi used a similar tea to bathe burns, and in a poultice for treating warts, ringworms, fungal infections, chronic eczema and cancerous growths. To attract young maidens, the Omaha-Ponca warriors painted their bodies with the sap during spring mating rituals.

In 1612, John Smith said, "Pocones is a small roote that groweth in the mountaines, while being dried and beate in powder turneth red; and this they use for swellings, aches, anointing their joints, painting their heads and garments ...and at night where his lodging is appointed, they set a women fresh painted red with Pocones and oile, to be his bedfellow."

103

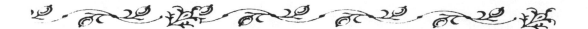

The settlers used a leaf tea to stimulate urination, expel intestinal parasites, to treat gout, and as a gargle to refresh the mouth. They used the roots in a decoction as an alterative, emetic, expectorant, stimulant and tonic to treat bleeding lungs, pneumonia, chronic bronchitis, whooping cough, cramps, colds, and sore throats. Bloodroot was used in a small dose as a gastrointestinal stimulant; in a medium dose as an expectorant; and in a large dose as an emetic. Externally, a poultice was used to treat skin irritations and minor wounds.

According to *King's American Dispensatory* (see *The People's Common Sense Medical Advisor, 1918*), bloodroot "stimulates digestive organs, increases action of heart and arteries ...stimulant and tonic ...very valuable as a cough remedy ...acts as a sedative ...further valuable as an alterative."

Bloodroot contains the active components an opium alkaloid, the alkaloids sanguinarine, berberine, sanguidimerine, cholerythrine, homochelidonine and protopine. Herbalists recommend using an infusion as an anesthetic, anti-cancer agent, antiseptic, cathartic, diaphoretic, emmenagogue and expectorant. The infusion is used to stimulate respiration, increase blood pressure, excite the flow of saliva, clear mucous from the respiratory system and relieve arrhythmic heartbeat due to protopine. Bloodroot is used commercially as a plaque-inhibiting agent in toothpaste and mouth washes.

Studies have shown that the alkaloid sanguinarine is an antiseptic that is an excellent plaque-inhibiting agent; protopine regulates irregular heartbeats; and, berberine lowers blood pressure, increases bile secretion, has a mildly sedating action, is an anti-convulsant and has a curare-like action in that it paralyzes muscles by blocking nerve impulses.

In large doses, bloodroot causes vomiting, vertigo and dimness of eyesight. Therefore, it should be used only under the supervision of a qualified medical or herbal practitioner.

Blue Cohosh
Caulophyllum thalictroides (L.) Michx

Common names
Blueberry road, blue ginseng, papoose root, squawroot.

Habitat
Rich woods throughout the Heartland.

Description
Blue cohosh is a member of the Berberidaceae (barberry) family. The generic name, *Caulophyllum*, is derived from the Greek words *caulos* (a stem) and *phyllum* (a leaf). The species name, *thalictroides*, is in reference to the resemblance of its leaf to those of meadow rue, *Thalictrum*.

Blue cohosh is a perennial with one aerial stem and one leaf, both blue-green in color. The leaf consists of two to three leaflets. The yellow-green flowers with six petals, six sepals, six stamens and one pistil are located in terminal clusters and bloom in April and May. It produces dark blue, pea-sized, berry-like-fruits with two seeds.

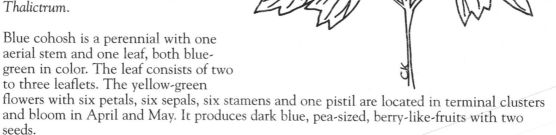

Medicinal Uses
Blue cohosh was discovered and primarily used by the American Indians. Cohosh is an Algonkin word meaning "rough," referring to the rhizome with its many old stem scars. Indian women (thus the name Squawroot) used blue cohosh as a powerful emmenagogue and dysmenorrhea to stimulate menstruation, to relieve cramps, to promote childbirth and for dropsical discharges. To facilitate childbirth, a root tea was drank daily during the week or two prior to childbirth to give rapid and comparatively painless childbirth. Blue cohosh was also used by American Indians for treating chronic rheumatism, bronchitis, colic, dropsy and nervous conditions. The Chippewa used the powdered root in a decoction to expedite parturition and menstruation. They also used the decoction for treating dyspepsia, lung and stomach ailments and as an emetic. The Meskwaki named the root "a woman" and from it brewed a tea for treating female genito-urinary disorders. The Cherokee used the roots for treating colic, labor, inflammation, nerves and rheumatism. They rubbed the leaves onto poison ivy to relieve itching and used the root sap to relieve toothaches.

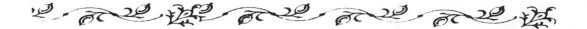

The settlers learned of the medicinal uses of blue cohosh from the Indian medicine man and used it for many of the same remedies. They also used blue cohosh to treat epilepsy and infant convulsions, thus earning it the common name, papoose root. Many physicians utilized blue cohosh for treating uterine leucorrhea, suppressed menstruation, painful menstruation and as an anti-abortive.

Blue cohosh was listed in *The United States Pharmacopoeia* from 1882 to 1905 as an emmenagogue and sedative. *The American Dispensatory* (see *The People's Common Sense Medical Advisor, 1918*) stated that blue cohosh was an emmenagogue (excites menstrual flow) and that its use as a parturient originated from the Indian squaws, who used a root decoction for two or three weeks prior to labor to facilitate childbirth. Dr. Ellingwood recommended using blue cohosh "at the commencement of the menstrual period, in chronic uterine disorders, in painful menstruation, threatened abortion, nursing sore mouth, rheumatism, whooping cough, and bronchitis."

Blue cohosh contains the active components caulophylline, the alkaloid methylcytisine and the glycoside caulosaponin. Herbalists recommend using an infusion of the leaves, seeds, and/or rhizomes as an antispasmodic, demulcent, diaphoretic, diuretic, emmenagogue and parturient. The infusion is used for stimulating delayed menses, and relieving menstrual pains and as a douche for uterine leucorrhea.

Studies have shown that methylcystine stimulates respiration, the motion of the intestines and raises blood pressure; caulosaponin is a uterine stimulant and also constricts the blood vessels of the heart.

In large doses, blue cohosh may have a toxic effect on the cardiac muscles and cause intestinal spasms. Blue cohosh should not be used for self medication except under the strict supervision of a qualified medical or herbal practitioner.

Blue Flag
Iris versicolor L.

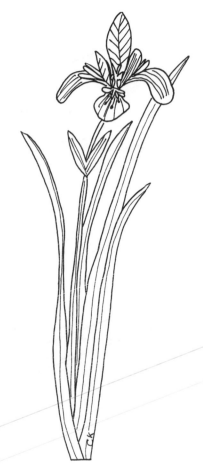

Common uses
Flag lily, flower de-luce, poison flag, wild iris.

Habitat
Marshes, swamps and lowland forests of Ohio, Indiana, Illinois, Missouri, Minnesota and Wisconsin.

Description
Blue flag is a member of the Iridaceae (lily) family. The generic name, *Iris*, is named for Iris, the golden-winged Greek goddess of the rainbow. According to Greek mythology, Iris carried the commands of the gods to man by traveling on the path of the rainbow. She was a virtuous woman, so Hera (Juno) commemorated her by giving her name to a flower that had blossoms bearing all colors of the rainbow.

Blue Flag is a perennial. The long leaves are swordlike. The violet-blue flowers have sepals that are violet at the outer edge and with papery sheaths. It blooms from May through July.

Medicinal Uses
The American Indians used the rhizomes in an infusion to treat sore eyes, as a strong laxative, an emetic and to stimulate bile flow. The infusion was used in a poultice to relieve the pain and swelling of sores, bruises and rheumatism. A paste from the fresh rootstock was applied as a poultice to treat sores and bruises by the Omaha-Ponca Indians. The Creek used a decoction of the rhizomes as a powerful cathartic. The Penobscot Indians of Maine considered the rootstock as a panacea and believed they could keep diseases away if the rhizomes were kept in their dwellings.

The pioneers adapted the medicinal uses of blue flag from the Indians. It was listed in *The United States Pharmacopeia* from 1820 to 1895 as a cathartic, emetic and diuretic as a remedy in the treatment of all blood diseases and chronic kidney and spleen disorders.

Blue flag contains the active components tannin, a volatile oil, salicylates, the alkaloid berberine and the resin irisin. Herbalists recommend using a very weak root decoction as an alterative, cathartic, diuretic, emetic, laxative, purgative, stimulant and vermifuge for constipation, dropsy, gastritis, liver ailments, rheumatism and as a blood purifier.

Boneset

Eupatorium perfoliatum L.

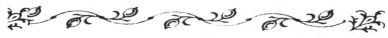

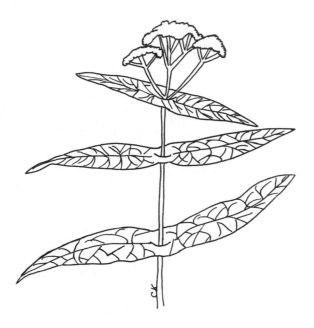

Common names
Feverwort, Indian Sage, thoroughwort.

Habitat
Marshes and low, wet soil near streams throughout the Heartland.

Description
Boneset is a member of the Asteraceae (sunflower) family. The generic name, *Eupatorium*, is named after Mithridetes Eupator, a King of Pontus 115 B.C. who used boneset as an antidote to poison. Legend has it that when captured by his enemies, Mithridetes preferred death to captivity. Because he had fortified himself with boneset against poisoning, Mithridetes had to have a slave stab him.

Boneset is a perennial herb with long, hairy, erect stems and stout rhizomes. Opposite, lanceolate leaves with the leaf base encircling the stems have coarsely-serrated margins. Small tubular white flowers with five lobes and protruding styles bloom in August and September. It has five-angled, hairy achene.

Medicinal Uses
Boneset was called "Indian Sage" by the settlers because it was so widely used by the Indians. The Indians considered it a panacea for all ills, aches and pains. The Cherokees, Menomini, and Mohegan Indians used boneset for treating colds, fevers, flu and sore throats. The Alabama used an infusion for relieving stomach pains. The Creek used an infusion for treating general body pains. The Iroquois used it for urinary disorders. Chippewa mothers bathed fretful children in boneset tea to bring restful sleep.

Boneset was one of the common North American Indian herbs that was quickly adopted by the White settlers for its use as a cough and fever herbal. In colonial America, a flu that caused severe body aches was called a "breakbone fever." The use of dried leaves and flowering tops as an anodyne and febrifuge was listed in *The United States Pharmacopoeia*, 1820 to 1916, and *The National Formulary*, 1926 to 1950.

Millspaugh said: "There is probably no plant in American domestic practice that has more extensive or frequent use ...almost every country farm house has its bunch of dried herb

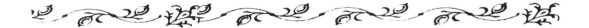

hanging ...for immediate use ...the use of a hot infusion of the tops and leaves to produce diaphoresis, was handed down to the early settlers of this country by the Aborigines."

During the Civil War, boneset was recommended as a febrifuge medicine for the Confederate troops. A boneset infusion, said one doctor "drank hot during the cold stage of fevers and colds as a tonic and antiperiodic, is thought by many physicians to be even superior to the dogwood, willow or popular, as a substitute for quinine. It is quite sufficient in the management of malarial fever that will prevail among the troops during the summer, and if it does not supply entirely the place of quinine, will certainly lesson the need for its use."

The Blacks of the South used boneset as an important remedy for fevers, a mild tonic for dyspepsia and general debility, and to aid indigestion of the elderly.

Boneset contains the active components volatile oils, the terpenoid sesquiterpine, resin, the flavonoids quercetin, kaempferol, rutin and eupatorin. Herbalists recommend using a flower and/or leaf infusion as a cathartic, emetic, febrifuge, laxative and stimulant. The infusion is used for indigestion, dyspepsia, rheumatism, snakebites, pneumonia, malaria, typhoid, female disorders, bladder ailments, and as a mild tonic stimulant in moderate doses to restore "the tone of the system."

Recent research indicates that the sesquiterpene lactones in boneset and Joe-Pye weed (*Eupatorium purpuerum*, a closely related species) are large polysaccharides that have significant immunostimulatory effects and may have anti-cancer activities.

Large doses of boneset may cause kidney and liver damage, internal hemorrhaging or severe intestinal problems and therefore, should only be used be internally under the strict supervision of a qualified medical or herbal practitioner.

Buckbean

Menyanthes trifoliata L.

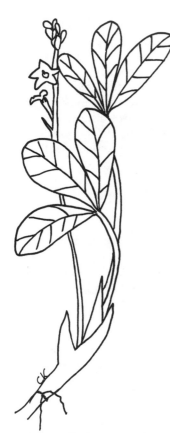

Common names

Bogbean, marsh trefoil.

Habitat

Bogs and shallow water in Indiana, Illinois, Iowa, Kansas, Nebraska, Missouri and Kentucky.

Description

Buckbean is a member of the Menyanthaceae (bogbean) family. The generic name, *Menyanthes*, is from two Greek words, *men* (month) and *anthos* (flowers), referring to the plant that remains in flower for a month and is used to regulate the menstrual cycle.

Buckbean is a perennial herb with thick, creeping rhizomes. It has alternate, trifoliate leaves with sheathing bases. The erect, leafless stem (scape) is topped by a raceme of numerous five-lobed white or pink flowers. The petals are fringed with white cottony hairs. It blooms in May and June. The fruit is a globose capsule.

Medicinal Uses

During the Middle Ages, buckbean or bogbean (referring to the habitat) was recommended as a cure for scurvy, rheumatism and gout. The bitter tasting leaves were once used in beer making and in herbal cigarettes. A dried leaf or root tea has traditionally been used to treat fevers, stomach, rheumatism, liver ailments, hemorrhages and to expel intestinal parasites.

Buckbean contains the active components tannins, the glycoside iridoid, the bitter compounds loganin and menyanthin, pectin, flavonoid glycosides and inulin. Herbalists recommend using a leaf infusion as a bitter tonic, cathartic, choleretic, emmenagogue, febrifuge, laxative and stomachic for fevers, constipation, delayed, painful menses and to stimulate the appetite and bile flow.

Recent research confirms that the phenolic acids found in buckbean may be responsible for the choleretic and bitter, digestive tonic qualities of buckbean.

Large doses of buckbean may cause vomiting and diarrhea, therefore, use with caution under the supervision of a qualified medical or herbal practitioner.

Burdock
Arctium lappa L.

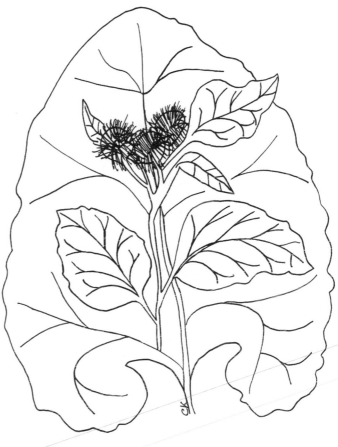

Common names
Beggar's buttons, greater burdock.

Habitat
Waste areas and shaded soil in Michigan, Ohio, Indiana, Illinois and Wisconsin.

Description
Burdock is a member of the Asteraceae (sunflower) family.

Burdock is a biennial herb with a brown, spindle-shaped taproot. Globose flowerheads with numerous hook-tipped green bracts and purple tubular disc-florets are arranged in terminal clusters. Mature flowerheads are spiny balls and bloom from July to September. Fruit is an achene with a pappus of short, rough hairs.

Medicinal Uses
The early settlers and Indians used burdock as an alterative, aperient, diaphoretic, diuretic and overall general tonic. A root infusion was taken for several weeks to cure syphilis and chronic skin aliments. The young leaves and dried roots were used in a compress or salve for treating bruises, inflamed, open sores and wounds, gout, burns and scalds. Juice from the leaves, mixed with honey, was drank to increase urine flow, and to rid one of kidney pain. A root tea was traditionally used by the settlers to treat rheumatism, gonorrhea, liver and kidney ailments. Externally, the tea was used as a wash for hives, eczema and other skin eruptions.

Burdock contains the active components inulin, the glycoside lappatin, polyacelyane, polyphenolic acids, mucilage, tannins, resin, the volatile acids: acetic, lauric, myristic, stearic, palmitic, propionic, and isovaleric acid. Herbalists recommend using a root decoction as an antiseptic, alterative, choleretic, diaphoretic, diuretic, hypoglycemic and stimulant for detoxifying the immune systems of the stomach, kidney, urinary tract, liver, lymph

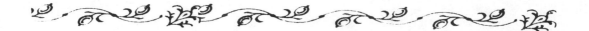

glands, and to stimulate weight loss. Fresh or dried wild burdock roots can be simmered in water for dinner, and the cooking water (tea) can be used for treating fevers, influenza, rheumatic pain and to soothe the upper respiratory tract. The tea can be used externally for bathing wounds, ulcers, eczema and to alleviate many acute and chronic skin problems.

Due to polyacelyane, burdock's anti-microbial actions make it excellent in the treatment of skin eruptions.

The seeds also contain the bitter glycosides arctiin and chlorogenic acid. Herbalists recommend using an infusion as an astringent and diuretic to soothe sores, insect and snakebites, mucous membranes, sore throats and to cleanse the skin. The infusion is also used to relieve flu symptoms, constipation and kidney ailments.

In France, the fresh roots are used to treat diabetes. A lotion containing the leaves and roots is massaged into the scalp to retard baldness. Japanese studies suggest that the roots may be anti-cancerous. In China, the seeds are used to treat the eruptions of measles, sore throats, tonsillitis, colds and flu. The roots and leaves are used to treat rheumatism and gout because they encourage the elimination of uric acid in the kidneys.

Bush Clover
Lespedeza capitata Michx.

Common name
Round-headed bush clover.

Habitat
Dry fields and prairies from Ohio to Florida, Texas to Minnesota.

Description
Bush clover is a member of the Fabaceae (pea) family.

Bush clover is a perennial. Alternate, compound, clover-like leaves have three lanceolate leaflets. Flowers are creamy white in crowded, bristly heads and bloom from July through September.

Medicinal Uses
The Fox Indians used the roots of bush clover as an antidote for poisons. The Omaha-Ponca Indians used the stems for moxa (burning sticks used to burn the skin as a counterirritant) to treat neuralgia and rheumatism.

Bush clover contains the active components tannin, the flavonoids lespecapitosine and kaempferitrin, two flavonoid derivatives apigenin and luteolin. Herbalists recommend using an infusion as an astringent and diuretic for tumors, urinary and kidney ailments.

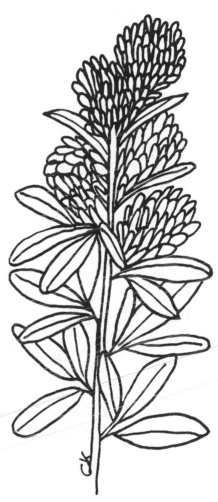

Research has demonstrated that bush clover lowers blood cholesterol levels, removes nitrogenous compounds from the blood, and is an effective anti-tumor agent for treating certain carcinosarcomas.

Buttercup

Ranunculus sp.

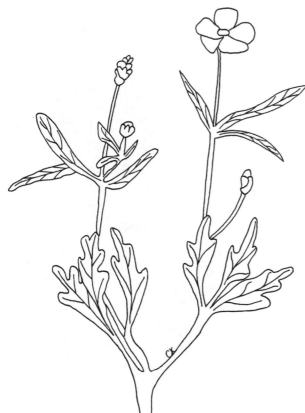

Common names
Bachelor button, blister plant, butter daisy, crowfoot, swamp buttercup, pilewort.

Habitat
Fields, moist woods, ditches, wet meadows and riverbanks throughout the Heartland.

Description
Buttercup is a member of the Ranunculaceae (buttercup) family.

Buttercup species (*Ranunculus abortivus, R. fascicularis, R. sceleratus* and *R. septentrianalis*) are erect perennials. Palmately-divided, five to seven lanceolate leaves have serrated segments. Shiny, golden yellow flowers bloom from May through September. Flat, smooth fruits have a distinct margin.

Medicinal Uses
Early physicians from the time of Dioscorides and Hippocrates used buttercup to cure tumors, chilblains and toothaches. Beggars of old placed the leaves of buttercup on their arms and legs to produce blisters and ulcers in order to increase pity for themselves, hoping to collect more money. Culpeper prescribed a decoction of the leaves and roots for the treatment of hemorrhoids, thus, the name pilewort.

Canadian Indians inhaled the smoke of crushed buttercup leaves to cure headaches. A preparation of the roots was used to stop persistent nosebleeds. Illinois-Miami Indians employed a decoction of crushed roots to treat gunshot or arrow wounds. The Cherokee used the juice from the leaves as a sedative or in a tea for treating sore throats and thrush. They also used the juice in a poultice for treating boils. The Fox applied the root as a styptic in epistaxis, an ulceration of the mucous membranes, especially those of the nose and lungs.

All buttercup species, with a clear, poisonous, acrid juice, contain the active component the glycoside ranunculin; *R. sceleratus* contains the highest level of ranunculin. Herbalists

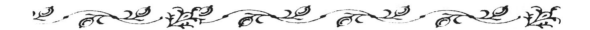

recommend using an infusion as an astringent. Applied directly, the infusion, or preferably in an ointment, is still a valuable remedy for hemorrhoids.

Research has shown that in dried plants, the glycoside ranuculin converts to anemonin. Anemonin (also found in the related species, *Anemone pulsatilla*, pasque flower), is used as an astringent, diuretic, expectorant and emmenagogue for nervous tension, neuralgia, earaches, inflammations and cramping of the reproductive system.

The fresh plants are extremely poisonous if ingested internally. Use caution when handling all buttercup species, because in addition to blistering, the juice may also cause a photodermatitis, a rash that develops when exposed to the sun.

Always consult a qualified medical or herbal practitioner before using any Ranunculus species for self medication.

Catmint
Nepeta cataria L.

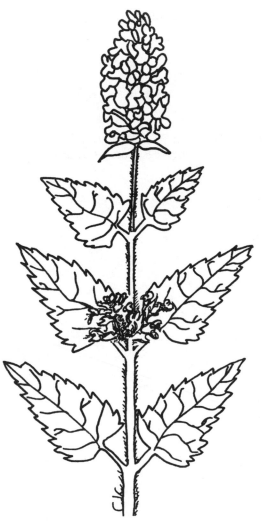

Common name
Catnip, catwort, field balm.

Habitat
Open woods, roadsides, railroads and occasionally cultivated throughout the Heartland.

Description
Catmint is a member of the Laminaceae (mint) family. The generic name, *Nepeta*, is named for the Eutruscian city Nepte in northern Italy.

Catnip is a perennial herb with tall, hairy, square stems that branch from the base. Leaves are opposite and oval with a cordate base, are coarsely dentate, whitish above and gray-green below. Flowers are clustered whorls in the upper leaf axils. The calyx tube has fifteen ribs and five unequal teeth; the corolla is two-lipped and white with purplish dots. It blooms from July through September. The fruit is four smooth nutlets.

Medicinal Uses
Catmint has an old reputation as a medicinal and seasoning herb. The dried leaves with a sharp balsam-like taste have been smoked for their mild hallucinogenic effects. Culpeper recommended that "the green leaves bruised and made into an ointment is effectual for piles …the head or other parts washed with a decoction taketh away scabs, scurf, etc."

According to an eighteenth century British horticulturalist, cats will not destroy catmint that has been sown from seed, maintaining "if you sow it, the cats won't know it.." Even so, catmint raised from seed is only protected from cats as long as it is intact.

Early settlers used catmint tea as a tonic for treating stomach disorders, fevers, infant colic, respiratory ailments, nervous disorders and to increase menstrual flow. The Cherokee, Chippewa and Menomini Indians adopted the medicinal remedies used by the settlers. They also used a poultice on painful boils and swellings.

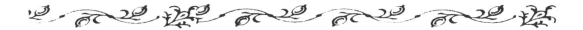

Catmint was an official medicine in The *United States Pharmacopoeia* from 1843 to 1882 and in *The National Formulary* from 1916 to 1950 as an antitussive, aromatic, carminative, diaphoretic, diuretic and stimulant. It was considered an excellent remedy for inducing perspiration without increasing body temperature.

Catmint contains the active component tannins, bitter compounds, and a volatile oil with carvacrol, nepetal, citronellol, geraniol, thymol and nepetalactone. Herbalists recommend using an infusion of the flowering stems as an antispasmodic, carminative, diaphoretic, emmenagogue and stimulant. The infusion is used for migraine headaches, nervous disorders, respiratory ailments and gastrointestinal ailments. Catmint is also used as an herbicide and insect repellent.

Studies have shown that nepetalactone, a non-addictive, mild sedative, is particularly useful in settling children down at night.

Chickweed
Stellaria media (L.) Vill.

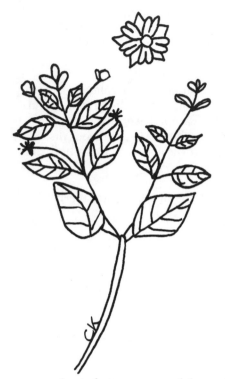

Common names
Adder's mouth, Indian chickweed, star chickweed.

Habitat
Roadsides, damp woods, and thickets throughout the Heartland.

Description
Chickweed is a member of the Caryophyllaceae (pink) family.

Chickweed is a lusty annual, growing to a foot high in matted to upright trailing stems. It thrives throughout the winter. The leaves are stemless with the lower and median leaves egg-shaped and the upper leaves varying in shape. White flowers have five deeply-notched petals and ten stamens and bloom from January through December.

Medicinal Uses
Chickweed is a traditional folk remedy for treating asthma, conjunctivitis, constipation, dyspepsia, obesity (an old wives' remedy), scurvy, stomach cancer and tumors. An infusion prepared from the entire herb was used to treat respiratory ailments and arthritis. A warm, fresh leaf poultice was used externally for treating inflammations, abscesses, wounds, infections, hemorrhoids, conjunctivitis, ulcers, boils, carbuncles, swollen testicles and venereal diseases.

Chickweed contains the active components rutin, choline, inositol, large amounts of vitamins C, D, and B-complex, beta carotene, minerals and steroidal saponins. Herbalists recommend using a tincture or infusion as a demulcent, diaphoretic, diuretic, emollient, expectorant, stimulant and tonic for anemia, arthritis, asthma, gout, irritated skin conditions, respiratory ailments (including tuberculosis), stomach, liver, kidney or bladder ailments. Due to its excellent diuretic properties, chickweed is an important ingredient in many popular all natural weight loss pills.

Studies show that the steroidal saponins increase the absorptive ability of all membranes and eliminate congestion from the liver, kidneys and lungs.

Chicory
Cichorium intybus L.

Common names
Blue daisy, blue sailors, coffee weed, wild succory.

Habitat
Waste areas throughout the Heartland.

Description
Chicory is a member of the Asteraceae (sunflower) family

Chicory is a perennial herb with erect, branched, furrowed stems. Basal rosette leaves are stalked, deeply pinnately serrated and hairy beneath. The stem leaves are sessile and lanceolate. Flowerheads consist of clusters of two or three bright blue florets They bloom from June to October. The fruit is an achene.

Medicinal Uses
Chicory was used as a medicinal herb, vegetable and salad plant in ancient Egyptian, Greek and Roman times. Since the seventeenth century, dried, roasted, ground roots have been used as a coffee substitute or adulterant.

Chicory is a gentle, but effective, bitter tonic which increases the flow of bile and is a specific remedy for gallstones. Galen called it "a friend of the liver" and prescribed it as a liver remedy. In accordance with the Doctrine of Signatures, the milky sap was used to ease the pain in the breasts of nursing mothers with too much milk.

Chicory contains the active components inulin, tannin, cichoriin, esculetin, taraxasterol, fructose, pectin, the bitter compounds lactucin and intybin (lactucopictin). Herbalists recommend using an infusion as an anti-inflammatory, choleretic, digestive tonic, laxative, mild diuretic and stomachic for anemia, liver disorders, kidney and gall stones, and inflammations of the urinary tract. The infusion is also used as an aid in eliminating uric acid in the treatment of rheumatism and gout.

Research has shown that an alcoholic extract of chicory has anti-inflammatory activity in rats and may be useful for treating rapid heart beat and heart arrhythmias. The action of the alcoholic extract mimics the action of quinidine in cinchona in depressing the heart rate.

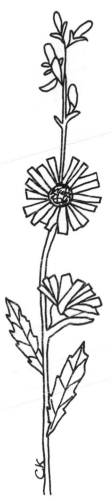

119

Clover

Trifolium pratense L. and *T. repens* L.

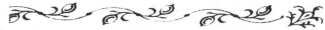

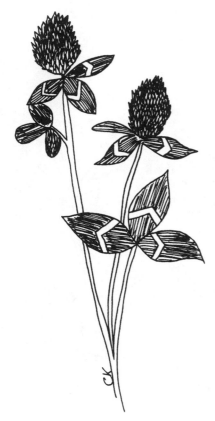

Common name
Dutch clover, purple clover, red clover, trefoil, white clover.

Habitat
Open fields and waste areas throughout the Heartland.

Description
Clover is a member of the Fabaceae (pea) family.

Clover is a perennial herb with erect, angled stems and branched rhizomes. The trifoliate, alternate, oval leaves and entire leaflets have a characteristic white crescent band on the upper surface. Red-purple or white flowers are in a dense terminal, globose, sessile flowerhead and bloom from May to September. The fruit pod contains one or two seeds.

Medicinal Uses
Clover contains the active components proteins, isoflavones, phosphorus, tannin, phenolic glycosides, salicylates, cyanogenic glycosides, coumarin, mucilage, organic acids and calcium. Herbalists recommend using an infusion of the flowerheads as an antiseptic, anti-inflammatory, antispasmodic, astringent, expectorant and vulnerary. The infusion is used for bronchitis, coughs, hoarseness, diarrhea, chronic skin diseases, gastritis, enteritis, severe diarrhea and rheumatic pains. Clover blossom tea, with mint and dandelion, is an excellent appetite suppressant for the dieter. Externally, a poultice is used in compresses or bath preparations for rashes, ulcers, burns, skin cancer, athlete's foot and sores.

Recent studies show that the isoflavones in clover are both estrogenic and a cancer preventive.

Comfrey
Symphytum officinale L.

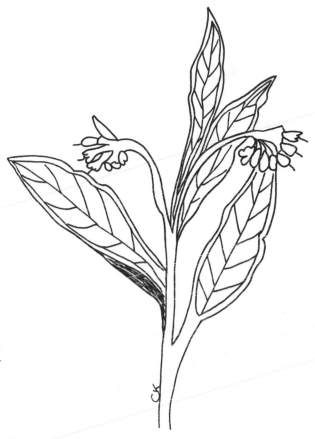

Common names
Ass's ear, boneset, healing herb, knitbone.

Habitat
Waste grounds and often cultivated throughout the Heartland.

Description
Comfrey is a member of the Boraginaceae (borage) family.

Comfrey is a perennial herb with a square stem branched near the top and a black turnip-like root. Alternate lower leaves are ovate to lanceolate. Higher leaves are narrower, with the bases continuing as wings down the stem to the leaf below. Bell-shaped white, cream, purple or pink flowers in nodding cymes in the upper leaf axils bloom from June to August. It produces four ovoid, glossy-black nutlets. The entire plant is roughly hairy.

Medicinal Uses
Comfrey has been used for over two thousand years. The Greek physician, Dioscorides, prescribed comfrey to heal wounds, mend broken bones, stop bleeding and for bronchial problems. The Romans made a poultice to use on wounds. They also drank comfrey tea for treating ailments such as stomach disorders, diarrhea and internal bleeding. Culpeper claimed that comfrey root "is said to be so powerful to consolidate and knit together, that if they be boiled with dissevered pieces of flesh in a pot, it will join them together." Historically, herbalists have used comfrey in poultices, liniments and ointments. Bath preparations made from the leaves are an excellent remedy to help reduce and relieve painful joint swellings, gout, bruises, thrombosis, stubborn wounds, and varicose ulcers.

Comfrey contains the active components tannin, mucilage, allantoin, beta-sitosterol, triterpenoids, vitamin B_{12}, starch, traces of pyrrolizioline alkaloids, an essential oil and calcium. Herbalists recommend using an infusion of the roots and/or leaves as an astringent, emollient, mild sedative and vulnerary for diarrhea, dysentery, coughs and bronchial irritations.

121

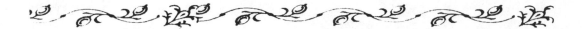

The infusion is also used in poultices, liniments, ointments and bath preparations for arthritis, gout, bruises, stubborn wounds and varicose veins.

Recent American studies have shown that comfrey breaks down red blood cells, thus aiding in dissolving bruises. Allantoin, a nitrogenous crystalline substance and a cell proliferant that promotes the growth of connective tissue, bone and cartilage, is easily absorbed through the skin, increasing the speed at which wounds heal and broken bones knit.
A recent London study showed that comfrey inhibits prostaglandin, the cause of inflammations of the stomach lining. Japanese scientists reported that the entire herb in vinegar is useful for treating cirrhosis of the liver. Several studies have shown that the steroidal saponins in comfrey stimulate the ovaries and testes.

Comfrey has been reported to cause serious liver damage if taken in large amounts over a period of time. Therefore, comfrey should be used only under the strict supervision of a qualified medical or herbal practitioner.

Compass Plant
Silphium laciniatum L.

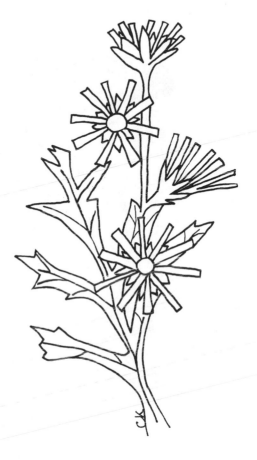

Common names
Gum weed, rosin weed.

Habitat
Prairies throughout the Heartland.

Description
Compass plant is a member of the Asteraceae (sun-flower) family. The generic name, *Silphium*, comes from the Greek for "silpion," a plant of the carrot family used as medicine by the Greeks. In 1753, Linnaeus transferred the name to this genus. The species name, *laciniatum*, describes the leaves which are "cut" into narrow strips or lobes. The common name, compass plant refers to the leaves twisting edgewise north and south at midday whenever it grows in full sun.

Compass plant is a coarse perennial herb with erect, stiff, hairy stems and massive rootstocks. It has alternate, stiff-stemmed leaves. The basal leaves with deep pinnate segments are mostly linear and coarsely serrated. Bell-shaped flowerheads are in a spike-like group above the basal leaves. Numerous yellow ray and disk flowers bloom from June through September. Fruits are broad, flattened achenes.

Medicinal Uses
The compass plant was used by physicians during the nineteenth century as an astringent, antispasmodic, diaphoretic, diuretic, emetic, emollient, expectorant, febrifuge, stimulant and tonic. An infusion was used to treat liver and spleen ailments, fevers, ulcers and debility. As an emollient, it was used to soothe chapped, sore skin and mucous membranes.

Early settlers and Indians used the juice of the compass plant as a general tonic, anthelmintic and as a sedative. A leaf infusion was used by new mothers to encourage milk flow. From the macerated root, the Pawnee Indians made a tea for general debility. The Omaha Indians used the dried root in a decoction to alleviate head colds or pain. Many Indian children chewed the resin as a chewing gum.

Coneflower

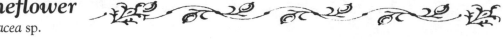

Echinacea sp.

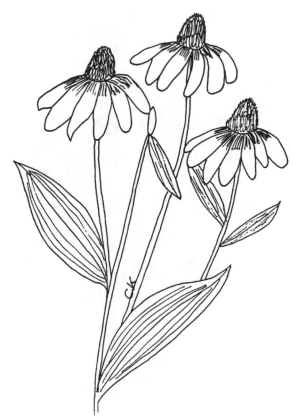

Common names
Black Sampson, echinacea, pale cone-flower, purple coneflower.

Habitat
Open woods, prairies and occasionally cultivated throughout the Heartland.

Description
Coneflower is a member of the Asteraceae (sunflower) family. The generic name, *Echinacea*, comes from the Greek word *echinos*, for hedgehog, referring to the spiny bracts between the disk flowers.

Echinacea species (*Echinacea augustifolia, E. pallida, E. purpurea*) are perennial herbs with a woody taproot. One to several stems are mostly unbranched, rough and hairy. Alternate, narrow lanceolate leaves are egg-shaped at end of long stalks. Light pink to pale purple ray flowers are spreading or tapering. Three-lobed, brown-purple disk flowers are situated on stiff bracts. The plant blooms in June and July. Dark fruits are small, four-angled achenes.

Medicinal Uses
Coneflower, native to the prairies of North America, was the most widely used medicinal plant of the Plains Indians. They used all coneflower species interchangeably for the same remedies. Macerated roots were used to treat snakebites, stings, spider bites, cancer, toothaches, burns, hard-to-heal wounds, flu and colds by all Indian tribes of the Upper Missouri River Region. The Lakota and Sioux used freshly scraped roots for treating hydrophobia, putrefied wounds and blood poisoning. The Kiowa and Cheyenne chewed the roots for treating colds, sore throats and toothaches. The Cheyenne also made a tea from the leaves and/or roots for treating sore throats, gums, rheumatism, arthritis, mumps and measles. Some Indians used the juice from purple coneflower on their hands, feet and mouth to make them insensitive to burns during sacred ceremonies.

Coneflower was the only native prairie plant to be widely accepted as a medicinal remedy by folk practitioners and doctors. This "blood purifier" was used to cure rheumatism, bee

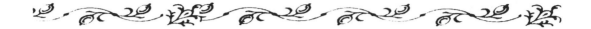

stings, *Streptococcus* infections, cholera, respiratory infections, bronchitis, measles, chicken pox, scarlet fever, gonorrhea, boils, abscesses, acne, poisonous snakebites, dyspepsia, tumors and syphilis. Many American herbalists still regard coneflower as one of the very best blood purifiers, as well as an effective antibiotic.

Coneflower contains the active components resin, betain, inulin, an essential oil with humulene and caryophylene, a caffeic acid glycoside, the polysaccharide echinacin B, poly-actylenes, isobutylalklamines, and sesquiterpene. Herbalists recommend using a root decoction as an antiseptic, alterative and aphrodisiac for the same remedies (listed above) as the Plains Indians and early settlers.

Research has shown that the root of coneflower possesses mild antibiotic properties against *Streptococcus* and *Staphylococcus aureus*. In 1971, the essential oil from coneflower was found to be inhibitory to certain forms of carcinoma and lymphatic leukemia. The wound-healing and anti-viral effects were attributed to echinacin B and caryophylone. Other researchers have also shown that coneflower possesses immuno-stimulatory properties (dependent on dose level) that produces an anti-inflammatory effect and neutralizes acid conditions in the blood characteristic of lymphatic stagnation. Coneflower has therapeutic value in treating tumors, syphilis, gangrene, eczema, hemorrhoids, and a host of pains and wounds.

More than two hundred pharmaceutical preparations are made from *Echinacea* species in Germany. These preparations include extracts, salves and tinctures that used are for treating chronic wounds, herpes, sores, throat infections, flu and colds.

Wild coneflower is slowly being over-harvested in many areas. At least one state, Tennessee, has placed *E. pallida* on its rare plant list. Cultivated varieties of coneflower, which have the same medicinal properties as the wild varieties, are available in herbal stores throughout the Heartland.

Cornflower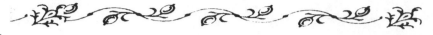
Centaurea cyanus L.

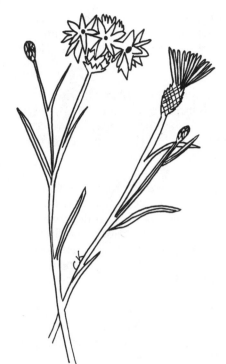

Common names
Bachelor's button, star thistle.

Habitat
Waste grounds and open fields throughout the
Heartland.

Description
Cornflower is a member of the Asteraceae (sunflower)
family. The generic name, *Centaurea*, refers to a Greek
legend that cornflower healed a wound on the foot of
Chiron, one of the centaurs; the species name, *cyanus*,
is from Latin after a youthful devotee of the goddess
Flora (Cyanus), whose favorite flower was the blue
cornflower.

Cornflower is an annual herb with an erect, branched,
wiry stem. It has alternate, grayish, linear-lanceolate
leaves. Solitary terminal flowerheads with large, bright
blue tubular florets are on long stalks and bloom from
July through September. The fruit is a flattened silver
achene.

Medicinal Uses
Culpeper said of cornflower: "seeds or leaves taken in wine good against plague, all infectious diseases and pestilential fevers. The juice put on wounds doth quickly solder up the lip
of them together and heals ulcers and sores in the mouth. The juice dropped into the eyes
take away heat and inflammation."

Cornflower contains the active components anthocyanins, centaurin and/or cyanidin, the
glycoside cichorlin, saponins, mucilage and tannins. Herbalists recommend using an infusion or tea mixture of the florets as an astringent, weak diuretic, dyspepsia and tonic for
indigestion, dyspepsia, gout disorders and as an eye wash. The florets are also used in compresses or bath preparations to treat wounds, skin disorders and as an ingredient in hair
tonics.

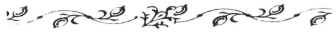

Culver's Root
Veronicastrum virginicum (L.) Farw.

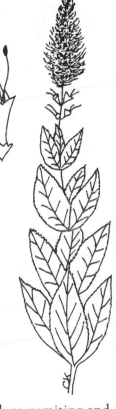

Common names
Black root, Culver's physic.

Habitat
Woods and prairies throughout the Heartland.

Description
Culver's root is a member of the Scrophulariaceae (figwort) family.

Culver's root is a perennial herb, often found in colonies. The erect stems are smooth to hairy and sometimes branched. Simple, lance-olate leaves, with serrated margins, are in whorls. Flowers are in a dense spike at the end of branches and bloom from June through August. White to pale pink petals are fused at the base into a short tube with the lobes separate. Fruits are woody, egg-shaped capsules. It produces numerous light brown seeds.

Medicinal Uses
The Cherokee drank a root tea for treating backaches, fever, hepatitis and typhus. They chewed the root for relieving colic. The Chippewa, Fox, Menomoni and Ojibwa steeped the root tea to treat fits, gravel, labor and other gynecological problems.

Culver's root contains the active components tannin, resin, the glycoside leptandra, a volatile oil and a crystalline principle. Herbalists recommend using a dried root and/or rhizome decoction as an alterative, antiseptic, cathartic, cholagogue, diaphoretic, diuretic, emetic, mild laxative and tonic. The decoction is used as a very effective laxative, to induce sweating, to stimulate the liver, to induce vomiting and for treating pleurisy and dyspepsia.

Use dried roots, because fresh roots are a violent laxative, and are potentially toxic.

Cup-plant
Silphium perfoliatum L.

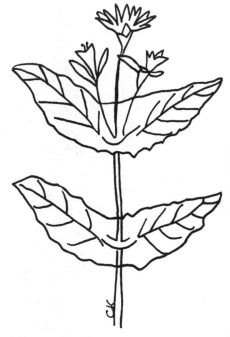

Common names
Carpenter's weed, Indian cup, rosin weed.

Habitat
Rich, medium to wet soils of open woods and meadows throughout the Heartland.

Description
Cup-plant is a member of the Asteraceae (sunflower) family. The generic name, *Silphium*, comes from the ancient Greek name of a resinous African plant.

Cup-plant is a coarse, tall perennial with smooth, square, erect stems that are four-angled, from which the common name carpenter's weed originates. Triangular, opposite leaves are single or branched. The larger lower leaves have winged petioles, and the smaller upper leaves, paired without petioles, join at the stem to form shallow cups which catch rain water, hence the name cup-plant. Showy yellow flowerheads on a center disc have twenty to thirty slender petal-like ray flowers that bloom from July through September. Seeds are small, winged, slender and oblong.

Medicinal Uses
The American Indians used a root tea for treating lung hemorrhages, back or chest pain, profuse menstruation and to induce vomiting. The Omaha, Winnebago and Missouri River Indians used cup-plant in smoke treatments for head colds, neuralgia, rheumatism and stomach ailments. The Chippewa used a root poultice for bleeding wounds. A root decoction was used for treating backaches and amenorrhea. The Fox drank a root tea for morning sickness.

According to Grieve, cup-plant is an alterative, diaphoretic and tonic. An infusion was used for treating liver and spleen ailments, fevers, ulcers, internal bruises and general debility.

Dandelion
Taraxacum officinale Weber

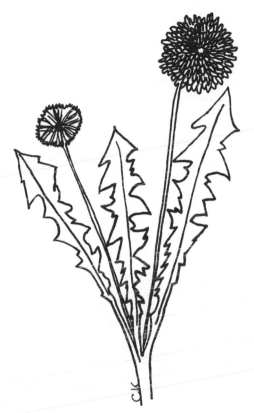

Common names
Blowballs, fairy clock, piss-a-beds, lion's tooth, puffball.

Habitat
Fields, lawns and waste grounds throughout the Heartland.

Description
Dandelion is a member of the Asteraceae (sunflower) family. The generic word, *Taraxacum*, comes from the Greek words, *taraxis* meaning disorder and *akas*, meaning remedy.

Dandelion is a perennial with a deep white taproot. The leaves in a basal rosette are nearly erect to reclining and the coarse margins are indented with irregular teeth. The golden flowerhead on a hollow flower stalk is a large "button" head of strap-like ray flowers. Dandelions bloom from March through frost. The tiny, pin-head seeds have a distinct beak. As the seed matures, the bracts re-open, allowing the white hairs to form a "puffball."

Medicinal Uses
Since ancient times, dandelion leaves have been used for salads and cooked greens. The flowers were made into a wine which may also have been used as a diuretic. The fleshy, tap root was cooked as a vegetable, and roasted as a caffeine-free coffee substitute. Medicinally, it was regarded as a treatment for jaundice, constipation, indigestion and urinary problems. It was the use as a bladder stimulant (diuretic) which earned dandelions the French nickname 'pissenlit' (wet-a-bed).

The European settlers introduced the medicinal uses of dandelion as a diuretic, tonic and gentle laxative to the Indians. An infusion of the leaves was used for cleansing the liver, gall bladder, spleen, kidney and urinary tracts. The infusion was also used for treating fevers, insomnia, gout and rheumatism. The roots were roasted and made into a non-caffeine coffee substitute.

Dandelion is one of nature's great medicines. Dandelions contain the active components amino acids, tannin, inulin, choline, the terpenoids taraxol and taraxasterol, the bitter compounds taraxacin and taraxacerin, phenolic acids, the phanolic glycoside asparagin,

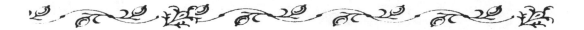

minerals, rubber, beta carotene, iron, calcium provitamin A, vitamins B and C. When collected before the plant flowers, the leaves contain more beta carotene than carrots, and more iron and calcium than spinach. Herbalists recommend using an infusion as a choleretic, diaphoretic, diuretic, laxative and tonic to reduce an enlarged liver and jaundice from hepatitis, aid poor digestion due to insufficient bile, and to treat skin diseases and rheumatism.

Dandelion has been traditionally used as a tonic to cleanse and strengthen the blood and tissues, especially the liver and gallbladder since it promotes bile flow, reduces inflammation of the bile duct and prevents the formation of gallstones. Pressed juice from the stalks or leaves is an effective cure for warts. The leaves are a gentle diuretic that cleanses the blood and recycles nutrients. The rich potassium content replaces that which the body loses. People who are overweight due to excessive fat, carbohydrates or concentrated sweeteners would benefit from a daily cup of dandelion tea. The flowers, boiled with honey, are excellent for relieving coughs and sore throats. The root, a mild laxative, is valuable in treating dyspepsia and constipation.

Dandelion juice or tea gently massaged on stiff joints relieves aches and swelling. A strong infusion added to bath water generally improves circulation, tones and revitalizes the skin. For the same effect, tie a muslin bagful of crushed leaves to the faucet under a hot water flow.

Dandelions are high in vitamins and iron, and the ethylene gas which they emit encourages fruit crops to ripen more quickly. Believe it or not, some farmers deliberately encourage the growth of dandelions in order to ensure an early harvest.

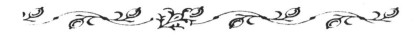

Dayflower
Commelina communis L.

Common names
Asiatic dayflower, wandering Jew.

Habitat
Waste area, roadsides, open fields throughout the Heartland.

Description
Dayflower is a member of the Commelinaceae (spiderwort) family. Dayflower was named by Linnaeus for three Dutch brothers named Commelin. Two of the brothers, well-known botanists, are represented by the two brilliant blue petals, and the third, a ne'er-do-well, is represented by the insignificant translucent petal.

Dayflower is a perennial with weak slender stems. The lanceolate leaves are thick and fleshy. The flowers have two conspicuous, deep blue petals and one inconspicuous white petal with three large anthers and three small yellow anthers in the form of a cross with brown spots in the center.

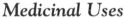

Medicinal Uses
Latin Americans use dayflower to treat conjunctivitis, dermatitis, dysmenorrhea, enteritis, gonorrhea, kidney ailments, leucorrhea, malaria and venereal diseases. The Chinese use the leaves in an infusion for treating acute tonsillitis, urinary infections, dysentery, abscesses, bleeding, boils, insect bites, colds, conjunctivitis, diarrhea, acute intestinal enteritis, fever, flu, gonorrhea, hypertension, malaria, mumps, snakebites and tonsillitis. They also use the infusion as a gargle for sore throats and laryngitis. The Navajo Indians used a tea to increase sexual potency in both humans and livestock.

In herbal medicine, dayflower is currently used in an infusion to treat burns, coughs, cramps, cystitis, leprosy, female disorders, nosebleeds, hemorrhoids and tuberculosis. The tender young leaves and flowers, with a taste similar to string beans, are excellent in salads or soups.

Devil's Shoe String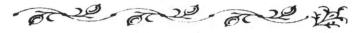
Tephrosia virginiana (L.) Pers.

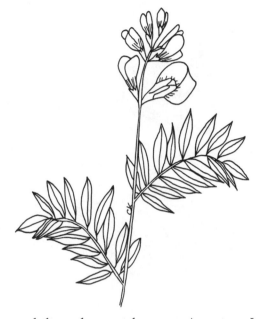

Common names
Goat's rue, rabbit pea.

Habitat
Prairies throughout the Heartland.

Description
Devil's shoe string is a member of the Fabaceae (pea) family.

Devil's shoe string is a silky-haired perennial. The pinnate leaves have seventeen to twenty-nine leaflets. The flowers have a yellow base and pink wings and bloom from May through August. The fruit is a hairy seed pod.

Medicinal Uses
As a folk herb, the roots of devil's shoe string were used for treating cholecystosis, coughs, syphilis and to expel worms. American Indians used a root tea as a children's tonic, and to treat tuberculosis, bladder ailments and male potency. The Creek Indians used the roots for treating consumption, bladder disorders and loss of manhood.

Devil's shoe string contains the active components deguelin, dehydrorotenone, rotenone and tephrosin. Herbalists recommend using a root tea as an anthelmintic, cathartic, diaphoretic, purgative, stimulant and tonic for fevers, bladder disorders, indigestion, constipation and general debility.

Devil's shoe string is an ornamental wild flower from which is derived rotenone, the insecticide and piscicidal compound used to poison fish. In the United Kingdom, rotenone is also used as a rat poison.

Research has shown that rotenone has anti-cancer activity in lymphocytic leukemia and nasopharyngeal tumor systems.

The crude plant preparation may cause dermatitis, conjunctivitis, and rhinitis. Deguelin, rotenone and tephrosin can cause paralysis and death, but they are not as toxic to man as they are to fish, insects and rats. Devil's shoe string should never be used internally except under strict supervision of a qualified physician or herbal practitioner.

Dutchman's Breeches

Dicentra cucullaria (L.) Bernh.

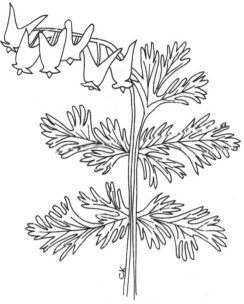

Common names

Boy britches, boys and girls, colic weed, white heads.

Habitat

Rich, moist woods throughout the Heartland.

Description

Dutchman's breeches is a member of the Papaveraceae (fumitory) family. The generic name, *Dicentra*, means "two spurs", and the species name, *cucillaria*, means "hooded." The common name refers to the beautiful flowers shaped like pairs of miniature pantaloons hung upside down.

The flower of Dutchman's breeches is unusual, having four petals with the two larger outer petals enclosing two smaller inner petals which adhere by their tips. The closed inner petals envelop the sexual parts, anther and pistils, of the flower. The smooth, slender stems arise from a common point. Each stem, actually a leaf petiole, is topped with a smooth, thrice-divided leaf. A leafless flower stalk arches higher than the leaves and carries four to ten flowers that bloom in April and May. The elongated seed capsule contains ten to twenty tiny, crested seeds.

Medicinal Uses

The Iroquois used Dutchman's breeches in an ointment to make athlete's legs more limber. The settlers used a root tea as a diuretic to treat urinary problems and to promote sweating. A leaf poultice was used for skin diseases. Dried tubers of Dutchman's breeches and a close relative, Squirrel corn (*D. canadensis*), were used in a tonic to treat venereal diseases and in a poultice to treat skin diseases.

Dutchman's breeches contains the active components fumeric acid, protopine, the alkaloids isoquinoline and corydaline. Herbalists recommend using a root infusion as an alterative, astringent, diaphoretic, diuretic and tonic for fevers, urinary aliments and skin disorders.

Research has shown that the alkaloid isoquinoline is a central nervous system depressant that is useful in the treatment of paralysis and tremors.

All parts of Dutchman's breeches may cause skin rashes if used over a prolonged time.

Elecampane

Inula helenium L.

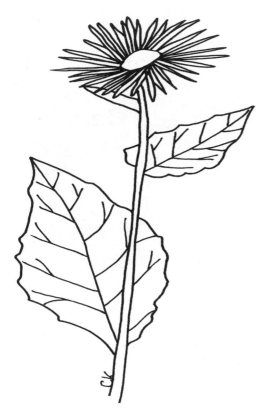

Common names

Inula, scabewort, wild sunflower, yellow star-wort.

Habitat

Fields and roadsides throughout the Heartland.

Description

Elecampane is a member of the Asteraceae (sunflower) family.

Elecampane is a perennial herb with large, branched, tuberous roots. The large, serrated leaves are hairy above and downy below. It has large terminal yellow flowerheads and blooms from June to August. The hairless fruit is a four-ribbed achene with a reddish pappus.

Medicinal Uses

Historically elecampane has been used to promote menstruation, and for treating respiratory disorders and anemia. In ancient Greece, elecampane was used as a stimulant to the brain, stomach, kidneys and uterus.

Elecampane contains the active ingredients inulin, sterols, resin, pectin, mucilage, and the volatile oils alantolactone, isolantalactone and azulene. Herbalists recommend using a warm decoction of the roots and/or rhizomes as an anthelmintic, antiseptic, diaphoretic, diuretic, expectorant, stimulant and tonic for respiratory ailments such as asthma and bronchitis, and as a digestive tonic. Externally, the herb, in a wash or ointment, is used for scabies, herpes and other skin ailments.

Research shows that the volatile oils are powerful anti-bacterial and anti-fungal agents. Alantolactone is an anthelmintic agent that is used to expel worms.

Evening Primrose
Oenothera biennis L.

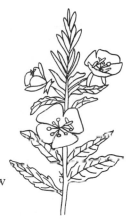

Common name
Tree primrose.

Habitat
Roadsides and fields throughout the Heartland.

Description
Evening primrose is a member of the Onagraceae (willowherb) family.

Evening primrose is a perennial with numerous lanceolate leaves
The roots and leaves smell and taste like peppers and radishes. The yellow
flowers have four broad petals, reflexed, drooping sepals and an X-shaped
stigma; they bloom from June through September.

Medicinal Uses
Evening primrose was a popular herb for many American Indian tribes. They used a root infusion for treating obesity and intestinal pains. The infusion was used in a poultice for treating hemorrhoids, bruises and various skin disorders. The macerated root was rubbed on muscles to give athletes strength. When the plant was taken to England in the seventeenth century by returning settlers, it was called the "King's cure-all" by herbalists, who considered it a panacea for treating most ailments.

Evening primrose seeds yield primrose oil containing the fatty acids linoleic acid (LA) and gammalinoleic acid (GLA). Research has demonstrated that GLA is used by the body to produce prostaglandins. Prostaglandins are hormone-like compounds that control every organ in the body. Each tissue must make short-lived prostaglandins as they are needed, since they are quickly inactivated by various enzymes and are not stored. Prostaglandins control the physiological responses that regulate blood pressure, reduce the risk of thrombosis, stimulate the immune system and regulate brain function. Moderate use of alcohol, diabetes, deficiencies of zinc and vitamin B_6, cancer-causing viruses and radiation treatments block the ability of the body to produce GLA.

Evening primrose oil has been shown to have beneficial effects in the treatment of premenstrual syndrome, treatment of hyperactive children, to counteract alcoholic poisoning, to aid alcohol withdrawal and to ease post-drinking depression. Recent studies have also shown that the oil is an effective agent against coronary artery disease, is a powerful anti-coagulant, reduces high blood pressure, that people ten percent or more above their ideal body weight lose weight without dieting when taking the oil daily, and that it stimulates liver tissue damaged by alcohol to regenerate. Studies also show that people with rheumatoid arthritis who were treated with primrose oil were able to stop their normal anti-arthritic drugs. When fish oil is also taken, the effect is enhanced.

135

False Solomon's Seal

Smilacina racemosa (L.) Desf.

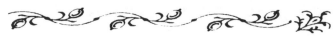

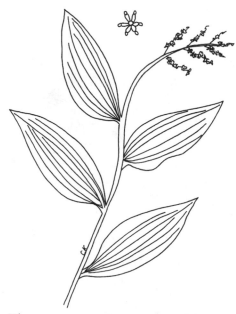

Common names
False spikenard, Job's tears, Solomon's phone, treacle berry.

Habitat
Rich, moist woods throughout the Heartland.

Description
False Solomon's seal is a member of the Liliaceae (lily) family. The generic name, *Smilacina*, comes from Greek meaning "small and thorny."

False Solomon's seal is a perennial with stiff, arching stems. The elongated thick, fleshy, knotted rootstock is light brown. The spreading, alternate leaves resemble those of Solomon's seal, *Polygonatum biflorum* and *P. commulatum*, with smooth margins, prominent parallel veins, and extremely short petioles pointed toward the tip. The numerous, tiny creamy-white star-shaped flowers with six petals are in branched clusters at the end of the stem. They bloom from April through June. The ruby-shaped fruits, have a molasses-like bittersweet taste.

Medicinal Uses
The Indians and early settlers used false Solomon's seal as a food source and in medicinal preparations. The berries were eaten to treat and prevent scurvy. The young shoots were used as a substitute for asparagus. The root stocks were prepared like potatoes. Blackfoot, Meskwaki and Potawatomi Indians used the dried, powdered roots to stop bleeding and to relieve itching rashes. They used a decoction to treat convulsions, constipation, female disorders, rheumatism, stomach ailments and as a light tranquilizer to hush a crying child. Early settlers used the leaves of false Solomon's seal in an infusion as a treatment for headaches and sore throats.

Herbalists use false Solomon's seal as a diaphoretic and diuretic. An infusion is drunk to induce sweating and cleanse the blood of toxins.

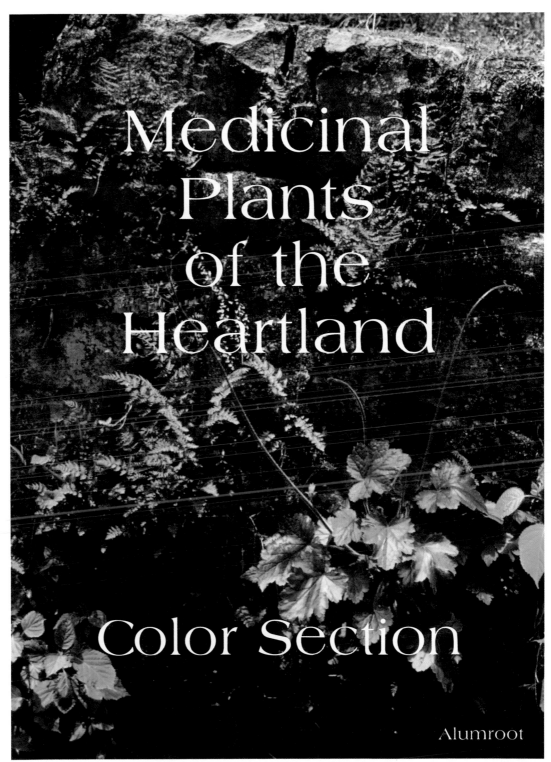

Medicinal Plants of the Heartland

Color Section

Alumroot

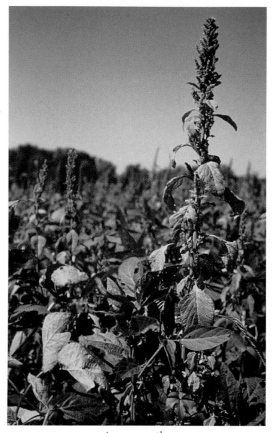

Amaranth

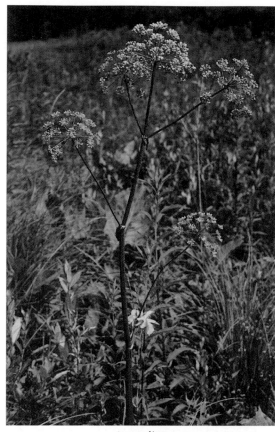

Angelica

American
Ginseng

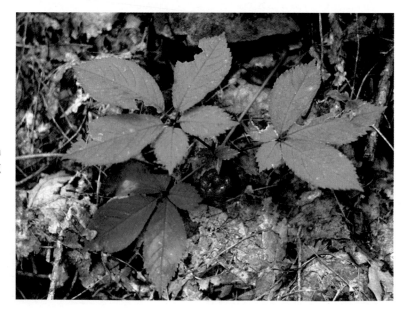

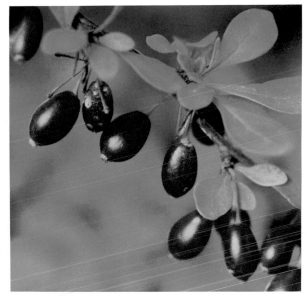

Barberry

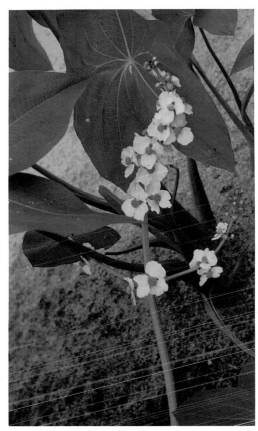

Arrowhead

Bearberry

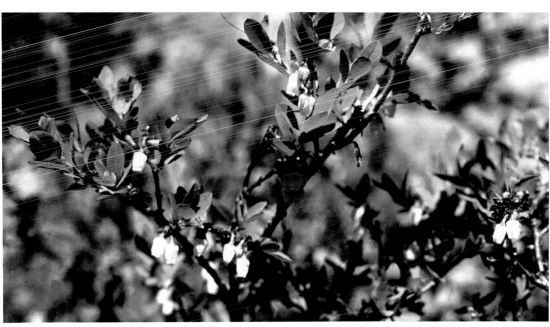

Blackberry

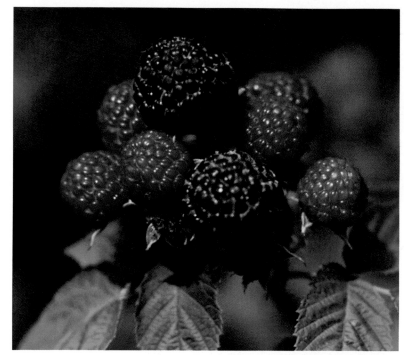

Blue Cohosh

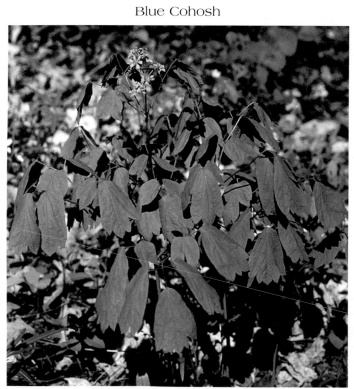

Bloodroot

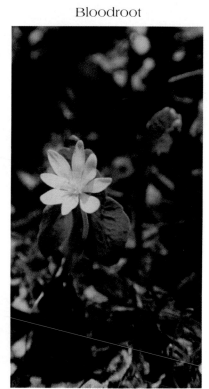

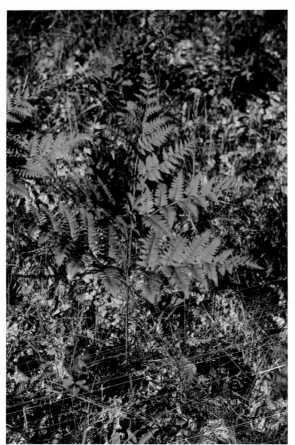

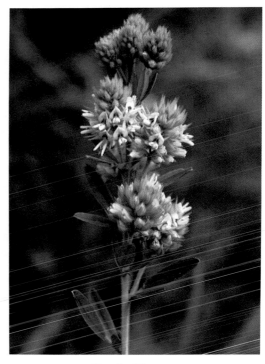

Bush Clover

Bracken Fern

Buttercup

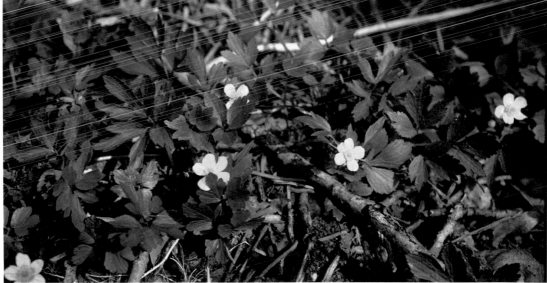

141

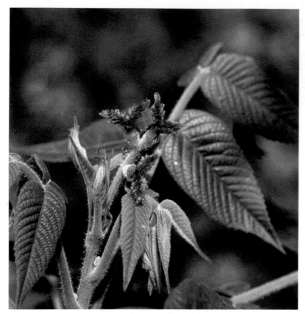

Butternut

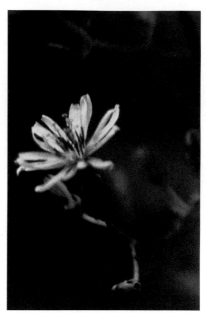

Chicory

Clover

Cramp Bark

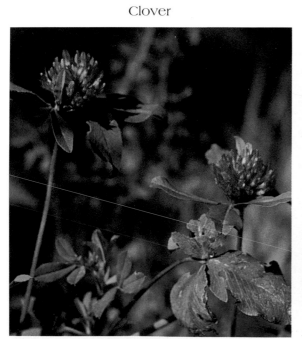

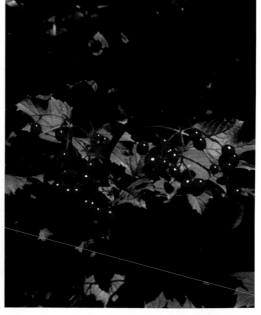

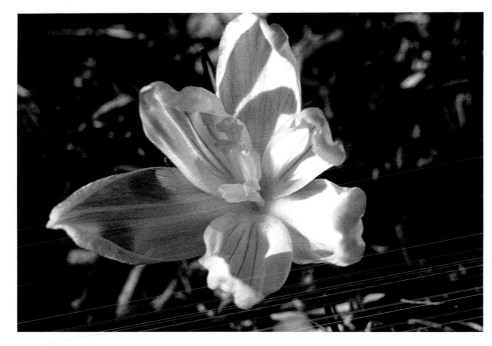

Crocus/
Saffron

Coneflower

Culver's Root

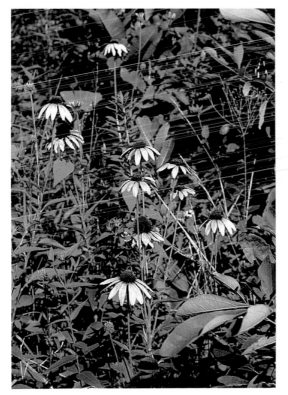

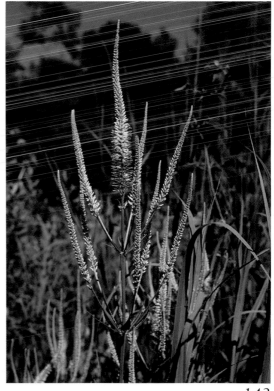

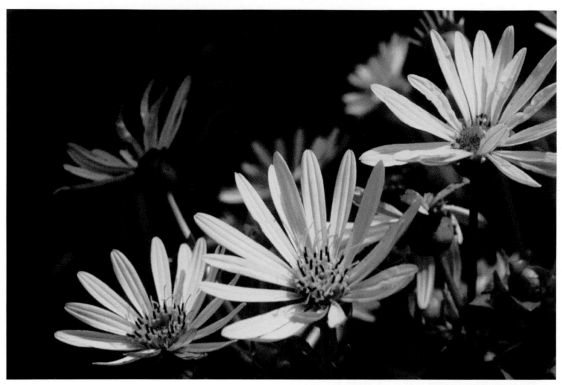

Cup Plant

Devil's Shoe String

Dayflower

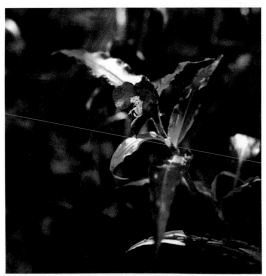

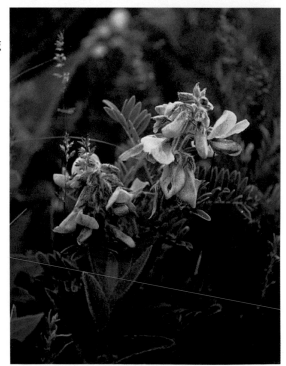

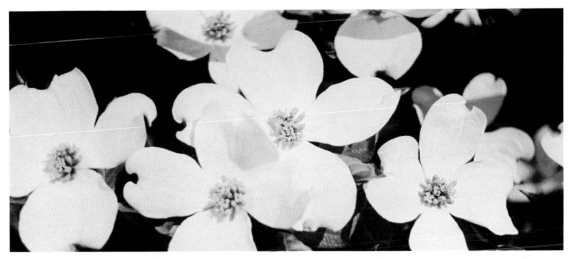

Dogwood

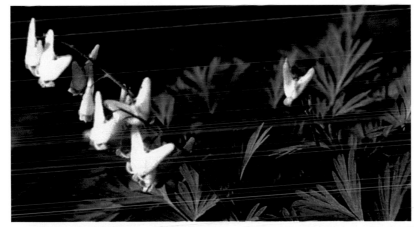

Dutchman's
Breeches

Elderberry

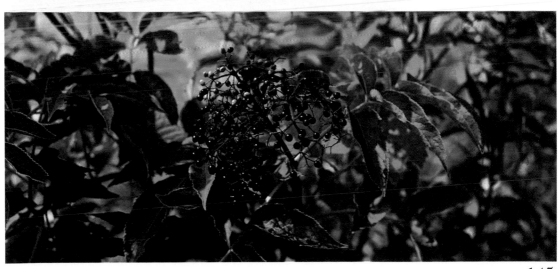

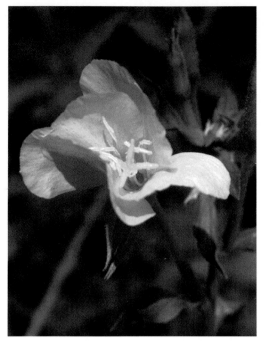

Evening Primrose

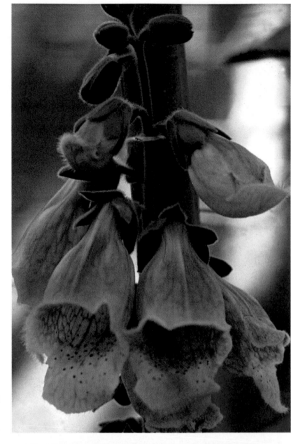

Foxglove

False Solomon's Seal

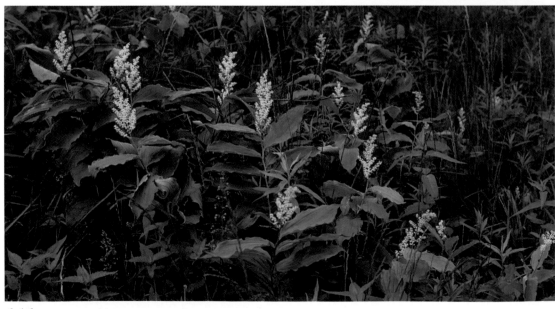

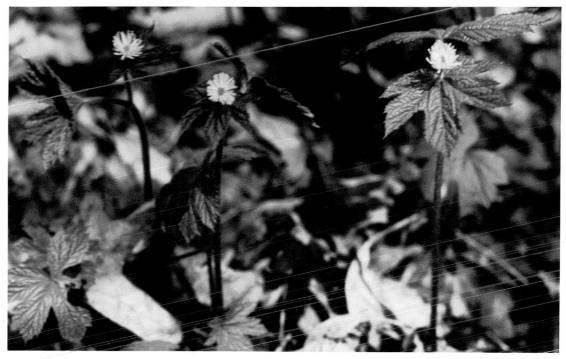

Goldenseal

Gum Plant

Hawthorne

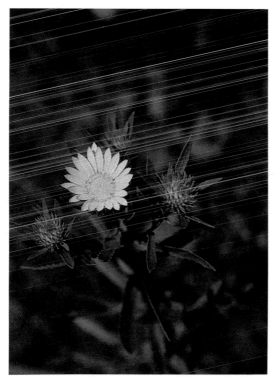

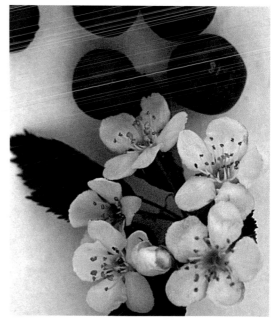

Hepatica

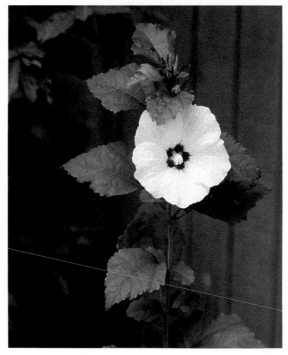

Hercules' Club

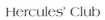

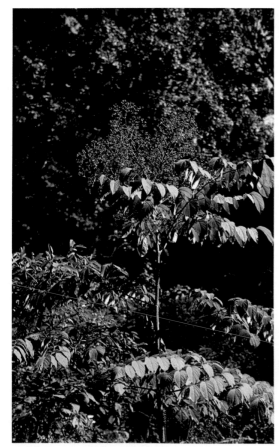

Hollyhock

148

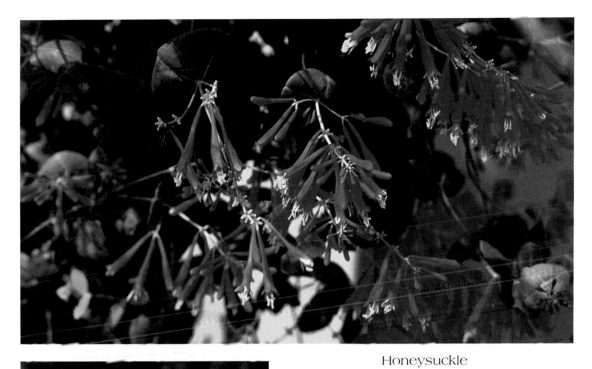

Honeysuckle

Horsemint

Hops

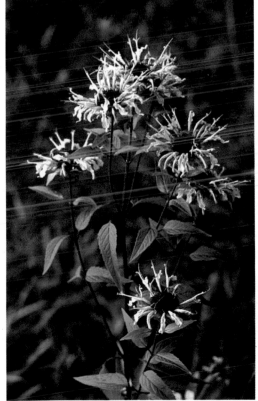

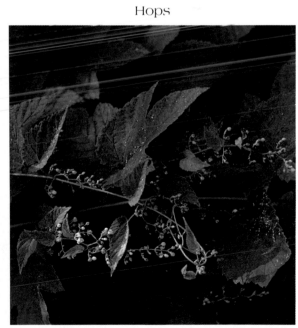

Horsenettle

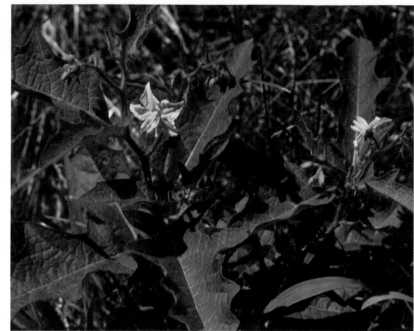

Indian Hemp

Jack-in-the-Pulpit

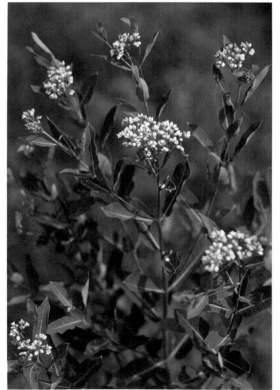

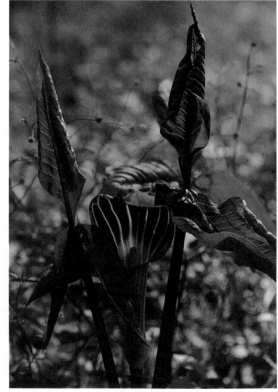

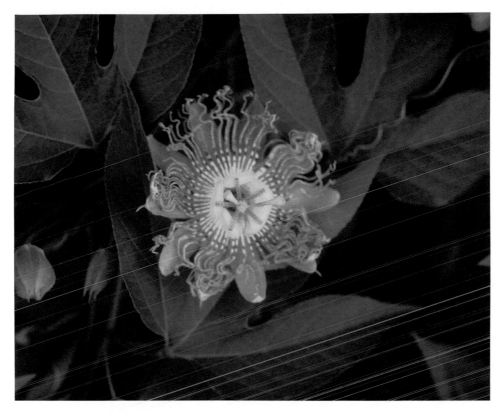

Passion
Flower

Plantain

Pleurisy Root

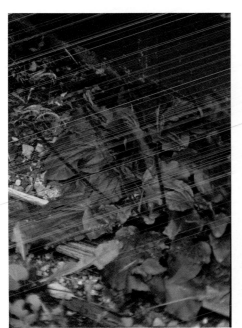

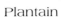

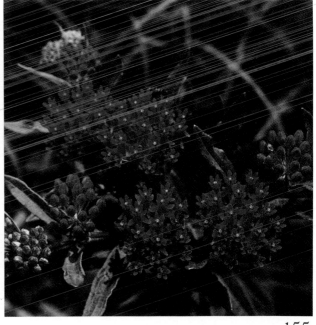

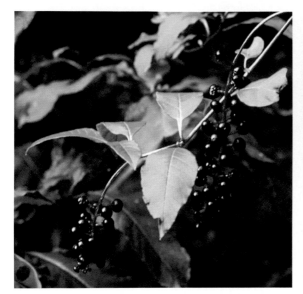

Poke

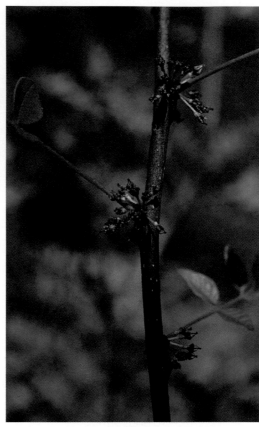

Prickly Ash

Prickly Pear

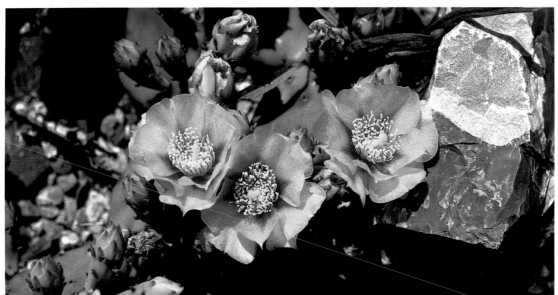

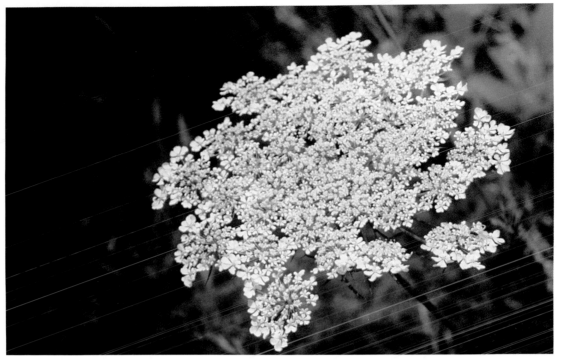

Queen Anne's Lace

Rattlesnake Master
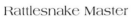

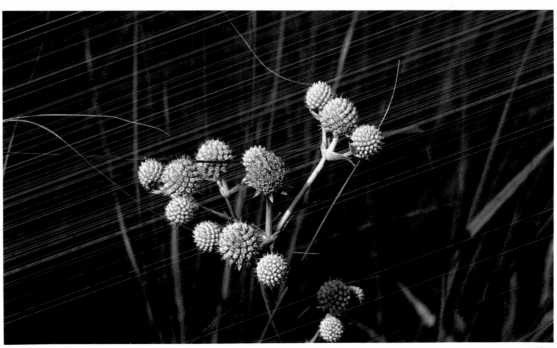

Red Cedar

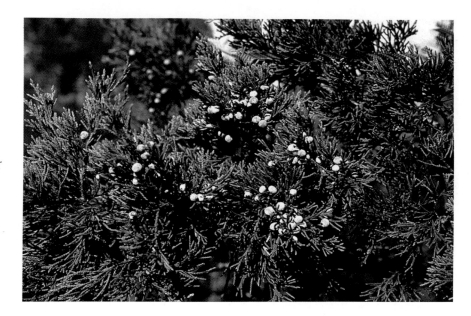

Sarsaparilla

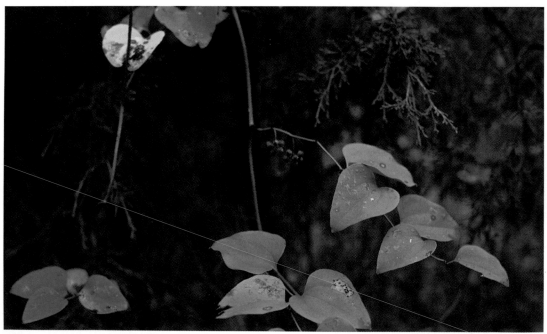

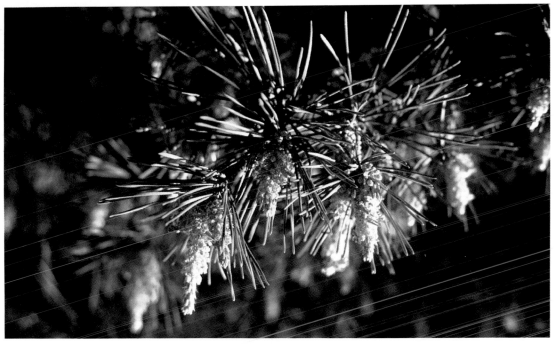

Scotch Pine

Self-Heal

Seneca Snakeroot

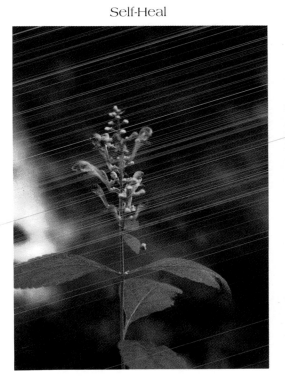

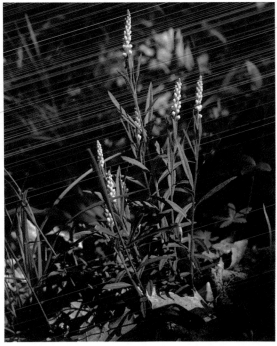

Senna

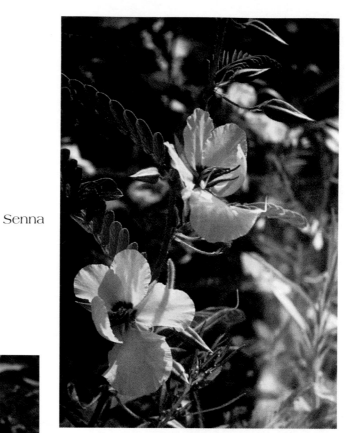

Skunk Cabbage

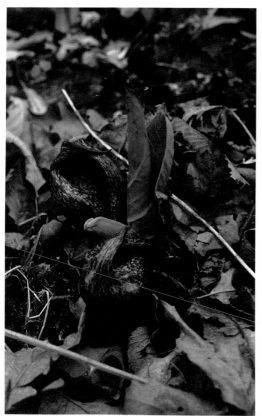

Smartweed

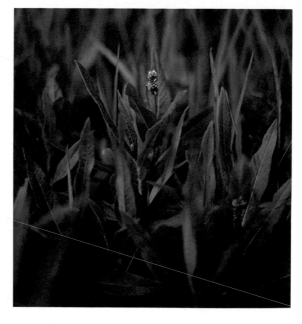

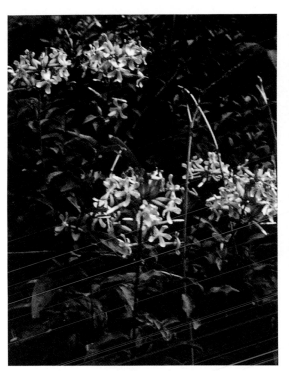

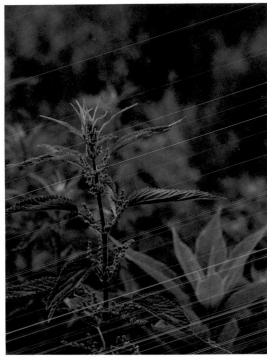

Soapwort

Stinging Nettle

Spicebush

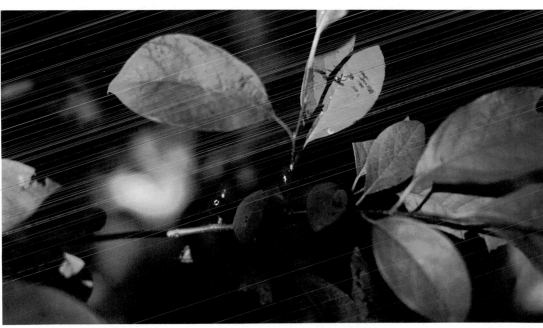

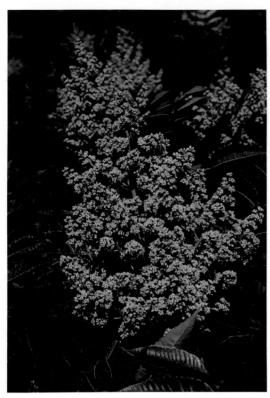

Sumac

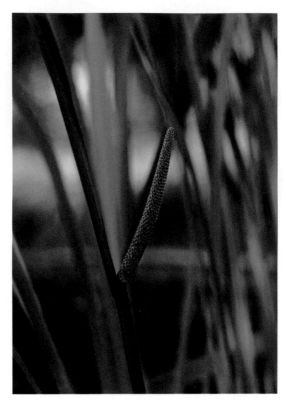

Sweet Flag

Sunflower

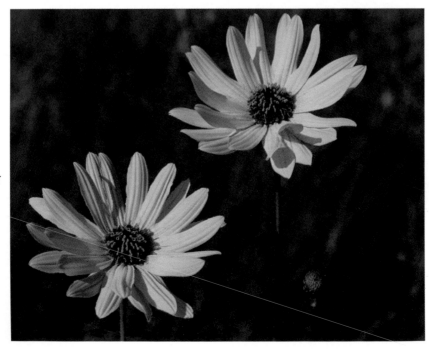

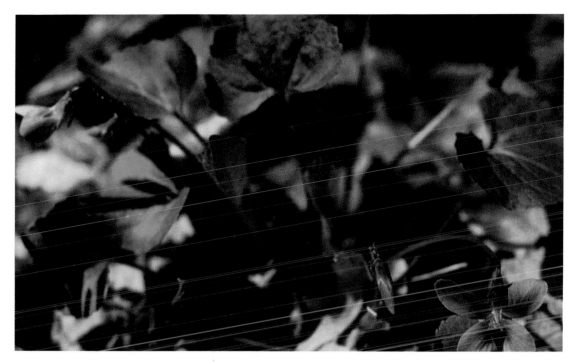

Sweet Violet

Trillium

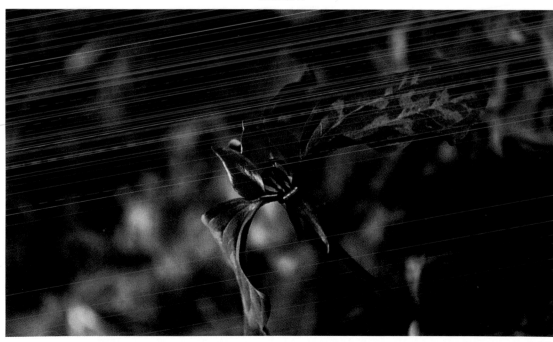

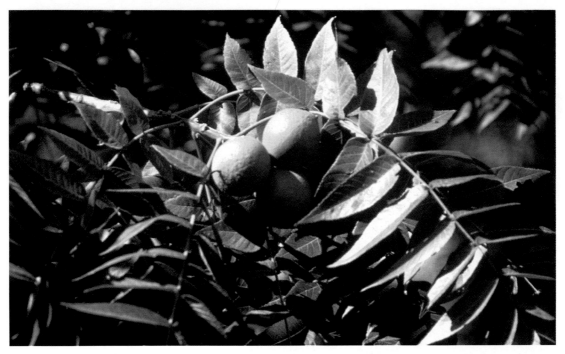

Walnut

Water Hemlock

White Trillium

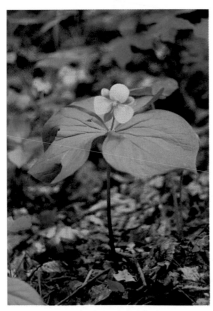

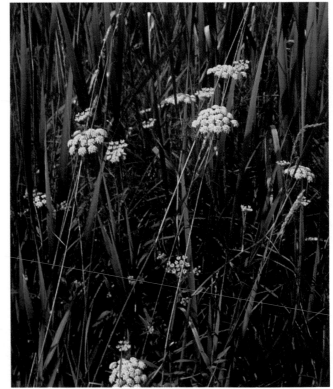

164

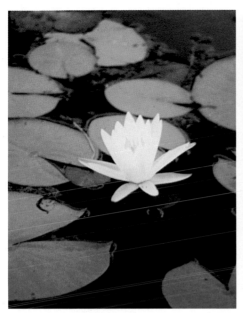

White Pond Lily

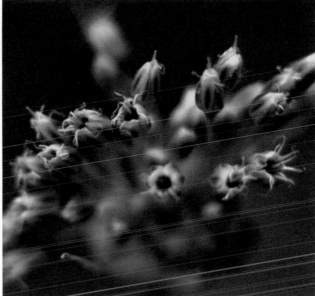

Wild Garlic

Wild Coffee

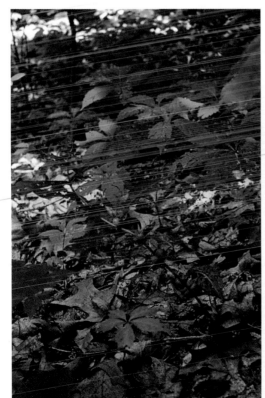

Wild Geranium

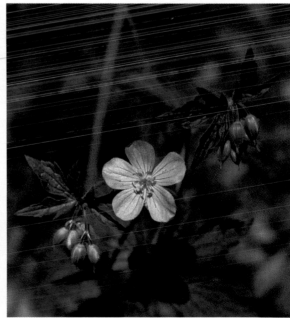

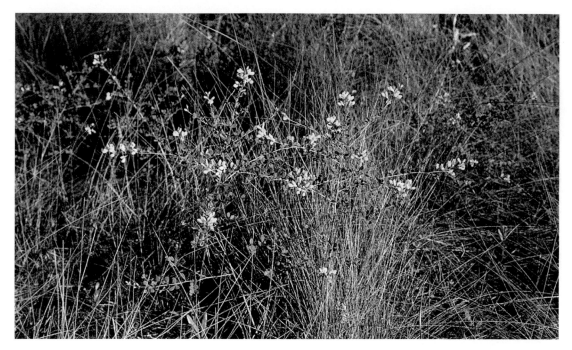

Wild Indigo

Wild Ginger

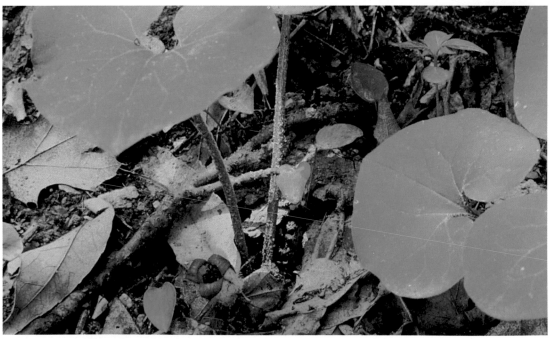

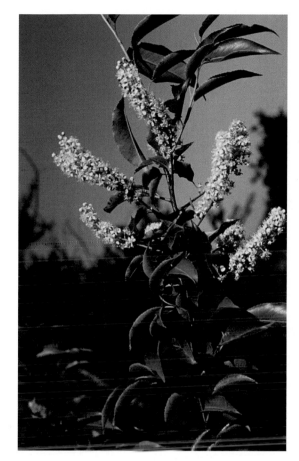

Wild Plum

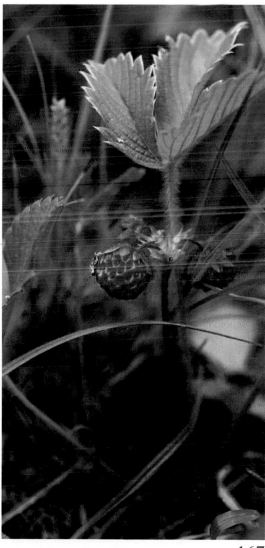

Wild
Strawberry

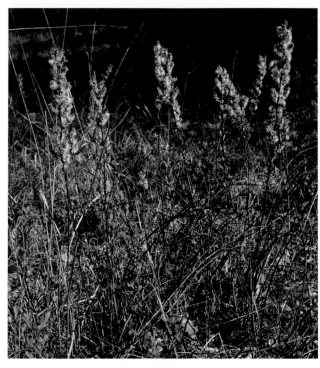

Willow

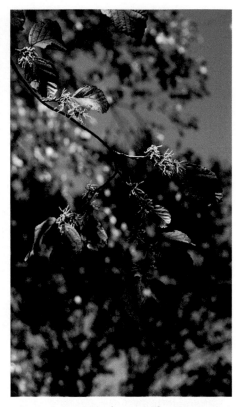

Witch Hazel

Wood
Sorrel

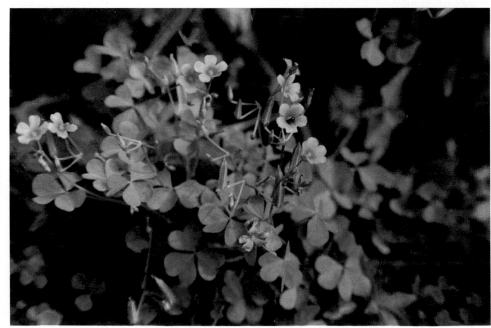

Feverfew

Tanacetum parthenium Bernh.; *cv. Chrysanthemum parthenium* (L.) Bernh.

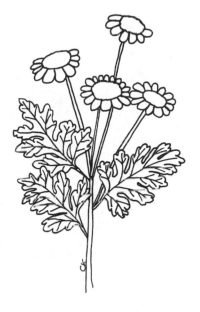

Common name
Bachelor's button.

Habitat
Roadsides throughout the Heartland

Description
Feverfew is a member of the Asteraceae (sunflower) family.

Feverfew is a perennial with erect, branched, downy leafy stems and yellowish, pinnate to bipinnate, alternate leaves. Terminal flowerheads with short, broad white ray-florets and yellow, tubular disc florets are arranged in loose corymbs, and bloom in July and August. The fruit is a ribbed achene.

Medicinal Uses
Dioscorides used feverfew for treating stomach ailments, fevers, menstrual irregularities and headaches. Culpeper recommended boiling the herb in wine, as it "cleanses the womb, expels afterbirth and does a woman all the good she can desire of any herb. A decoction with honey helps cough or chest colds, cleans the reins and bladder and to help expel the stone." He also recommended using the decoction in a poultice for treating and soothing swellings and open wounds, and as a mouth rinse after tooth extraction. Planted around dwellings, feverfew purifies the atmosphere and wards off disease.

Feverfew contains the active components camphor, bitter compounds, the sesquiterpene lactones parthenolide and santamarine, tannins and mucilage. Herbalists recommend using an infusion as an antispasmodic, carminative, emmenagogue, mild anthelmintic, mild sedative, stimulant, stomachic and tonic to soothe the digestive tract, treat arthritis and promote sleep. The infusion with honey is good for coughs, wheezing and difficulty breathing. A tincture applied locally relieves pain and swellings from insect and snakebites. The dried herb has a penetrating aroma and must always be stored well away from other herbs.

British research has shown that feverfew is an excellent remedy for migraines, nausea and vomiting, it relieves the inflammation and pain of arthritis, promotes restful sleep, improves indigestion and relieves asthma attacks. Sesquiterpene may act to inhibit prostaglandin and histamine which are released during inflammatory processes. This action prevents the spasms of blood vessels in the head that trigger migraine headaches.

Some people may develop mouth blisters from overexposure to the herb.

Fleabane
Erigeron philadelphicus L.

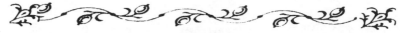

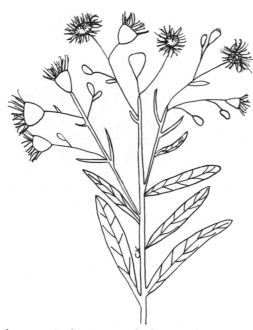

Common names
Daisy fleabane, horseweed, lace buttons, marsh fleabane.

Habitat
Open woods, fields, roadsides and waste grounds throughout the Heartland.

Description
Fleabane is a member of the Asteraceae family. The generic name, *Erigeron*, comes from two Greek words meaning "spring" and "old man," referring to early blooming and to the gray-white hair appearance.

Fleabane is an annual herb with leafy, stiff, erect, hairy stems that branch toward the top. Small daisy-like flowerheads are on stalks in a cluster at the tip of the upper branches. Individual flower heads have yellow disk centers encircled by two or three sets of white rays which may be tinged with pink or purple. They bloom from May through October. It produces tiny, wedge-shaped seeds.

Medicinal Uses
According to legend, fleabane was used to protect man and beast. During the Middle Ages, an oil from the leaves and flowering tops was used by physicians for hastening uterine contractions. Millspaugh stated that fleabane was useful in the treatment of urinary disorders, diabetes, dysentery, hemorrhoids and diarrhea. Supposedly, the flowerheads also repel fleas, hence, its common name.

The Cherokee and Chippewa Indians used fleabane for treating amenorrhea, stomach disorders, dysentery, colds, coughs, epilepsy, gout, hemorrhages, headaches and kidney ailments. The Ojibwa drank a flower infusion for treating fevers. They also inhaled the smoke from dried flowers for relieving head colds.

Fleabane, a diuretic and astringent, is a traditional folk remedy for treating diarrhea, kidney stones, and hemorrhages of the intestines, bladder, kidney and stomach.

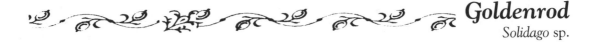

Goldenrod
Solidago sp.

Common names
Early goldenrod, grass-leaved goldenrod, tall goldenrod.

Habitat
Moist, open woods, fields and waste ground throughout the Heartland.

Description
Goldenrod is a member of the Asteraceae (sunflower) family.

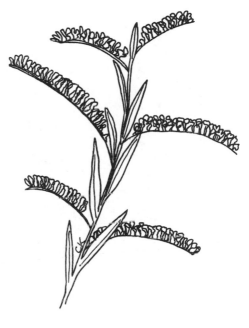

Goldenrod species (*Solidago canadensis, S. graminifolia, S. juncea*) are perennials with slender, downy erect stems. Alternate, ovate to elliptic leaves have serrated margins. The short-stalked flowerheads are arranged around the stem in a terminal raceme or panicle. The ray florets are female and the tubular disc-florets are bisexual. They bloom from August through October. The fruit is a hairy, brown, ribbed achene with a pappus of white hairs.

Medicinal Uses
Several Indian tribes have used goldenrod species medicinally for treating burns, fevers, snakebites and sore throats. The Chippewa used a root tea for treating respiratory ailments and convulsions. The Ojibwa and Potawatomi used a flower infusion for relieving chest pains. They used the roots in a poultice for treating boils. The Mohawk used an infusion of the entire herb for treating snakebites.

All goldenrod species contain the active components saponins, quercetin, flavonoids, tannin and an essential oil. Herbalists recommend using a pleasant tasting tea as an aromatic, astringent, carminative, diaphoretic, diuretic, emmenagogue and stimulant for colic, stomach cramps, respiratory and urinary ailments, dysentery and to regulate the menses. The tannins make goldenrod a useful remedy for diarrhea, and for cleansing mucus from the upper respiratory system. Goldenrod is also excellent for treating urinary and kidney disorders. Externally the tea is used as a wash for hemorrhoids, rheumatism, neuralgia and headaches. Recent studies have shown that quercetin is useful in treating hemorrhoids and nephritis.

The pollen of goldenrod species may cause allergic reactions in some people.

171

Goldenseal
Hydrastis canadensis L.

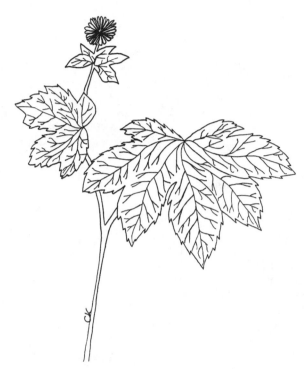

Common names
Ground raspberry, tumeric root, yellow puccoon, yellow root.

Habitat
Rich, moist shady woods throughout the Heartland.

Description
Goldenseal is a member of the Ranunculaceae (buttercup) family.

Goldenseal is a perennial herb with a thick, hairy stem. The thick, oblong rhizome has yellow-brown bark and a bright yellow interior. There is a single basal leaf with a long petiole and two small stem leaves, called bracts. Each deep, green leaf has five to nine deep lobes with coarse teeth. The terminal, small, green-white erect flower has no petals, three sepals, numerous stamens and pistils and forms a dense head. It blooms in April and May. Small fleshy, raspberry-like berries, hence the name ground raspberry, contains one to two shiny, black seeds.

Medicinal Uses
Goldenseal was one of the favorite plants of the Northeastern Indians who used the root medicinally, and its yellow juice to stain their faces and dye their clothing. Goldenseal was used by various tribes for treating dyspepsia, eye ailments, gonorrhea, inflammations, skin ailments, blisters, dropsy and jaundice. The Cherokee mixed powdered goldenseal root with bear grease to use as an insect repellent. They used the root in an infusion as a bitter tonic for treating stomach and liver ailments. The infusion was also used as a wash for sore mouths, inflamed eyes, diseases of the skin and as a douche. The Meskwaki and Potawatomi used goldenseal to treat eczema, and as an inhalant for asthma.

The settlers adopted the numerous medicinal remedies of goldenseal from the Indians. They used the plant as an astringent, diuretic, stimulant and tonic. Crushed rhizomes and roots were used in a decoction for treating of skin diseases, sore throats, sore eyes, mouth ulcers and bleeding. They also sniffed the powdered root for catarrhal conditions of the sinuses and nose. The root sap was used to dye wool and silk yellow, and cotton a fine green.

172

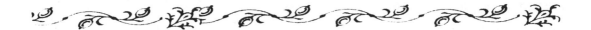

An American folk healer wrote in nineteenth century, "this root is one of the Indian's favorite remedies; and medical men of the present age recognize it as one of the standard remedies for many pathological conditions or diseases of the human body. Too much cannot be said of this valuable agent, that has been veiled in darkness to the medical world so long, I consider it one of the kings of diseases of the mucous membrane. It is unsurpassed by any known remedy." He considered goldenseal extremely valuable as a tonic for disordered and debilitated states of the digestive and mucous tissues, and useful in combination with capsicum as a remedy for chronic alcoholism.

Goldenseal contains the active components resin, lignin, and the alkaloids hydrastine, berberine and canadine. Herbalists recommend using an infusion as an alterative, anti-fungal, anti-inflammatory, antiseptic, astringent, catarrhal, choleretic, laxative and tonic for morning sickness, dyspepsia, internal hemorrhage, liver, stomach, urinary and uterine ailments. Externally, the infusion is used as a mouthwash or gargle for infected gums and sore throats. The infusion is also used as a wash to treat ringworm, canker sores and poison ivy. The powdered roots sprinkled directly onto cuts or wounds, disinfects and promotes rapid healing.

Like ginseng, goldenseal is used for treating stress, anxiety, asthma and allergic reactions. This marvelous natural drug is a nontoxic, non-irritating antiseptic that both heals and soothes the surfaces of the body. Many modern herbalist consider goldenseal one of the best herbs available in North America. Goldenseal is an ingredient in many soothing and healing eye lotions and eye drops .

It has been shown experimentally that berberine lowers blood pressure, increases bile secretion, acts as a mild sedative and is an anti-convulscent.

Berberine has cumulative effects on the system and stimulates the uterus; therefore goldenseal should not be used during pregnancy or for a period of more than a week without the advice of a qualified medical or herbal practitioner.

Ground Ivy

Gleocoma hederacea L.

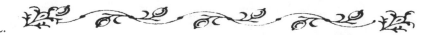

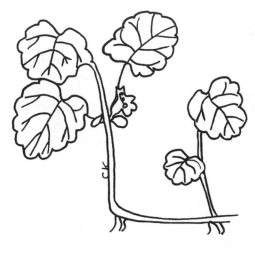

Common names

Cat's foot, alehoof, Gill-over-the-ground, Creeping Charlie.

Habitat

Moist, shaded areas, roadsides, woods and waste areas throughout the Heartland.

Description

Ground Ivy is a member of the Laminaceae (mint) family. The generic name, *Gleocoma*, is a Greek word *glaukos* (gray-green), a reference to the leaf color; the species name, *hederacea*, refers to the ivy-like creeping habit of the plant on the ground.

Ground ivy is a perennial herb with a long creeping rooting rhizome and ascending or erect flowering stems. Cordate to reniform opposite leaves are long-stalked and have serrated margins. Large blue-violet flowers have a straight corolla tube and two notched lips is in loose whorls at the base of the leaves. It blooms from March through June. The fruit is four, one-seeded nutlets.

Medicinal Uses

At one time ground ivy was the primary seasoning used in brewing ale to flavor, preserve and keep it clear. It was, that is, until the German's discovered the value of hops. During the days of witchcraft, garlands and headpieces of ground ivy were worn on Midsummer's Eve, June 24th, to ward off spells cast by witches. Ground ivy was considered potent for witches because it grew in graveyards. Europeans used ground ivy to treat headaches, kidney ailments, and to aid digestion. A leaf tea was used to bathe ulcerous wounds. The juice was inhaled to relieve nasal congestion and headaches. Prior to the nineteenth century in the United States, a leaf tea was drunk to prevent "painter's colic."

Ground ivy contains the active components tannin, rutin, the bitter compound gleocomin, saponin and potassium salts. Herbalists recommend using a flowering stem infusion as an astringent, anti-inflammatory, stimulant and tonic for gastritis, enteritis, diarrhea, dyspepsia, abscesses, eye problems, kidney disorders, sore throats, respiratory ailments and to stimulate the appetite. Externally, the infusion is used in compresses for sores and wounds, and in bath preparations for skin disorders. The fresh shoots and leaves can be added to salads and soups, or prepared and eaten like spinach.

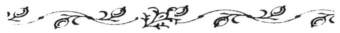

Gum Plant
Grindelia squarrosa (Pursh) Dunal.

Common names
Curly top, gum weed, rosin weed, tar-weed.

Habitat
Roadsides, railroads and pastures throughout the Heartland.

Description
Gum plant is a member of the Asteraceae (sunflower) family. The generic name, *Grindelia*, is named after David Hieronymus Grindel (1776-1836), a professor from Estonia, who wrote on pharmacological and botanical subjects.

Gum plant is a biennial herb with spreading to erect smooth stems. Simple, spatulate to ovoid, alternate, leaves have gland dotted, entire to coarsely serrated margins. It produces few to many flowerheads with yellow ray flowers and sticky disk flowers, and the resinous bracts are strongly curled. It blooms from July through October.

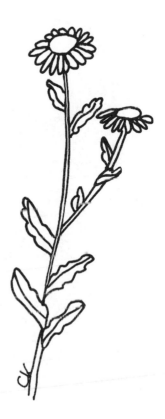

Medicinal Uses
The Indians made a root tea of gum plant for treating liver ailments. A poultice was applied to relieve the pain and swelling of rheumatic joints. The Cree used the herb combined with chamomile, for relieving kidney pains. They also used the flowering tops in an infusion for treating gonorrhea.

Gum plant contains the active components tannin, choline, selenium, a volatile oil, resin and the alkaloid grindeline. Herbalists recommend using a leaf and/or flowering-top infusion as an antispasmodic, cathartic, expectorant, and stimulant for gonorrhea, pneumonia, smallpox, lung ailments, stomachaches and urinary ailments. The infusion is also used as a wash to relieve the skin rash of poison ivy.

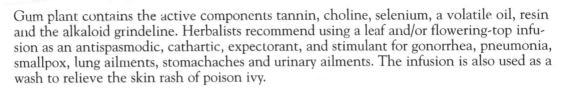

Hemlock
Conium maculatum L.

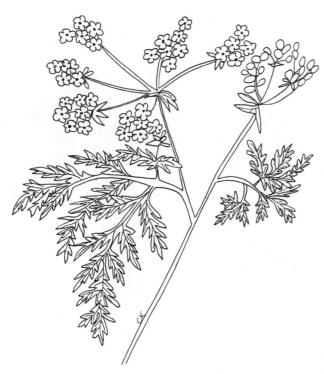

Common name
Poison hemlock, poison parsley, snake-weed, spotted parsley.

Habitat
Waste ground, fields, thickets and along roads throughout the Heartland.

Description
Hemlock is a member of the Apiaceae (parsley) family.

Hemlock is a biennial herb with tall, furrowed, branched hollow stems. The lower part of the stems are smooth and purple spotted. Alternate, finely pinnate or coarsely serrated leaves are dark green above and gray-green below. The leaves are on long petioles that surround the stem at the base. Small white flowers with unnotched petals are in terminal compound umbels and bloom from May through August. The round fruit is a double achene with waxy ribs.

Medicinal Uses
The poisonous effects of hemlock were known to the ancient Greeks, who used it for executions. Socrates was put to death in 399 B.C. by being given hemlock juice. Greek and Arabic physicians considered hemlock an effective treatment for tumors, pains in the joints and skin infections. Hemlock was praised by Avicennia as a cure for breast cancer.

According to Rafinsque in 1828, the valuable medicinal qualities of hemlock varied according to the area and climate where it was grown, time collected and preparation. "It is never dangerous in very small doses often repeated and gradually increased." He considered hemlock an effective anodyne and antispasmodic useful in relieving pain in cancer, epilepsy and syphilis.

Hemlock contains the active components, an essential oil, organic acids, the poisonous alkaloids coniine, methyl coniine and conhydrine. Herbalists recommend using a leaf or fruit infusion as an analgesic, antispasmodic and sedative. Small amounts (large doses can

176

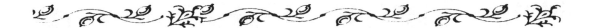

cause death) of the powdered leaves can be used as a sedative and painkiller for ulcers, gout and arthritis, and as an antidote to strychnine poisoning. Hartwell in *Plants Used Against Cancer*, reports that hemlock is useful for treating intestinal, nose, skin, sternum and uterine carcinomas. A tincture of hemlock is used by qualified practitioners in homeopathy for treating enlarged prostates. The isolated pure coniine is contained in a few proprietary ointments and suppositories to relieve severe pain.

All parts of the hemlock, especially the green, almost ripe seeds, are deadly poisons, and may also cause contact dermatitis. Hemlock should never be collected and used for self medication.

Hepatica
Hepatica nobilis Schreb.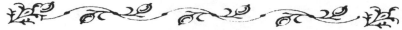

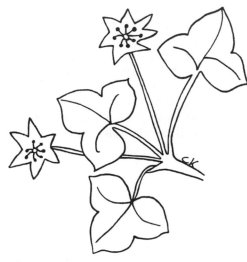

Common names
American liverwort, liver ear, noble liverwort, golden trefoil.

Habitat
Rich woods throughout the Heartland.

Description
Hepatica is a member of the Ranunculaceae (buttercup) family. The generic word, *Hepatica*, comes from Latin word *epatikos*, meaning "affecting the liver," referring to the color and shape of the dead leaves.

Hepatica is a perennial with three oval lobed, light green leaves that are light green and hairy when young, turning dark green with age. The leaves persist through the winter becoming purplish or liver colored. The individual flowers are on individual hairy stalks. The six to ten white to pink or blue-purple petals are actually colored sepals; below each flower is a whorl of three small unlobed leaves which may easily be mistaken for sepals. It blooms from March through June.

Medicinal Uses
Culpeper considered hepatica to be excellent herb for treating all diseases of the liver: "It is a singular good herb for all diseases of the liver, both to cool and cleanse it ...being bruised and boiled in beer, if drank it cools the heat of the liver and kidneys, and helps the running of the reins in men and the whites in women, it is a good remedy to stay the spreading of tetters, ringworm, and other fretting or running sores and scabs."

Millspaugh, valued hepatica for treating liver diseases as well as lung ailments: "The liver-leaf has held a place among medicinal plants from ancient times until the present. It is now falling into disuse on account of its mild properties, forming as it does simply a slightly astringent, mucilaginous infusion. It was used in haemoptysis, coughs and other lung affections, as well as all diseases of the liver, and in hemorrhoids; in the latter troubles its exhibitor must have met with no very flattering success."

Hepatica contains the active component the glycoside hepatilobin. Herbalists recommend using a leaf infusion as an astringent, diuretic, mild mucilaginous, and vulnerary for coughs, bronchitis, gallbladder, kidney and liver disorders. An infusion is a useful gargle for relieving chronic irritations of the throat and pharynx.

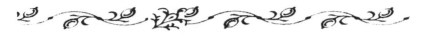

Hollyhock
Althaea rosea (L.) Cav.

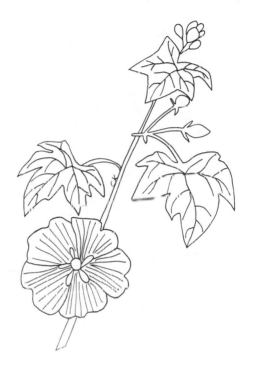

Common names
Purple or blue malva.

Habitat
Open fields, fence rows and often cultivated throughout the Heartland.

Description
Hollyhock is a member of the Malvaceae (mallow) family. The generic name, *Althea*, comes from the Greek word *altheirn* (to heal), referring to its healing properties.

Hollyhock is a perennial herb with tall erect, leafy stems. It has alternate, palmate leaves with blunt, dentate lobes. Large showy flowers are white, pink, red or deep purple, in leaf axils arranged in a spike-like cluster. They bloom from July through October. The disc-shaped fruit, a schizocarp, separates into a one-seeded nutlet, a mericarp. All parts of the plant are coarsely hairy.

Medicinal Uses
Hollyhock contains the active components, tannin, abundant mucilage and the pigment anthocyanin in dark flowers only. Herbalists recommend using an infusion (the herb must be free of the mallow rust *Puccina malvaccarum*) as an anti-inflammatory, diuretic and demulcent for inflammations of the mucous membranes, coughs, asthma, chronic gastritis, urine incontinence, diarrhea and enteritis. Herbal compresses and bath preparations are used for skin disorders, cuts and bruises. A leaf infusion may be used as a gargle to soothe swollen tonsils, inflamed mucous membranes, spongy gums, loose teeth and sore mouths. The dried, macerated leaves, boiled in wine, can be drank to prevent miscarriage and to kill worms in children. The flowers are used in cosmetics as an emollient. The violet colored variety can be used to dye cloth and color medicine and foodstuffs. The lovely pale periwinkle-blue and pink dried flowers are used in sachets and potpourris.

Horehound
Marrubium vulgare L.

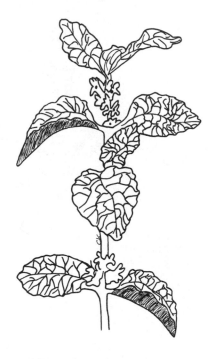

Common name
White horehound.

Habitat
Fields and roadsides throughout the Heartland.

Description
Horehound is a member of the Laminaceae (mint) family.

Horehound is a perennial herb with erect, square, branched stems and short, stout rhizomes. Opposite, ovate leaves are wrinkled, bluntly serrated and long-stalked. Small white tubular flowers are in dense whorls in the axils of the uppermost leaves. The flowers are a calyx tube with ten veins, ten hooked teeth; the corolla is two-lipped with the upper lip flat. It blooms from May through September. The fruit is four nutlets. All parts of the plant have an apple-like smell.

Medicinal Uses
Horehound takes it name from Horus, the Egyptian god of sky and light. Egyptians called it the seed of Horus, bull's blood and eye of the star. Ancient Greeks used horehound as an anti-spasmodic and antidote for mad dog bites. Among the Hebrews, it was one of the ritual bitter herbs of Passover. Culpeper called horehound the "herb of Mercury," and claimed that the herb "helpeth to expectorate tough phlegm from the chest being taken with the roots of the Iris or Orris"; in addition "purges away yellow jaundice; and with the oil of roses, dropped into the ears, eases the pain of them."

Horehound contains the active components marrubiin, a sesquiterpene, tannin, saponin, resin, and the diterpene alcohols marrbiol and marrubenol. Herbalists recommend using an infusion of the flowering stems as an antispasmodic, cholagogue, emmenagogue, expectorant, mild sedative and stomachic. The infusion is used for chronic hepatitis, tumors, tuberculosis, typhoid, parathyroid, snakebites, asthma, menstrual complaints, liver and gallbladder complaints, itches, jaundice and bronchitis. Horehound has been traditionally used as a reliable liver and digestive remedy. Large doses will expel worms.

Studies have shown that small amounts of marrubiin have a normalizing effect on irregular heartbeats. As marrubiin breaks down in the body, it is a strong stimulator of bile production.

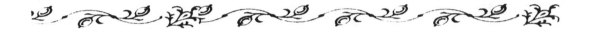

Externally, horehound is used in compresses to treat painful and inflamed wounds. With honey, this green herb is a good remedy for all chest complaints and coughs. It is used in candies and lozenges for hoarseness, coughs and catarrh. For smokers' cough, make a decoction of hyssop (*Hyssopus officinalis*), coltsfoot (*Tussilago farfara)*, marshmallow root (*Althaea officinalis*), and horehound in equal parts and drink as often as needed.

To make horehound lozenges, steep one and one-third cup dried leaves in two cups boiling water, strain. Add to the liquid two cups honey, four cups brown sugar and one teaspoon cream of tartar. Heat to a temperature of 220° F. Add one teaspoon butter and heat to 312° F. Remove from the heat, add one teaspoon lemon juice and pour into hot, buttered pans, mark into squares and cool.

Horsemint

Monarda fistulosa L., *M. punctata* L.

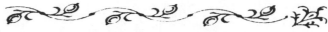

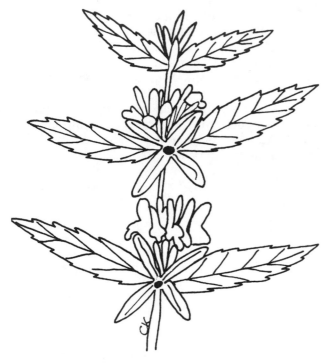

Common names
Purple bee balm, wild bergamot.

Habitat
Dry woods, fields, prairies, and road-sides throughout the Heartland.

Description
Horsemint is a member of the Laminaceae (mint) family. The generic name, *Monarda*, is in honor of the sixteenth Spanish physician and botanist, Nicolas Monardas; and the species name, *fistulosa*, is from Latin meaning "like a reed or pipe."

Horsemint is an aromatic, erect perennial with a square, hairy stem. Opposite, narrow to ovate, gray-green leaves are pointed towards the tip and have serrated margins. Pink to lavender flowers have a distinct upper lip or lobe, and the stamens protruding from the tubes are found in clustered, dense ragged heads. It blooms from July through September.

Medicinal Uses
Many Indian tribes used the water from boiled, fresh horsemint leaves to bathe patients suffering from chills. They boiled the dried herb to produce vapors to treat bronchial ailments. A root tea was drank for treating stomach disorders. A tea of the leaves and flowers was used for respiratory ailments. Chippewa and Navajo Indians used horsemint to treat colds, burns, fevers, flu, coughs, gastritis, headaches and intestinal parasites. Winnebago and Blackfoot Indians used a decoction of the leaves as a cure for pimples, eczema and other skin eruptions. The Creek Indians used an infusion for deafness, delirium, dropsy and rheumatism.

Horsemint was officially listed in *The United States Pharmacopoeia*, 1820 to 1882 and *The National Formulary* since 1950 as a carminative, diuretic, emmenagogue and stimulant. The American medical profession of the nineteenth century prescribed the leaves and tops of horsemint to check vomiting, induce perspiration, alleviate arthritis, regulate menses and to release gassy colic.

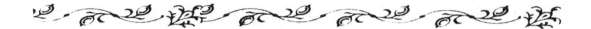

Horsemint contains the active components thymol, a crystalline phenol and a pungent, aromatic oil. Herbalists recommend using an infusion as an anthelmintic, antiseptic, carminative, diaphoretic, diuretic and fungicide for respiratory ailments, fevers, diarrhea and to expel worms. A poultice is used to relieve itchy skin disorders and hemorrhoids.

Thymol is listed in *The United States Pharmacopoeia* as an anthelmintic and antiseptic. During World War I when the thyme fields were destroyed in Europe, horsemint was grown in the United States as the source for thymol. Thymol is used in many pharmaceutical preparations.

Horsenettle

Solanum carolinense L.

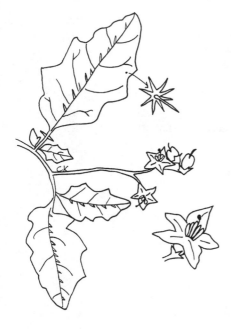

Common names
Bull nettle, sand briar, apple of Sodom, Devil's tomato.

Habitat
Open woods, roadsides and waste areas throughout the Heartland.

Description
Horsenettle is a member of the Solanaceae (nightshade) family.

Horsenettle is a bushy, dark green perennial. The stems and underside of the leaves are prickly. A beautiful flower with five violet or white pink petals is a umbel-shaped blossom with five bright yellow anthers and one pistil. It blooms from June through October and produces a small, orange-yellow, smooth tomato-like fruit.

Medicinal Uses
Cherokee Indians used the wilted leaves to treat poison ivy. They gargled a seed tea for soothing sore throats, and drank a tea made from the seeds and leaves for treating goiters and to expel intestinal parasites. The settlers took five or six berries, in increasing quantities, as a treatment for tetanus. The berries, leaves and rootstock were used as an anodyne and diuretic for treating epilepsy, asthma, bronchitis and convulsions. Southern Blacks used horsenettle in the treatment of epilepsy. Horsenettle was listed in *The National Formulary* from 1916 to 1936.

Horsenettle contains the active components the alkaloids solamine and solanidane. Herbalists recommend using a berry infusion as an anti-spasmodic, diuretic and sedative. When properly prepared, the berries are an excellent remedy for epilepsy, infantile convulsions and menstrual hysteria. The dried berries have been found to produce antibacterial activities against *Pseudomonas* species.

The horsenettle berries are extremely poisonous and should only be used under strict supervision of a qualified medical or herbal practitioner.

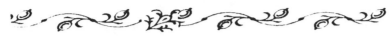

Horseradish
Armoracia rusticana Gilib.

Common names
Mountain radish, red cole.

Habitat
Open fields, waste areas, and occasionally cultivated throughout the Heartland.

Description
Horseradish is a member of the Brassicaceae (mustard) family. The generic name, *Armoracia*, was used by Pliny, the first physician to recommend horseradish for its medicinal properties.

Horseradish is a perennial herb with an erect branched stem and a thick, long cylindrical fleshy root. The long, oblong basal leaves have undulate and serrate margins. The stem leaves are smaller, narrower, short-stalked or sessile, serrated or smooth. Numerous white flowers are arranged in a compound, terminal panicle and bloom from May through August. The fruit is an oval silicula.

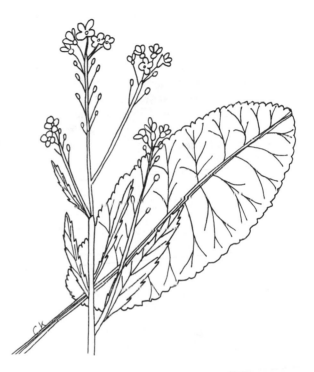

Medicinal Uses
Many an early doctor used the fiery, pungent roots as a diaphoretic, diuretic (it is one of the most potent herbal diuretics), expectorant, rubefacient, and vermicide. Rich in vitamin C, horseradish was used to treat scurvy-plagued individuals. A syrup of grated horseradish, honey and water was a standard remedy for hoarseness, and every mother's remedy for stimulating the appetite. The Cherokee Indians used horseradish for treating amenorrhea, asthma, colds, dyspepsia, gravel and rheumatism.

Horseradish contains the active components vitamin C, allylisothiocyante, the glycoside sinigrin and asparagin. Herbalists recommend using horseradish root (fresh root is more potent than dried) as an antiseptic, diuretic, expectorant, mild laxative, rubefacient and stimulant. When sinigrin is combined with water, it yields mustard oil, a powerful circulatory stimulant and antibiotic A tea is an excellent remedy for all respiratory ailments. A healthy spoonful of horseradish sauce will quickly open the sinuses. Horseradish is contained in a few proprietary medications used for treating influenza and infections of the urinary tract. Externally, horseradish is used in a poultice for relieving respiratory congestion,

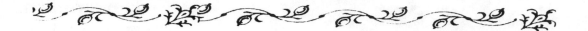

pain and inflammation of rheumatism, arthritis, aching joints, chilblains, insect bites and stings.

Studies have confirmed the antibiotic properties of horseradish against gram-negative, gram-positive bacteria and some pathogenic fungi. Horseradish has also been shown to have anti-tumor activity. Asparagin is a known diuretic.

Care must be taken because large doses may irritate the digestive and intestinal tract. Do not use if taking thyroxin for low thyroid function. Frequent application of horseradish to the same spot may irritate the skin.

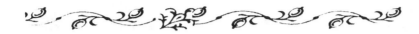

Indian Hemp
Apocyum cannabinum L.

Common names
Dogbane, Indian physic, milkweed, dropsy weed.

Habitat
Prairies, fields and rocky woods throughout the Heartland.

Description
Indian hemp is a member of the Apocyanaceae (dogbane) family. Dioscorides named the plant apokynon, referring to "the plant with milky juice." The species name, *cannabinum*, means "of cannabis" or "of hemp," referring to the woody outer fibers.

Indian hemp is a perennial with erect, smooth or hairy, waxy stems with a milky sap and creeping rhizomes. It has opposite, lanceolate to egg-shaped leaves. Flowers with white to pinkish petals are bell-shaped with flaring lobes and in loose to dense clusters at the ends of branches. It blooms from June through September. Slender, tapering cylindrical pods occur in pairs.

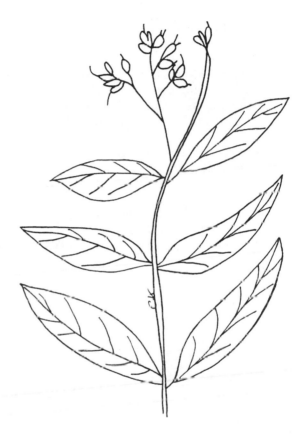

Medicinal Uses
Indian hemp fibers have been found in an Ohio-Hopewell fabric, Adena fabric, and a Sauk-Fox bog dating from 1000 to 3000 B.C. According to Rafinesque, Indian hemp was highly valued by southern Indians as a tonic, emetic, alterative and anti-syphilitic. "The root is the most powerful part; but it must be used fresh, since time diminishes or destroys its power ...Chickasaw and Choctaw Nations considered Indian hemp a specific for syphilis. They chewed the fresh root and swallowed only the juice ...this use later introduced into Tennessee and Kentucky as a great secret." Many Indian tribes have used the root of Indian hemp in a tea for treating ague, cold, dropsy, fevers, headaches and sore throats, as a diuretic during pregnancy, as an oral contraceptive and to expel worms. The milky sap was used for treating venereal warts. Cherokee, Meskwaki and Fox Indians used a root tea or strong infusion for treating asthma, Bright's disease (nephritis), respiratory ailments, rheumatism and uterine obstructions. The Chippewa boiled the roots for treating heart palpitations, convulsions, dizziness, headaches, insanity and nervousness.

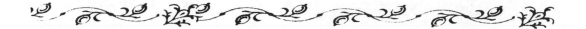

South Carolina Blacks steeped the roots in whiskey for treating colds, constipation and fevers. A root decoction was used by midwives to induce abortion.

Indian hemp contains the active components cardiac glycosides cymarin, apocannoside, K-strophanthin, cynocannoside and genistroplanthidin. Herbalists recommend using an infusion as a diaphoretic, diuretic and expectorant for asthma, respiratory ailments, fevers, headaches, incontinence and venereal warts.

Recent research has shown that both cymarin and apocymarin have anti-tumor activity. Apocymarin also elevates blood pressure. The toxic cardioactive glycosides are a very valuable remedy for dropsy caused from heart failure and hepatic cirrhosis.

Indian hemp has properties similar to digitalis, but is more powerful, often causing nausea, diarrhea and irritation of the mucous membranes. Indian hemp should not be used for self medication unless under the strict supervision of a qualified medical or herbal practitioner.

Indian Physic
Euphorbia corollata L.

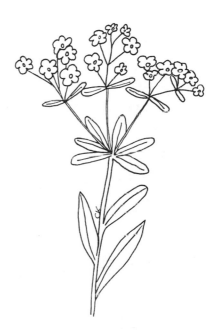

Common names
Spurge, emetic root, flowering spurge, milkweed, tramp's spurge.

Habitat
Prairies, woods, fields and roadsides throughout the Heartland.

Description
Indian physic is a member of the Euphorbiaceae (spurge) family. The generic name, *Euphorbia*, comes from the Greek "euphor bean," a plant named after Euphorbos, a Greek physician of the first century B.C.; and the species name, *corollata*, comes from the Latin *coralla*, which means little crown or garland.

Indian physic is a perennial herb with a milky sap in the erect stems and hairy, spreading branches above. Its has alternate, simple, lanceolate-shaped to elliptical leaves. Numerous small, flower-like cups at the end of branches contain many male flowers and one long female flower with five white petal-like appendages. It blooms from June through October. Fruits with three lobed capsules contain three gray seeds.

Medicinal Uses
As the name implies, Indian physic was widely used by the Indians, including the Meskwaki, as an emetic and purgative. A leaf or root tea was used to treat chronic constipation, rheumatism and diabetes. The root was used in a poultice for treating snakebites. Meskwaki Indians mixed Indian physic with sumac (*Rhus* sp.) berries to get ride of pinworms. They also combined the root with mayapple (*Podophyllum peltatum*) as a cathartic.

Indian physic was listed in *The United States Pharmacopoeia* from 1820 to 1882, as a diaphoretic and expectorant in small doses, and as an emetic and laxative in large doses.

Herbalists use Indian physic containing flavonoids, alkaloids and triterpenoids as an emetic and purgative.

The diterpenes in the latex are an irritant to the skin and may cause blistering. Care must be taken when handling.

Indian Tobacco

Lobelia inflata L.

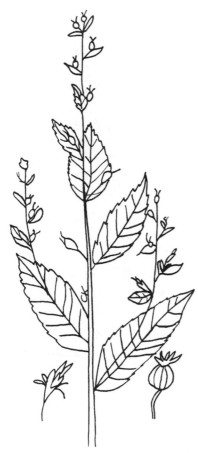

Common names
Asthma weed, pukeweed.

Habitat
Rich woodlands and open woods throughout the Heartland.

Description
Indian tobacco is a member of the Lobeliaceae (bluebell) family. The generic name, *Lobelia*, is named after Mathiew de Lobel (1538-1616), a Flemish physician and herbalist; the species name, *inflata*, means "puffed-up or swollen," in reference to the enlarged seed capsule.

Indian tobacco is a perennial herb with stems that are hairy below and smooth above. Simple, alternate, elliptic to lanceolate leaves with serrated margins. Inconspicuous flowers, with three petals, fused into a short, whitish tube which opens into two blue lips, are in a short spike-like group extending above leaves. They bloom from July through October. An egg-shaped fruit with numerous minute seeds is enclosed by the fused, inflated sepals.

Medicinal Uses
Indian tobacco, called 'pukeweed' by the American Indians, was used to empty the stomach and to heal during the Indians' great councils and sacred ceremonies. Cherokee Indians used Indian tobacco for treating headaches, asthma, boils, colic, croup, syphilis, pertussis, sore throats, stiff necks and to expel intestinal parasites. They smoked the herb to break the tobacco habit.

Indian tobacco was used by early physicians as an expectorant, anti-asthmatic, emetic and stimulant to treat asthma, nerves, respiratory ailments, convulsions, diphtheria, epilepsy and tonsillitis. Indian tobacco was adopted by the Physiomedical School of Herbalists as a major relaxant remedy to treat pain caused by muscle spasms.

Millspaugh emphasized that in large doses, lobelia is a narcotic poison. "Its principle sphere of action seems to be upon the pneumagastric nerve, and it is to the organs supplied by this nerve that its toxic symptoms are mainly due, and its 'physiological' cures of pertussis, spasmodic asthma, croup and gastralgia gained. Its second action in importance is that of

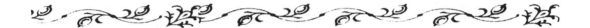

causing general muscular relaxation ...it cures of strangulated hernia (by enemata), tetenic spasms, convulsions, hysteria and may help hydrophobia. Its third action is upon mucous surfaces and secretory glands increasing their secretions ...death is usually preceded by insensibility and convulsions."

Indian tobacco contains the active components resin, chelidonic acid, the bitter glycoside lobelacrin, the pungent, volatile oil lobelianin, the alkaloids lobeline, isolobinine, lobelanidine, and lobinaline. Herbalists recommend using an infusion as an astringent and expectorant for respiratory ailments, chronic bronchitis and spasmodic asthma. The infusion gives almost instant relief from suffocating phlegm and mucus that has collected in the respiratory tract.

Studies show that isolobinine is a respiratory relaxant and that lobeline stimulates the respiratory system. It is used by physicians to resuscitate newborn infants. Lobeline also has pharmacological properties similar to nicotine. First it stimulates the central nervous system and then strongly depresses it. It is therefore used to aid tobacco withdrawal symptoms.

The plant has a mildly euphoric, marijuana-like quality, while conferring a great sense of clarity. Taken as a tea, its is even more pronounced, acting both as stimulant and relaxant.

Indian tobacco is poisonous in large doses because it is a nerve depressant. Therefore should never be used for self-medication without supervision from a qualified medical or herbal practitioner.

Jack-in-the-Pulpit

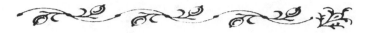

Arisaema triphyllum (L.) Schott

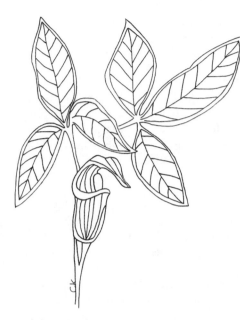

Common name
Indian turnip.

Habitat
Rich woods throughout the heartland.

Description
Jack-in-the-Pulpit is a member of the Araceae (arum or calla) family. The generic name, *Arisaema*, comes from two Greek words, *aris* (a kind or arum) and *haema* (blood); the species name, *triphyllum*, comes from Latin for "three leaves."

Jack-in-the-Pulpit is a perennial with two stalks that have three leaves. Between the stalks grows a third stalk topped with a green tubular spathe (the pulpit) which has a hood turned down over it that protects a greenish or dark purple tube, the spadix (Jack or preacher). Usually, there are both male and female flower on some spadix (one sex may abort). The male flowers consist of small white structure with four purple cup-like anthers. The female flowers are green, knob-like organs with purple stigmas. The male flowers are above the female on the base of the spadix near the point where it joins the spathe. It blooms from April through June. The brilliant crimson, berry-like fruit has four to six seeds.

Medicinal Uses
Chippewa Indians used an infusion of Jack-in-the-Pulpit to treat sore eyes. The Pawnee and Cherokee applied the rhizome or powdered root as a counter-irritant for relieving headaches, rheumatism and other similar pains. They also used a root infusion to treat snakebites, ringworm, stomach gas, colds, sore throats and asthma. The Osage and Shawnee used a corm (root) decoction to treat coughs, fevers and malaria.

Jack-in-the-Pulpit contains the active components mucilage, a volatile acrid principle and calcium oxalate crystals. Herbalists recommend using the corms in an infusion as a diaphoretic, expectorant, irritant and stimulant for laryngitis, headaches and respiratory ailments. Externally, a poultice was used for treating rheumatism, sores, abscesses, boils and swellings from snakebites.

Chewing fresh Jack-in-the-pulpit can irritate the mucous membranes and burn the mouth and throat. Taken internally in large doses or over a prolonged time it may cause violent gastroenteritis, which may result in death.

192

Jewelweed
Impatiens biflora L. and *I. pallida* L.

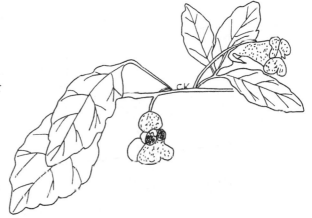

Common names
Pale touch-me-not, touch-me-not, wild balsam.

Habitat
Wet soil, open woodlands, especially near streams throughout the Heartland.

Description
Jewelweed is a member of the Balsaminaceae (touch-me-not) family. The generic name, *Impatiens,* comes from Latin for "impatient," referring to the explosive action of the fruit which distributes the seeds.

Jewelweed is an annual plant with pale green branched stems that appear translucent. The stem joints are enlarged. Pale blue-green, oval to egg-shaped thin leaves, with coarsely serrated margins, alternate along the stem. (*I. pallida* has leaves that are narrower). Orange flowers (*I. pallida* has yellow flowers) with red-brown dots, with a funnel-like shape are partially closed at a larger end and smaller end that is a curved spur holding nectar, are single or in loose clusters. A slender flower stalk curves from the leaf axial and attaches to the center of the funnel. It blooms from July through September. The fruit is a slender capsule. The seeds have a delicious, butternut-like taste.

Medicinal Uses
The Potawatomi Indians used the juice of the fresh plant on many skin irritations, nettle stings (a remedy used even today) and poison-oak and -ivy for instant relief. The settlers used the leaves as a general tonic. They also rubbed the fresh juice on aching foreheads to ease headache pain.

Jewelweed contains the active component naphtholoquinone. Herbalists recommend using a tea as an aperient (gentle laxative) and diuretic to relieve nervous tension. The fresh juice boiled in oil is good for treating fresh mosquito bites, bee and wasp stings, warts, bruises, athlete's foot, ringworm, nettle stings, minor burns, cuts, eczema and sores.

Naptholoquinone, an anti-inflammatory and fungicide, is an active ingredient of Preparation H and other commercial ointments used for treating hemorrhoids.

Jimsonweed
Datura stramonium L.

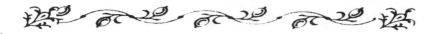

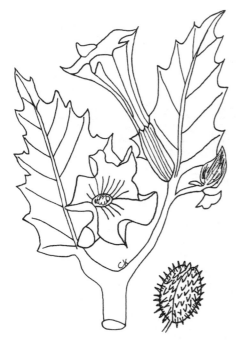

Common names
Devil's apple, thorn apple, yerba del diable.

Habitat
Fields, prairies and waste grounds throughout the Heartland.

Description
Jimsonweed is a member of the Solonaceae (nightshade) family.

Jimsonweed is a large annual with yellow-green, stout stems that branch freely. The large leaves with waxy, coarsely-serrated margins, are dark green on top and paler beneath. Large, pure white flowers have an upright, long, sharp five-angled, tubular calyx surmounted by five sharp teeth and a funnel-shaped corolla. It blooms from June through October. The fruit is a large egg-shaped green capsule covered with numerous sharp spines.

Medicinal Uses
Jimsonweed was used by the priests of Apollo to produce prophecies. Priests of Delphi were said to be inspired by inhaling jimsonweed smoke before delivering their oracles. Gypsies, who introduced the plant into Europe, smoked the leaves for intoxicating visions. Witches inhaled the fumes, and used it during their incantations. Gamblers nibbled on the seeds in attempts to become clairvoyant and able to read their opponent's cards.

In the Southwest, jimsonweed was part of many Indian rituals conducted by the Shaman or medicine man. Carlos Castaneda gives a beautiful, detailed description of a Shaman teaching his student how to use jimsonweed in *The Teachings of Don Juan: A Yaqui Way of Knowledge*. Jimsonweed was used by South American Indians as an anesthetic for setting bones, as part of puberty rites and an aphrodisiac for women.

American Indians used a poultice made from the blossoms to treat wounds and kill pain, and smoked the dried leaves in a pipe to relieve asthma. The Zuni Indians of New Mexico drank a decoction for its anesthetic qualities. Toloache, an Aztec tribe of Indians, used the entire plant to produce hypnotic states. Carolina Indians used the seeds in an ointment for treating burns and scalds. The Cherokee used a poultice of flowers, roots, and/or wilted leaves on wounds. They also smoked the leaves for treating asthma. The Rappahannock used the herb for congestion, fever, inflammation, pneumonia and sore throats.

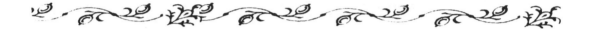

According to legend, the common name is a corruption of "Jamestown weed." In 1676, a detachment of British troops sent to Jamestown, Virginia, ate some shoots of the weed and went berserk for eleven days.

Jimsonweed contains the active components tropane, hallucinogenic actins, the alkaloids hyoscine, hyoscyamine, atropine and scopolamine. Herbalists recommend using an infusion of the leaves and/or seeds as an antispasmodic, anodyne and narcotic. A tincture or proprietary preparation is used for asthma, bronchitis, dyspepsia and Parkinson's Disease to check secretions, stimulate breathing and circulation, and overcome muscle spasms.

Externally, a poultice is used for treating hemorrhoids, skin eruptions, wounds, painful joints and muscles. The leaves can be smoked for asthma and colds. The crushed plant can be bound to bruises and swellings or used as an ingredient in bath herbs. Jimsonweed is the best source of atropine, a drug used by ophthalmologists to dilate the pupils of the eyes. The herb can be smoked, drank, boiled or simmered in oil to cause deliriums, hallucinations, intense prophetic dreams and to give the "illusion" of flying. It is said to increase one's sexual desires.

Research has shown that actins inhibit granular secretions and dilate the airways. It is this action that makes actin an excellent remedy in conventional medicine for stimulating breathing during asthma attacks

Jimsonweed is still used in conventional and homeopathic medicine. Jimsonweed is rarely, if ever, used by herbalists because of its toxicity.

An overdose of jimsonweed can be fatal; a fatal dose for a child is about twenty seeds. Jimsonweed induces symptoms of poisoning similar to those of deadly nightshade. All parts of the plant are EXTREMELY POISONOUS, especially the seeds. Jimsonweed is a dangerous plant: it should never be collected and used for self medication.

Joe-Pye Weed

Eupatorium purpurem L

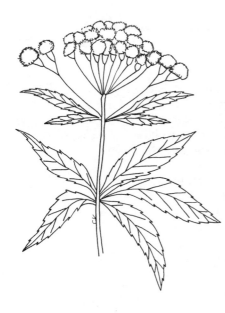

Common names
Kidney wort, Purple boneset, Queen of the meadow.

Habitat
Open woods, fields and prairies throughout the Heartland.

Description
Joe-Pye weed is a member of the Asteraceae (sunflower) family.

Joe-Pye weed is a perennial. The large, thin, opposite leaves with sharp, serrated margins are in whorls of three or four. The bruised leaves and stem have a sweet vanilla odor. The tiny, fragrant creamy white, pale pink or pale lilac flowers are in a dome-like cluster. Long stamens and pistils extending beyond the petals give a characteristic fuzzy appearance. It blooms from July through September.

Medicinal Uses
Many Indian tribes used Joe-Pye weed as a fever remedy. The Iroquois, Menomoni and Cherokee Indians used it as a diuretic for treating genito-urinary ailments. Chippewa mothers bathed fretful children with a root infusion to induce restful sleep.

In Colonial times, European settlers relied on the Indian medicine man for the knowledge of local herbs and their use. Joe Pye, a physician in New England in the late 1700s, gained fame by using the plant to treat typhus fever. His preparation of the roots produced profuse sweating, breaking the fever. Consequently, the plant is called Joe-Pye weed.

Millspaugh recommended using Joe-Pye weed as an excellent diuretic and stimulant for treating chronic renal and cystic disorders, dropsy, hematuria, gout and rheumatism. Early herb doctors used a decoction of the roots to produce a heavy urine flow that would flush out kidney stones (gravel). The root was officially listed in *The United States Pharmacopoeia*, from 1820 to 1842, as an astringent, emetic, cathartic and diaphoretic.

Joe-Pye weed contains the active components resin, the flavonoid eupatorin and a volatile oil. Herbalists recommend using a rhizome and/or root decoction as a diuretic for prostate and pelvic inflammations and painful periods. The decoction is also used to encourage the excretion of excess uric acid in the treatment of rheumatism, gout, kidney and urinary disorders.

196

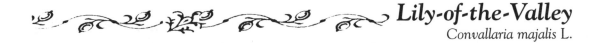

Lily-of-the-Valley
Convallaria majalis L.

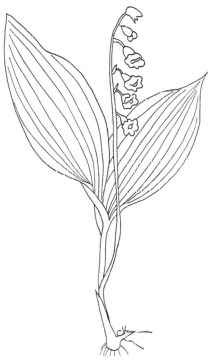

Common names
May lily, Jacob's ladder.

Habitat
Open fields, roadsides and occasionally cultivated throughout the Heartland.

Description
Lily-of-the-valley is a member of the Liliaceae (lily) family.

Lily-of-the-valley is a perennial herb with two broad elliptic leaves on each stem. A scape with a cone-sided raceme of drooping white, sweet-scented bell-shaped flowers appears later. It blooms in May and June and produces a bright red, globose berry.

Medicinal Uses
Lily-of-the-valley yields a yellow dye that is used in dyeing clothes. Lily-of-the-valley has a long history of medical use for treating heart conditions. A decoction of the plant was thought to strengthen the brain. Externally, it was applied locally for bruises, and as a wash for irritations of the mouth. At one time the dried ground roots were an ingredient in snuff.

Lily-of-the-valley contains the active components saponins, flavonoids, asparagin, the poisonous cardiac glycosides convallotoxin, convalloside and gluconvalloside. Herbalists recommend using a flowering stem and/or leaf infusion as a cardiac tonic and diuretic. The individual cardiac glycosides are isolated and included in proprietary medications prescribed for various heart conditions. They are considered as effective and safer than digitalis for regulating the heartbeat without putting demands on the coronary blood supply. The cardiac glycosides are released sequentially, are non-cumulative and are readily excreted by the kidneys. The flavonoids encourage the arteries to dilate. Asparagin acts as a diuretic.

Children should be warned not to eat the attractive berries since they may cause paralysis and respiratory failure. Medical help should be sought immediately if a child eats them. All parts of the plant are extremely poisonous and lily-of-the-valley should never be collected and used for self medication.

Mallow
Malva sylvestris L.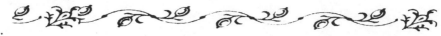

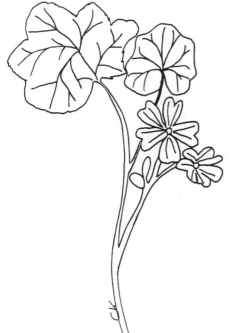

Common name
High mallow.

Habitat
Waste areas throughout the Heartland.

Description
Mallow is a member of the Malvaceae (mallow) family.

Mallow is a biennial or perennial herb with an erect ascending or decumbent stem and a spindle-shaped taproot. Both stems and leaves are softly hairy. The basal leaves are round and shallow-lobed. The alternate deep, palmate-lobed stem leaves are serrated. Large rose-purple flowers with five notched petals and prominent velvet stems are in clusters in leaf axils. They bloom in August and September. The disc-shaped fruit (schizocarp) splits into a one-seeded, wrinkled mesocarp when ripe.

Medicinal Uses
The Indians and early settlers used a decoction with mallow leaves and roots to increase the milk in nursing mothers, to speed delivery, to ease the pain of urination and as an antidote to poisons. The leaves and stalks were used to relieve the pain of gonorrhea. Steeped in white wine vinegar, the roots and seeds were used to ease the pain of the swollen breasts of nursing mothers. The bruised leaves were laid on itchy insect bites to relieve the itching. The juice in oil, was used as an ointment to relieve rough, dry skin, scalds, burns or dry scabs.

Mallow contains the active components anthocyanin, abundant mucilage, the organic pigment provitamin A, vitamins B and C. Herbalists recommend using a flower and/or leaf (free of mallow rust, *Puccina malvacearum*) infusion as an anti-inflammatory, astringent, emollient and expectorant for treating bronchitis, laryngitis, gastritis, enteritis and constipation. Externally, the infusion is used in compresses and bath preparation for skin rashes, boils and ulcerous conditions. The infusion is also used as a gargle for relieving sore throats. Fresh leaves and young shoots can be added to salads and soups or cooked as a vegetable.

Marijuana
Cannabis sativa L.

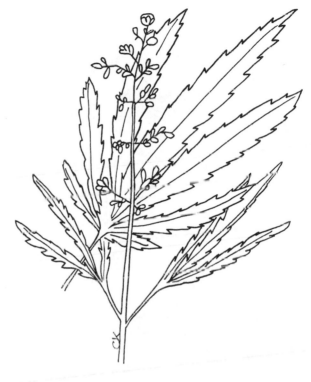

Common names
Grass, hemp, pot, reefer, weed.

Habitat
Open fields, prairies and roadsides throughout the Heartland.

Description
Marijuana is a member of the Cannabaceae (hemp) family.

Marijuana is an annual herb with an erect, hairy stem. The palmately divided, long-stalked leaves have serrated margins. The plant is dioecious with the male flowers arranged in panicles and female flower growing in a leafy spike in the leaf axils. It blooms from June through October. The fruit is a shiny, gray-green achene.

Medicinal Uses
Seeds of marijuana have been found in Northern European funerary as early as the fifth century B.C. Grieve reports that the principle use of marijuana was for easing pain, inducing sleep, soothing nervous disorders, neuralgia, gout, rheumatism, tremors, and infantile convulsions and insomnia.

Marijuana contains the active component a dark resin with tetrahydro-cannabinol, cannabinol, cannabidiol, cannabidiolic acid and cannabigerolic acid. Herbalists recommend using a leaf and/or flowering-stem infusion as an analgesic, antispasmodic and sedative. Marijuana is used in proprietary medicines for glaucoma, nausea in cancer therapy, insomnia, depression, neuralgia, migraines, asthma and as a local anesthetic in dentistry. A tincture is used to aid parturition, senile catarrh, gonorrhea, female disorders, chronic cystitis and painful urinary disorders. The resin is combined with an ointment or oils for treating inflammations and neuralgia complaints. The leaves are dried to yield the drug known as hashish, cannabis or marijuana, which is smoked, drunk or chewed for hallucinogenic effects.

In the United States it is illegal to grow, possess or sell marijuana without a government permit.

Mayapple
Podophyllum peltatum L.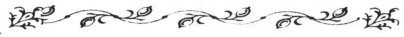

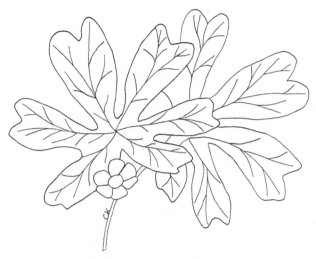

Common names
American mandrake, duck's foot, hog apple, Indian apple, raccoon berry.

Habitat
Moist, rich woods and lowlands throughout the Heartland.

Description
Mayapple is a member of the Berberidaceae (barberry) family. The generic name, *Podophyllum*, is derived from two Latin words *podos* (foot) and *phyllon* (a leaf), referring to the resemblance of the palmate leaf to a web-footed aquatic bird.

Mayapple is a distinctive perennial herb with a large horizontal root. One or two large, broad-circular leaves have five to nine deep lobes that are veined and a coarsely-serrated margin that top a smooth, brittle stem. The saucer-shaped flower is on a short stout stalk arising from the stem axil has six to nine white, waxy petals. It blooms in May and produces a large, green-yellow, pulpy berry.

Medicinal Uses
Early New England Indians used the roots as a slow-acting but powerful laxative, a liver cleanser, and an emetic. Many tribes chewed the raw root to commit suicide. Native folklore stated that a woman who dug up mayapple would soon find herself pregnant. Cherokee and Delaware Indians used a root tea for treating constipation, deafness, rheumatism, sores, ulcers and expelling intestinal parasites. The Cree used a powdered root tea for treating liver ailments. The Potawatomi and Meskwaki used a root tea for treating snakebites. The Menomoni sprinkled an herbal infusion on potato plants to kill potato bugs. The Osage used an infusion as an antidote for poisons. The Penobscot Indians of Maine used the root as a cure for warts.

Early settlers used the powdered rhizomes in an infusion to treat a wide range of common diseases including typhoid, cholera, rheumatism, jaundice, dysentery, hepatitis, gonorrhea, syphilis, amenorrhea, prostate problems, urinary, liver, bowel and skin disorders. They boiled the entire plant and splashed the liquid over potato plants to control insects.

As early as 1897, physicians in Missouri used podophyllin to treat venereal warts. Podophyllin still remains the most widely used treatment for venereal warts.

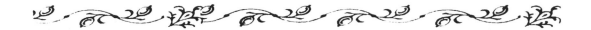

Pioneers used the fruits to make a preserve. Ripened fruits lose their toxicity and become edible, either raw or cooked. They also used mayapple as the "slowest acting purges." Mayapple was highly regarded as a treatment for summer diarrhea of children.

Mayapple contains the active components podophyllum and the two semisynthetic glycosides etoposide and teniposide which are FDA approved for testicular and small-cell lung cancers. Herbalists recommend using an infusion for venereal warts and various cancerous tumors. Etoposide and teniposide are used to treat testicular tumors, small-cell carcinomas of the lung and breasts, Hodgkin's disease, non-Hodgkin's lymphomas, acute granulocytic leukemia and Kaposi's sarcoma which is a malignant vascular skin disease often associated with AIDS. These glycosides affect cellular growth and are blamed for deformities in the children of mothers who took laxatives or dieting tablets containing them during pregnancy.

Mayapple is a powerful irritant to the intestine, acting as an emetic and purgative. The powdered root and resin are possible skin and eye irritants. If misused it can be dangerous, even fatal. Pregnant women should never use laxatives or dieting tablets containing mayapple. Mayapple should never be collected and used for self-medication without the supervision of a qualified medical or herbal practitioner.

Melilot
Melilotus officinalis (L.) Pallas

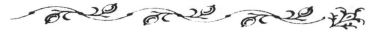

Common names
Melilot trefoils, yellow sweet clover.

Habitat
Roadsides and fields throughout the Heartland.

Description
Melilot is a member of the Fabaceae (pea) family. The generic name, *Melilotus*, is from two Greek words *meli* (long) and *lotos* (fodder or clover).

Melilot is a biennial herb with a tall, angled branched stem. Alternate, trifoliate leaves with oblong, serrated leaflets and stipules are joined to the stem. The yellow flowers are a long slender spike in the upper leaf axils. It blooms from June through September. The hairless, ovoid, brown pod is wrinkled when ripe.

Medicinal Uses
According to Gerard, melilot mixed with wine, "it mitigateth the paine of the eares and taketh away the paine of the head." Culpeper recommended the use of this mixture for inflammations of the eyes and other parts of the body.

Melilot is a very sweet honey-like smelling weedy herb that gets much of its odor from coumarin. It is cultivated for forage and hay, used to flavor cheeses, and is an ingredient in tobacco snuff. The seeds are used as a substitute for Tonka beans, to give a pleasant fragrance to tobacco, a delicate scent to toilet soaps, as a flavoring to liqueurs and as a moth repellent.

Melilot contains the active components melilotin and other coumarin glycosides. Herbalists recommend using a flower and/or flowering stem infusion as an anti-inflammatory, antispasmodic, aromatic, anti-thrombic, astringent, carminative, emollient and expectorant. The infusion is used for headaches, colic, diarrhea, painful urination and menstruation.

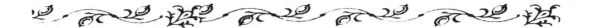

Externally, the infusion is used in poultices, plasters, salves, compresses or bath preparations for skin ulcers, wounds, rheumatism, headache pains and arthritis. The flowering herb is and ingredient in some pharmaceutical preparations used in the treatment of thrombosis and varicose veins.

All parts are slightly poisonous and should always be taken internally only under professional supervision. Large does may cause bleeding, headache, vertigo and vomiting.

Mexican Tea

Chenopodium ambrosiodes L.

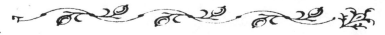

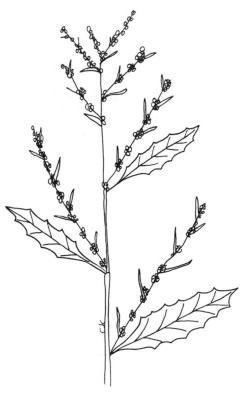

Common name
American wormseed, Jesuit's tea.

Habitat
Waste grounds throughout the Heartland.

Description
Mexican tea is a member of the Chenopodiaceae (goosefoot) family. The generic name, *Chenopodium*, is derived from two Greek words *khen* (goose) and *pous* (foot), referring to the shape of a foot.

Mexican tea is an annual herb with branched, reddish stems. Alternate, oblong to lanceolate leaves are coarsely serrated. Numerous, small, yellow-green flowers are in small globose clusters in the leaf axils on the lateral stems. It blooms from August through November. The fruit is an achene. All parts are strongly aromatic.

Medicinal Uses
Mexican tea is native to tropical America and can probably be found in the anthelmintic recipes of the Maya and Natchez Indians. The Houma Indians of the Southwest used the leaves, boiled in a mild tea, as a vermifuge to expel intestinal parasites. They also used a crushed leaf tea in a poultice on the forehead to relieve a headache. In the seventeenth century, Mexican tea was taken from the Americas to Europe.

Mexican tea contains the active components saponins, an essential oil with ascaridole, tannins and bitter compounds. Herbalists recommend using a flowering stem infusion as an anthelmintic, antispasmodic, a cardiac stimulant, diaphoretic and stomachic for asthma, nervous disorders and menstrual disorders. Today, Mexican tea is the source of chenopodium oil (obtained by distillation from fresh plants) used in preparations for treating roundworm and hookworm (*Ankylostos duodenale*). Chenopodium oil is listed in *The United States Pharmacopoeia* as a vermifuge. It is perhaps the best children's vermifuge remedy because it is easy to administer and is relatively non-toxic.

Mexican tea is poisonous in large doses and should be used only under the supervision of a medical or herbal practitioner.

204

Milk Thistle
Silybum marianum L.

Common name
Marian thistle.

Habitat
Open fields, roadsides, lawns and occasionally cultivated throughout the Heartland.

Description
Milk thistle is a member of the Asteraceae (sunflower) family.

Milk thistle is an annual or biennial. The sharp spined leaves are mottled or streaked with white veins. The flowers are purple tufts with a dense, bristle-spined receptacle and bloom from June through September. The fruit is an egg-shaped achene.

Medicinal Uses
Milk thistle has been used for treating liver diseases since antiquity. Pliny recommended using the juice mixed with honey for "carrying off bile." Culpeper considered milk thistle to be as efficient as blessed thistle (*Cnicus benedictus*; also known as *Carduus benedictus*) for treating ague, preventing and curing the plague, and for removing obstructions of the liver and spleen. He also recommended boiling the young tender plant after removing the spines and eating it as a spring blood purifier.

Milk thistle contains the active components silymarin, the flavonoids silybin, silydranine and silychistin. Herbalists recommend using a seed infusion as a bitter tonic and cholagogue in the treatment of gallstones accompanied by colic, chronic inflammation of the liver and cirrhosis.

Studies show that silymarin helps to stabilize liver cell membranes by altering the receptor sites of the outer membrane cell structure so certain toxins cannot enter the cell. It accelerates liver tissue regeneration by stimulating protein synthesis, and acts as a liver-specific antioxidant in hepatitis, cirrhosis, mushroom poisoning, and liver poisoning from chemical, drug or alcohol abuse.

German research suggests that silybin is clinically useful in treating severe Amantain mushroom poisoning. Research has also proven its efficiency in human liver disease. Commercial preparations of the seed extracts are now manufactured in Europe.

Milk thistle should be used for self medication only under the supervision of a qualified medical or herbal practitioner.

Motherwort
Leonurus cardiaca L.

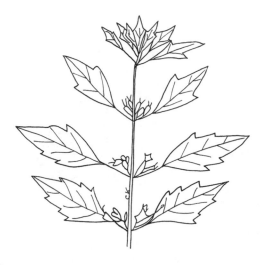

Common name
Lion's tail.

Habitat
Pastures, waste areas and roadsides throughout the Heartland.

Description
Motherwort is a member of the Laminaceae (mint) family.

Motherwort is a perennial herb with an erect, rough, square, branched leafy stem and stout rhizomes. Opposite, oval, palmately-lobed leaves are green above, white-felted beneath and are irregularly serrated. White or pink hairy flowers (bell-shaped calyx with five equal teeth; the corolla, two-lipped with purplish spots on the lower lip) are located in whorls in the upper axils. It blooms from July through September. The fruits are four nutlets.

Medicinal Uses
The Cherokee, Delaware and Mohegan Indians used motherwort bark for treating hysteria, nerves, stomach disorders and female disorders.

Old herbalists recommended motherwort for strengthening the heart and easing palpitations, asthma, cholecystitis, convulsions, insomnia, neuralgia, rabies, rheumatism and stomach aches. Motherwort is an excellent remedy for female disorders (hence its common name) such as emmenorrhea, dysmenorrhea, hysteria, palpitation, urinary cramps and general debility.

Motherwort contains the active components saponin, an essential oil, the bitter compound leonurin, the bitter glycosides leonurine and leonuridin, the alkaloids leonurinine and stachydrine and the tannins pyrogallal and catechins. Herbalists recommend using a flowering stem infusion as an analgesic, antispasmodic, astringent, diaphoretic, diuretic, emmenagogue, expectorant, febrifuge, laxative, nervine, sedative, tonic and vermifuge. The infusion is used for migraine headaches, hysteria, anxiety, diarrhea, menstrual irregularities, nervous heart disorders, irregular heart beat and high blood pressure.

Care must be taken when handling the plant. Dry plants can cause contact dermatitis, and the fragrant lemon-scented oil from the plant can cause photo sensitivity.

Mugwort
Artemisia vulgaris L.

Common names
Artemisia, Carline thistle, sailor's tobacco.

Habitat
Open sandy soil and dry slopes.

Description
Mugwort is a member of the Asteraceae (sunflower) family.

Mugwort is a perennial herb with a reddish, furrowed, angled, sparsely-hairy stem. Alternate, pinnately-lobed leaves are dark green above and wool-ly-white beneath. Small, oval, yellow flowerheads have dense leafy panicles. They bloom in August and September. The fruit is a cylindrical achene. All parts of plant are slightly aromatic.

Medicinal Uses
Hippocrates used mugwort to treat female disorders. In the Middle Ages, mugwort was called *Cingulum Saneti Johannis*, referring to the belief that

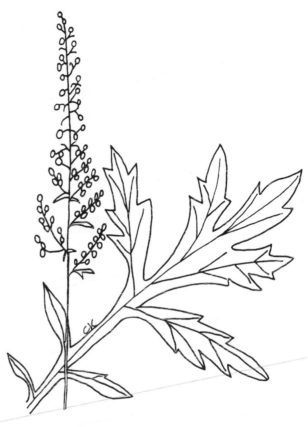

John the Baptist wore a girdle of mugwort into the wilderness. It was believed to preserve the wayfarer from fatigue, sunstroke, wild beasts and evil spirits. A crown was worn on June 23rd, St. John's Eve, to protect against evil possession.

American Indians used a leaf decoction of mugwort for treating bladder ailments, pneumonia, rheumatism, ringworm, sores, tumors, ulcers and wounds. The Cherokee used mugwort for treating backaches, gravel, mastitis and venereal diseases. Rafinesque reported that mugwort was used as a laxative, diuretic and emmenagogue. It was also used as a "moxa" (a burning stick famous in Chinese medicine) to stimulate acupuncture points in the treatment of rheumatism.

Mugwort contains the active components tannin, a volatile oil with cineole and thujone, flavonoids and the bitter principle absinthin. Herbalists recommend using a flowering stem (leaves and/or flowering top) infusion as an anthelmintic, diuretic, emmenagogue, expectorant, opium antidote and tonic. The infusions is used for nervous disorders,

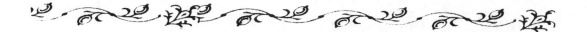

epilepsy, kidney ailments, insomnia, gynecological complaints and to promote digestion. The leaves can be smoked to alleviate asthma. To have vivid dreams, steep mugwort in vinegar and use the mugwort flavored vinegar as a salad dressing. In Sumatra, mugwort is smoked as an opium substitute. In China, mugwort twigs fashioned into rope are burned to repel mosquitoes. Mugwort is an effective moth repellent.

Mugwort may cause dermatitis and should always be used under the supervision of a qualified medical or herbal practitioner.

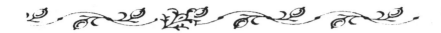

Mullein
Verbascum thapsus L.

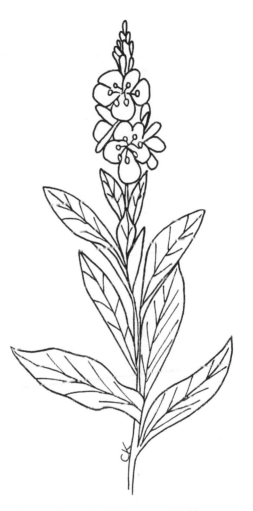

Common names
Aaron's rod, Jacob's staff, Witches taper, Woolly mullein.

Habitat
Roadsides, open fields and waste areas throughout the Heartland.

Description
Mullein is a member of the Scrophulariaceae (flax) family.

Mullein is a tall, unbranched biennial with soft, hairy, basal rosette-winged stems and soft, downy or woolly foliage. Single, alternate leaves are widely oblong or lanceolate with smooth unlobed margins. Dense yellow flowers have a five-part calyx, five-lobed corolla and five stamens. It blooms from June through September and has a high, club-like seed spike.

Medicinal Uses
In ancient Greece, the leaves were rolled, dried and made into wicks for oil lamps and candles. Medicinal usage dates back to Hippocrates. Dioscorides used mullein to treat lung diseases, diarrhea, insomnia and to relieve pain, He also used mullein in compresses for relieving the pain and swelling of hemorrhoids. Since the time of Pliny, heated mullein leaves have been used in a poultice for treating arthritis. Possession of a twig of mullein in the Middle Ages was said to protect a person from witchcraft and wild beasts. Mullein stalks were dipped in tallow and set on fire to frighten away witches.

The Potawatomi, Cherokee and Creek Indians used a fermentation of the leaves in hot water and vinegar for treating inflamed tumors. They drank a leaf tea for treating coughs, and applied the bruised leaves to rashes and glands swollen by mumps. Many a frontiersman, pioneer, woodsman and camper have used the woolly leaves as toilet paper.

As a substitute for rouge, Quaker women rubbed the woolly leaves of mullein on their cheeks to make them pink. The Amish smoked the leaves to relieve asthma attacks.

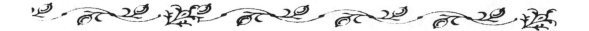

Mullein contains the active components saponin, mucilage, volatile oil, flavonoids, the glycoside aucubin, B-complex, vitamin D and hesperidin. Herbalists recommend using an infusion as an antibiotic, anti-inflammatory, demulcent, anti-fungal, antispasmodic, astringent, expectorant, laxative, sedative and tonic for convulsions, diarrhea, nervous stomachs, mucous membranes, respiratory ailments and diseases of the glands. Mullein tea is one of the safest, most effective herbal cough remedies. Mullein oil made of macerated flowers in olive oil, is an effective remedy for gum diseases, earaches and relieving the pain of hemorrhoids, frost bite and bruises. The dried leaves can be rolled into a cigarette or smoked in a pipe to relieve the irritations of respiratory mucous membranes, asthma, spasmodic coughs and to control the hacking cough of consumption.

Research has shown that mullein oil is an anti-inflammatory with antibiotic activity that inhibits the tuberculosis bacillus, *Mycobacterium tuberculosis*.

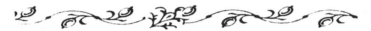

Mustard
Brassica nigra L. and *B. rapa* L.

Common names
Black mustard, wild mustard.

Habitat
Open fields, roadsides, waste grounds and occasionally cultivated throughout the Heartland.

Description
Mustard is a member of the Brassicaceae (mustard) family.

Mustard is an annual herb with erect branched stems and a slender taproot. Alternate, entire and lanceolate leaves are bristly (upper leaves are smooth) and pinnately divided with a large terminal lobe. Bright-yellow flower is prominently veined and in a raceme. It blooms from April through October. The fruit, with a narrow-beaked silicula, has globular black seeds.

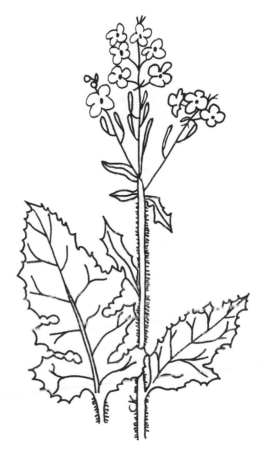

Medicinal Uses
The Ancient Greeks valued black mustard for its medicinal properties. Early Romans mixed wine with macerated seeds to make a version of table mustard. Preferred as a medicinal, Culpeper and early herbalists recommended taking black mustard internally to relieve digestive problems and toothaches. A poultice was applied externally to encourage blood flow.

Early settlers and Indians cultivated mustard for food and medicine. They ate the seeds and prepared the leaves, which are high in calcium, potassium, iron, vitamin A and C, riboflavin, niacin and thiamine, like spinach. A paste of powdered black mustard seeds mixed with bear or hog lard, or mutton tallow was applied as compresses to treat lumbago, arthritic and rheumatic joints, bad sprains and toothaches. Medicinally, a mustard plaster is a time-honored cure for treating congested chests. The plaster makes the skin warm and opens the lungs to make breathing easier.

Mustard contains the active components the glycoside sinagrin and the enzyme myrosin. Herbalists recommend using a seed and/or leaf infusion as an anti-bacterial, anti-fungal, laxative and stimulant. Powdered seeds, mixed with water, set free allylisothiocynate (mustard

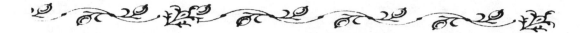

oil), the strong-smelling, hot tasting substance associated with the herb. In small doses, mustard is said to stimulate the mucous membrane of the stomach and increase the secretions of the pancreas, thereby improving digestion. A mustard infusion is a valuable emetic (induces vomiting) for ingestion of household cleaning agents.

Mustard preparations may irritate the stomach and intestines or cause skin blisters if used in large doses or over a prolonged period of time.

Ox-Eye Daisy
Chrysanthemum leucanthemum L.

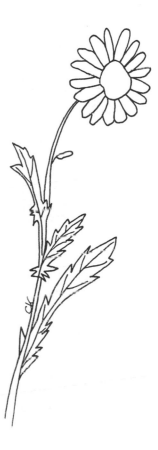

Common names
Butter daisy, daisy, Marguerite, poverty weed, white weed.

Habitat
Open woodlands, roadsides, fields and waste grounds throughout the Heartland.

Description
Ox-eye daisy is a member of the Asteraceae (sunflower) family. The generic name, *Chrysanthemum*, comes from two Greek words, *chrisos* (golden) and *anthos* (flower).

The ox-eye daisy is a perennial. The outermost white ray flowers (petals) are strap-shaped, and the minor yellow disk flowers are tubular. Yellow center florets contain both stamen and pistils and produce one-seeded fruit.

Medicinal Uses
In the Lore of Ancient Greece, ox-eye daisy was considered a sacred plant to the soldiers of Artemis (Goddess of Woman). Later the Roman Catholic Church dedicated the plant to St. Margaret and St. Mary Magdaline, hence the common name Marguerite. The practice of picking the petals one by one to find if one is loved, dates back to medieval times. Ox-eye daisy has always been thought of as a good luck charm for those in love.

Ox-eye daisy was traditionally used as a treatment for women's ailments. Gerard in his book, *The Herbal*, noted "that daisy negates all kinds of pains, especially in joints and gout (mixed with unsalted butter and applied as a poultice). The juice from the leaves and roots, snuffed into nostrils, clears the head. A decoction is good for ageing agues."

Ox-eye daisy contains the active components saponin, an essential oil, tannins, mucilage and a bitter compound. Herbalists recommend using a flower infusion as an antispasmodic, astringent, diuretic, expectorant and tonic. The infusion is an excellent remedy for gastritis, enteritis, diarrhea and infections of the upper respiratory tract. Externally, ox-eye daisy is used in compresses and bath preparations for skin disorders, wounds and bruises. The young leaves are used in salads and soups.

Passion Flower
Passiflora incarnata L.

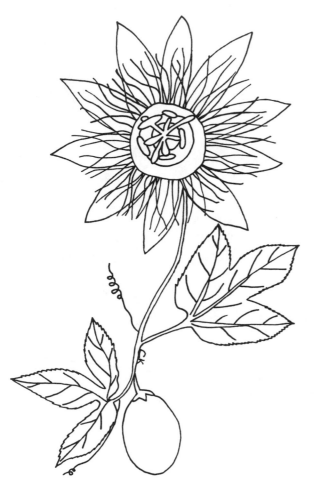

Common name
Maypop.

Habitat
Dry soil, fields, roadsides, and thickets from Pennsylvania to Florida, Oklahoma to Missouri.

Description
Passion flower is a member of the Passifloraceae (passion flower) family.

Passion flower is a perennial. Alternate leaves have three to five finely-serrated lobes and glands that are readily visible on the stalk. Solitary flowers have five white or lavender petals, five sepals, five stamens, a brilliant pink or purple corolla, and a series of rings bearing thread-like processes. It blooms in late summer. The fruit is a berry, called a granadilla or water lemon, and is round to ovoid with a thin yellow or orange skin. The edible yellow pulp is succulent and sweet.

Medicinal Uses
Centuries ago, Peruvian Indians discovered the sedative properties of passion flower fruit for treating insomnia and nervousness. Europeans took passion flower home from Peru, and later brought it to North America. When the plant was introduced into Europe, Catholics saw it as a symbolic representation of the Passion of Christ. The corona was the crown of thorns, the five sepals and five petals symbolized the ten Apostles (absent are Judas, the traitor, and Peter, who betrayed Christ); and the other parts of the flower represented the nails and the wounds. Children in the South love to stomp on passion flower fruit to make it pop, hence the common name maypop.

Passion flower has long been used for its quieting qualities as a carminative agent and sedative for treating menstrual cramps, tension headaches, insomnia, hysteria and other nervous disorders, without bad side effects. Early American Indians applied crushed leaves

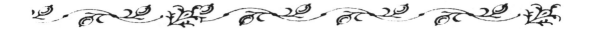

in a poultice to treat bruises and other injuries. A tea made from the woody vines was drunk to soothe the nerves. The Cherokee and Houma Indians used a root infusion for treating boils, cuts, earaches, inflammations, and as a liver and blood tonic.

Passion flower contains the active components flavonoids, sterols, the alkaloids harmol, harmane, harmaline, harmine and harmalol. Herbalists recommend using a flower and/or fruity-tip infusion as an antispasmodic and sedative. Passion flower has a non-addictive effect, and is an important remedy for relieving anxiety, tension, insomnia, and reducing high blood pressure. Smoking passion flower has been said to impart a marijuana-like high.

Research has shown that the plant extracts are mildly sedative and that they slightly reduce blood pressure, increase respiration rate and decrease motor activity.

Pennyroyal
Hedeoma pulegioides (L.) Pers.

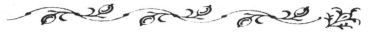

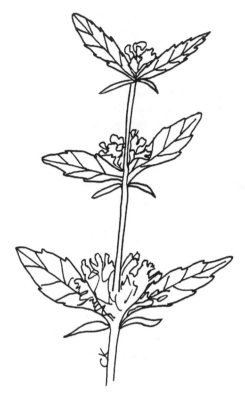

Common names
American pennyroyal, squaw mint, tick-weed.

Habitat
Rocky woods, fields, roadsides and occasionally cultivated throughout the Heartland.

Description
Pennyroyal is a member of the Laminaceae (mint) family. The species name, *pulegioides*, is from the Latin *pulex* (flea) referring to its reputed power of driving away fleas.

Pennyroyal is an annual herb. The opposite, elliptical or obovate leaves with a smooth or slightly-serrated margin with fine hairs. Blue-lilac, two-lipped tubular flowers are in whorls at the leaf axils. It blooms from July through September. The fruits are four nutlets.

Medicinal Uses
Pliny recommended using pennyroyal as a panacea for treating numerous disorders. He especially recommended hanging bundles of pennyroyal in sleeping rooms to purify the air. Culpeper reflected on the uses of European pennyroyal (American pennyroyal has similar medicinal uses): "The herb, boiled and drank, provokes woman's courses and expels the dead child and afterbirth. If taken in water and vinegar mingled together, it stops the deposition to vomit. Mingled with honey and salt, it voids phlegm out of the lungs and purges the stool ...The green herb bruised and put into vinegar, cleanses foul ulcers and takes away the mark of bruises and blows about the eyes, and burns in the face ...One spoonful of the juice sweetened with sugar candy is a cure for hooping-cough."

Pennyroyal was one of the plants introduced by the Pilgrims. Several tribes of native American Indians used pennyroyal leaves for kidney complaints, a menstrual regulator for young girls, and in a hot tea for diarrhea, bronchitis and rheumatism. A nineteenth century Indian medicine man wrote: "The hot tea of the plant is a very effective remedy for all cramps and pains and colic. It is an active sweat producer or in medical terms, an active diaphoretic. Good for colds and cramping ...I prefer the tea from the plant over and above all other forms and modes of preparation." The Chickasaw Indians soaked the plant in water and placed it on the forehead to relieve itchy, watery eyes. The Mohegans drank

216

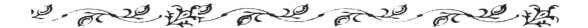

pennyroyal tea to soothe the stomach. The Catawbas used a tea to relieve colds. Both Indians and white settlers rubbed the distinctive-smelling leaves onto the skin to protect themselves from insects.

Pennyroyal contains the active components the essential oil with pulegone, pinene, limonene, menthone and salicylic acids. Herbalists recommend using a mild tea as an anti-spasmodic, aromatic, carminative, diaphoretic, rubefacient, and stimulant for respiratory ailments, fever, menstrual cramps, nausea and to aid digestion. Externally, a leaf poultice is used for relieving headaches, toothaches, and itching, burning skin. Pennyroyal oil is also an excellent insect repellent for wood ticks, fleas, flies, mosquitoes and gnats. Many common insect repellent sprays contain pennyroyal oil. To keep fleas away from your pet, try braiding the plant with a string to make a flea collar, or scatter some leaves on your pet's bed.

Large doses of pennyroyal may cause abortions and even death. Therefore it should not be used internally unless under the supervision of a qualified medical or herbal practitioner.

Periwinkle

Vinca minor L.

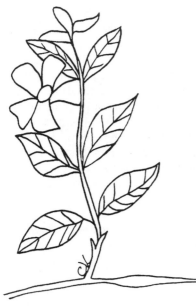

Common name
Lesser periwinkle.

Habitat
Woodlands, often found around old cemeteries and also cultivated as a ground cover throughout the Heartland.

Description
Periwinkle is a member of the Apoycynaceae (dogbane) family. The generic name, *vinca*, is from the Latin word *vincio* (to bind).

Periwinkle is a perennial herbaceous subshrub with creeping stems. Opposite short stalked, evergreen leaves are leathery and elliptic. It has a stout, ascending solitary flower (blue, mauve or white) with five petals. It blooms from April through July. The fruit is a follicle with tiny, rough black seeds.

Medicinal Uses
In the Middle Ages, periwinkle was used against "devil sickness and demoniac possessions," against snakes, wild beasts, poisons and for making various wishes, charms and love potions. Dioscorides and Galen recommended periwinkle for fluxes, the excessive flow of any body secretion. Culpeper used periwinkle to stop nasal and mouth bleeding. He also used it to treat hysteria, nervous disorders and insomnia. Grieve used an ointment made from the bruised leaves in all treatments of inflammatory ailments of the skin and to soothe bleeding piles.

Periwinkle contains the active components tannins, saponins, pectin, the alkaloids vincarmine and resperpine. Herbalists recommend using a flowering-stem infusion as an antiseptic, antispasmodic, astringent, cardiac stimulant, carminative, diuretic, emetic, hemostat, lactagogue and sedative. The infusion is used for bleeding, catarrh, diarrhea, dysentery, eczema, hypertension, female disorders, coughing spasms and hemorrhoids.

Research in eastern Europe has shown that vincarmine has weak antagonistic actions as a depressor of adrenaline gland activity in the treatment of arterial hypertension, and as a sedative effective against migraine headaches. Resperpine shows anti-cancer activity in certain tumor systems.

All parts of the plant are poisonous. Always consult a qualified medical or herbal practitioner before collecting and using for self medication.

218

Plantain
Plantago major L.

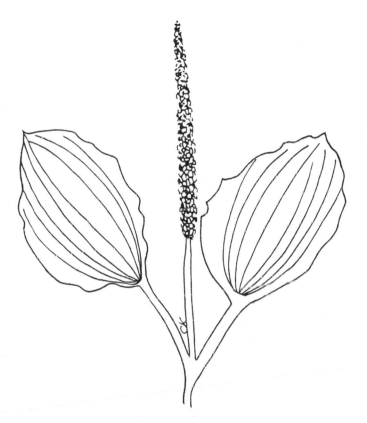

Common names
Broad-leaf plantain, soldier's herb, snakeweed.

Habitat
Open fields, roadsides and lawns throughout the Heartland.

Description
Plantain is a member of the Plantaginaceae (plantain) family.

Plantain is a perennial herb with a long, erect, fine-angled, furrowed, leafless flowering stem. Lanceolate, parallel-veined leaves are in a basal rosette. Stems and leaves are silky and hairy. Inconspicuous brown flowers with long white stamens are in a dense cylindrical spike. It blooms from April through August. The fruit is a two-seeded capsule.

Medicinal Uses
Europeans used plantain as a general tonic to treat scrofula, eye ailments, bronchial ailments (the extract slows respiration and reopens airways), and stimulate the mucous membrane of the trachea and secretory tissues of the digestive organs. The use of plantain leaves to treat cuts was mentioned by Shakespeare in Romeo and Juliet. The Chinese used the seeds as a panacea to treat asthma, respiratory ailments, gonorrhea, colic, coughs, hemorrhage, hemorrhoids and malaria. Colonists and Indians used a compress of hot, wet leaves on wounds, cuts, scratches and abrasions to reduce bleeding and to prevent or cure infection.

Plantain contains the active components mucilage, the glycoside aucubin, tannin, monoterpene alkaloids, triterpene, carotene, salicylic-, linoleic- and silicic-acid. Herbalists recommend using a seed and/or leaf infusion as an astringent, demulcent, emollient, expectorant and vulnerary for coughs, pertussis, gastritis, fever, inflammations, kidney and bladder disorders, hoarseness and respiratory disorders. Coughing in children is alleviated by a thickened syrup made from the leaves and sweetened with honey. The infusion is also used externally in a douche for treating leucorrhea.

219

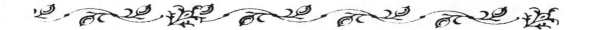

The astringent properties have been scientifically verified as a remedy for insect bites and skin irritations. The bruised leaves should be rubbed repeatedly on the bite or rash. The mucilage in plantain does reduce both low-density cholesterol and triglycerides, thus helping to prevent heart disease. The mucilaginous, fibrous seeds swallowed whole, are excellent for cleansing and soothing the intestines. The European plantain species is the main ingredient of Metamucil, which helps control appetite and reduces intestinal absorption of fat and bile.

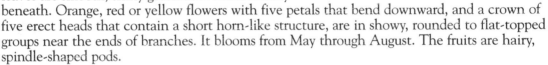

Pleurisy Root
Asclepias tuberosa L.

Common names
Butterfly milkweed, chigger flower, milkweed.

Habitat
Woods, open fields, roadsides and prairies throughout the Heartland.

Description
Pleurisy root is a member of the Asclepiadaceae (milkweed) family. The generic name, *Asclepias*, is named for the Greek god of medicine, Asklepios; the species name, *tuberosa*, means "full of swellings or knobs."

Pleurisy root is a perennial herb with erect, long, hairy, numerous, unbranched stems containing a watery sap and woody root stocks. Alternate, simple, lanceolate leaves are smooth, shiny green above and velvety beneath. Orange, red or yellow flowers with five petals that bend downward, and a crown of five erect heads that contain a short horn-like structure, are in showy, rounded to flat-topped groups near the ends of branches. It blooms from May through August. The fruits are hairy, spindle-shaped pods.

Medicinal Uses
Settlers used pleurisy root to relieve inflammations of the lungs and throat. Pleurisy root was listed as an official medicine in *The United States Pharmacopoeia* from 1820 to 1904 as an anti-rheumatic, cardiotonic, diaphoretic and expectorant.

American Indians, including the Omaha, Catawbas, Menomoni and Natchez, revered pleurisy root as a healer. They used the leaves to induce vomiting. The roots were used for treating dysentery, diarrhea, constipation, lung inflammations, pleurisy, rheumatism, fever and pneumonia. Externally, they applied a root poultice to bruises, swellings and wounds. The Cheyenne made a medicine of pleurisy root for snow blindness.

Pleurisy root contains the active components resins, a volatile oil, the cardiac glycosides asclepidian, uzarigenin and syriogenin which is toxic to humans. Herbalists recommend using a root decoction as an antispasmodic, carminative, cathartic, diaphoretic, expectorant and tonic for respiratory inflammations including pleurisy, consumption, diarrhea, dysentery, rheumatism and typhoid. In large doses, pleurisy root is an emetic and purgative.

Pleurisy root should never be used for self medication unless under the strict supervision of a qualified medical or herbal practitioner; this is especially important for people with cardiac problems.

221

Poke

Phytolacca americana L.

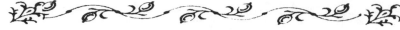

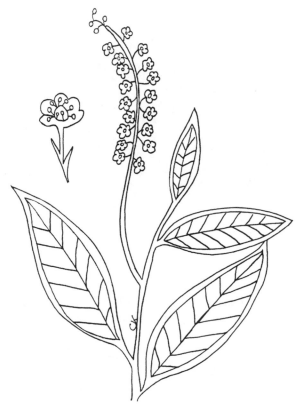

Common names
Pigeonberry, pokeweed.

Habitat
Roadsides, open fields, waste areas, and occasionally cultivated throughout the Heartland except in North and South Dakota.

Description
Poke is a member of the Phytolaccaceae (poke) family.

Poke is a perennial with thick, hollow, distinct red or purple stems and a fleshy root system. It has alternate, large dark-green, waxy lanceolate leaves with pointed ends, smooth margins and thick petioles. Small green-white flowers with four or five sepals are in cyme-like racemes arising opposite the petioles on the upper leaves. It blooms from May through September and produces dark purple berries with five to fifteen small seeds.

Medicinal Uses
The name poke, probably came from the Indians of Virginia who called it Pokan, meaning "red-juiced" plant, and who used it as a stain or dye. Connecticut Indians used the berries to stain sapling baskets a dark blue. Indians of the eastern states used a poultice of powdered poke root to treat tumors and skin eruptions. A salve for healing sores and granular swellings was made by combining roasted pokeroot, bittersweet (*Celastrus scandens*), moonseed (*Menispermum canadense*) and elderberry (*Sambucus canadensis*) bark, to a base of boiled lard and beeswax. The Cherokee and Delaware Indians used a root tea for treating nervous fevers, eczema and renitis. A berry wine was used to relieve rheumatism, a very dangerous remedy. The berries were used in a poultice to treat cancer, sores and swelling and in herbal steam baths for rheumatism. The Lumbee ate poke greens in the spring to cure boils and other "blood" diseases. Both the Indians and colonists cut the roots into small pieces and steeped a tablespoon with two cups boiling water (pokeberry tea). The tea was then drunk, sparingly, by the tablespoon, for relieving arthritis pain.

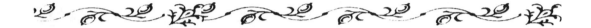

Young shoots up to six inches high, rich in vitamin C and fat soluble beta carotene, may be cooked like asparagus or eaten as a salad (poke salad is the subject of the Blues song "Poke Salad Annie"). Poke is regularly grown domestically and the shoots are canned and sold in some grocery stores, particularly in southern states.

Poke contains the active components phytolaccin, the triterpenoid saponin phytolacca-genin, the alkaloid phytolaccine, phytolaccic acid, resins and tannins. Herbalists recommend using a root decoction as an alterative, anti-fungal, antiseptic and stimulant for treating tonsillitis, swollen glands and mumps. In low doses, poke acts an alterative to stimulate metabolism and decongest the digestive tract, lymphatic system and various other organs. A poke root ointment is used externally for treating scabies, ringworm and fungal infection. A lotion and tincture is used for vaginal yeast infections.

The major medicinal actions of poke parallel the action of cortisone in stimulating the glandular network. Phytolaccagenin acts as a powerful molluskcide (kills mollusks) and paracide. The large poisonous poke roots at one time were collected in the fall by the pharmaceutical industry and utilized in small portions as an emetic and for treating arthritis. The dried roots are still used in Appalachia in the treatment of hemorrhoids. Also in Appalachia, pokeberry wine was thought to alleviate rheumatism. Today tinctures and ointments are used to reduce granular swelling, chronic arthritis and stiffness of joints. Poisonings were widespread in eastern North America during the nineteenth century when tinctures made from the root were popular as an anti-rheumatic.

The alkaloid phytolaccine causes severe vomiting, diarrhea, intestinal cramps, visual impairment, weakened respiration and pulse. Convulsions and death may follow. Poke should never be used internally for self-medication unless under the supervision of a qualified medical or herbal practitioner. Poke is mitogenic and handlers should always wear gloves.

Queen Anne's Lace
Daucus carota L.

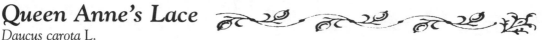

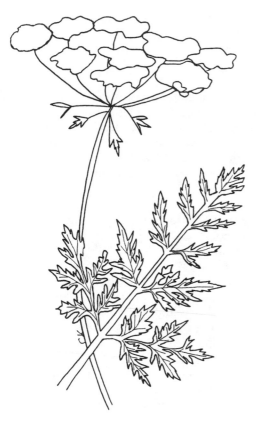

Common names
Bee's nest, carrot, Devil's plaque, wild carrot.

Habitat
Roadsides, open fields and waste areas throughout the Heartland.

Description
Queen Anne's lace is a member of the Apiaceae (parsley) family.

Queen Anne's lace is a biennial herb with a spindle-shaped taproot. In the second year, the plant produces an angled, branched, hairy, furrowed stem bearing alternate, bi- or tri-pinnate, finely divided leaves. White flowers with distinctive much-divided bracts, are in dense terminal, compound umbels. They bloom from May to October. The fruit, a double achene, is flattened and ribbed with hooked spines.

Medicinal Uses
The root of Queen Anne's lace is white, instead of orange, due to a lack of beta carotene. It is called Queen Anne's Lace because the finely-cut, lacy leaves were often used in fashionable headdresses and bouquets of the seventeenth to nineteenth centuries. The earliest known use of this plant, wild or cultivated, was for healing. A mixture of leaves, lemon peel and cornstarch was used as a surgical dressing by Germans during World War II, when regular medical supplies were unavailable. Grated roots were also used externally as a poultice for treating wounds, gangrene and cancer. In folk medicine, the seeds were a "morning-after" contraceptive (probably a day too late). The seeds were officially listed in *The United States Pharmacopoeia* from 1820 to 1882 to treat kidney aliments. Orientals consider wild carrots a potent aphrodisiac.

Queen Anne's lace contains the active components pectin, carotene (provitamin A), vitamins (C and B-complex), the alkaloid daucine which has a nicotine-like odor, sugar, a volatile oil with pinene, carotol, daucol, limonine, and geraniol. Herbalists recommend using the fully, grown, fresh root (carrot) as an anthelmintic, anti-cancer treatment, diuretic and stomachic. Fresh carrots effect the keenness of sight and ability to see in dim light. For children, carrots are effective for digestive ailments and tonsillitis. A carrot diet is said

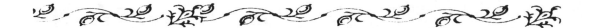

to alleviate pain in cancer patients and lowers blood sugar. An infusion is used as a diuretic to aid in eliminating uric acid in gout-prone people.

The seeds contain the active components the alkaloid daucine, the volatile oil with pinene, carratol, daucol, limonine and geranial. Herbalists recommend using the seeds as an aromatic, carminative, diuretic, emmenagogue and stimulant for dropsy, chronic dysentery, kidney aliments, and uterine pain. Research has confirmed the anti-bacterial, diuretic (due to high potassium salt content), hypertensive and vermifuge properties of the seeds.

The aerial parts of Queen Anne's lace are a useful antiseptic, diuretic for cystitis and prostate disorders, chronic coughs, dysentery, liver diseases, jaundice and to prevent or wash out urinary stones and gravel.

Carrot juice in excessive amounts induces toxic hypervitaminosis A.

Rattlesnake Master

Eryngium aquaticum L. and *E. yuccifolium* Michx.

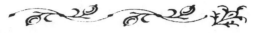

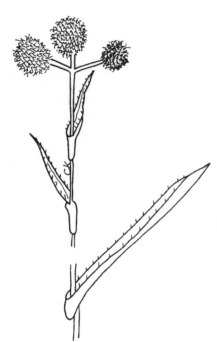

Common name
Button snakeroot.

Habitat
Prairies, rocky open woodlands, ponds and bogs from Michigan south to Florida, and Texas to Kansas.

Description
Rattlesnake master is a member of the Apiaceae (parsley) family. The genus name, *Eryngium*, is from the Greek meaning "a kind of prickly plant," referring to the spiny teeth along the leaf edges.

Rattlesnake master is a stout perennial herb with solitary, waxy, branched stems and thick, fibrous roots. Alternate, linear leaves are parallel-veined with bristly margins. Dense flowers with tiny white petals are in spherical clusters. It blooms from June to September and produces ovoid, slightly scaly fruit with two small segments.

Medicinal Uses

Eryngium species were used interchangeably by many American Indian tribes for treating rattlesnakes bites and various other venomous bites. The Meskquakie used rattlesnake master in the rattlesnake medicine ceremony and for treating bladder ailments. The Creek used it to treat neuralgia, rheumatism and kidney ailments and as an emetic. The Natchez chewed the stem and leaves to stop nosebleeds.

Settlers and physicians used the roots of rattlesnake master as an alterative, diaphoretic, diuretic, emetic and expectorant. A decoction of the root was used for treating dropsy, nephritis, calculus disorders, chronic laryngitis and bronchitis, irritations of the urethra, vaginal, uterine and cystic mucous membranes, gonorrhea, leucorrhea, mucoid diarrhea and local inflammations of the mucous membranes.

Rattlesnake master was listed in *The United States Pharmacopoeia* from 1820 to 1873. Millspaugh said that rattlesnake master was good for "exhaustion from sexual depletion with loss of erectile power."

Rumex
Rumex sp.

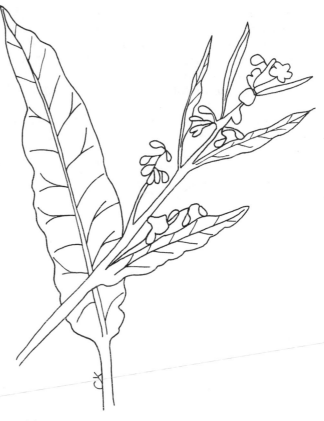

Common names
Bitter dock, broadleaf dock, curly dock, pale dock, sour dock, swamp dock.

Habitat
Fields, roadsides and waste grounds throughout the Heartland.

Description
Rumex is a member of the Polygonaceae (dock) family.

Rumex species (*Rumex acetosella, R. altissimus, R. crispus , R. mexicanus, R. obtusifolius, R. verticullatus*) are perennial herbs. The leaves are narrow to broad and green flowers are clustered in whorls or racemes. It blooms from May to October.

Medicinal Uses
Dioscorides recommended that rumex roots be eaten to ease the pain of scorpion stings. Millspaugh stated that rumex roots have been used since ancient times as a mild astringent, tonic and laxative for treating dyspepsia, gout, hepatic congestion, scrofula, syphilis and leprosy. They have also been used in an ointment to cure cancer and to eliminate skin parasites.

American Indians have used a root decoction of the various *Rumex* species interchangeably for treating a wide variety of remedies. They used a crushed root poultice on boils, bruises, swellings and sores. The Delaware and Shoshone used the decoction for treating liver complaints and venereal diseases. The Cherokee used the decoction for treating dysentery, skin rashes, ringworm, and rubbed the leaves onto sore throats. The Chippewa used a root decoction of broadleaf dock for treating children's eruptions. In the France of Louis XIV, the leaves were used as a poultice, in a manner similar to the Indians, for certain kinds of sores, especially venereal sores.

Rumex contains the active components vitamin C, beta carotene, potassium, oxalic acid, rumicin, emodin, anthraquinones, tannin and phosphorous. Herbalists recommend using a

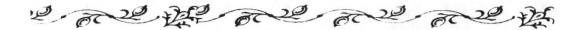

leaf infusion as an antiseptic, anti-coagulant, anti-fungal, astringent, "blood purifier," cathartic, choleretic, diaphoretic and emmenagogue. The infusion can be used for internal and external bleeding, especially excessive menstrual bleeding, and glandular inflammations. The infusion is an excellent coolant for hot days and fevers. The infusion is also used as a gargle for sore throats, or in a poultice for eczema, psoriasis, skin cancer. leprosy and nettle stings. The British say, "Nettles in, dock out."

Studies have shown that rumicin is a choleretic; emodin, a laxative; anthraquinone, an anti-fungal; and tannin, an anticoagulant and antiseptic.

Avoid using rumex if you have kidney disease or rheumatoid arthritis because overuse of rumicin may damage the kidneys and liver.

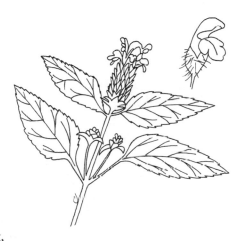

Self-heal
Prunella vulgaris L.

Common names
Carpenterweed, heal-all, hook weed, thimble flower.

Habitat
Lawns, fields and waste grounds throughout the Heartland.

Description
Self-heal is a member of the Laminaceae (mint) family.

Self-heal is a low perennial herb with erect or ascending, square, red-tinged stems and creeping rhizomes. Opposite ovate leaves are entire or serrate. Blue-violet, dense, two-lipped flowers are in terminal, oblong spike-like panicles. The corolla has a hooded upper lip. Self-heal blooms from May through September. The fruits are four smooth brown nutlets that are ridged apex to base.

Medicinal Uses
According to Gerard, "There is not a better wound barke in the world than that of Self-Heale ...The decoction of Prunell made with wine and water doth join togethern and make whole and sound all wounds, both inward and outward."

Many Indians, including the Algonquin, Cherokee, Chippewa, Cree, Delaware, Ojibwa and Mohegan, have used the aromatic, carminative herb for treating sore throats, hemorrhages, diarrhea, stomach troubles, fevers, boils, urinary disorders, liver ailments, gas, colic and female problems.

Self-heal contains the active components ursalic acid, tannin, bitter compounds, an essential oil, saponin and the glycoside aucubin. Herbalists recommend using a flowering stem infusion as an anti-coagulant, anti-inflammatory, antiseptic, astringent and diuretic for diarrhea, internal bleeding, peptic and duodenal ulcers. The infusion is also used as a mouthwash or gargle for throat and mouth infections. The tender leaves can be added to salads or prepared like spinach. Studies show that ursalic acid is an anti-tumor and diuretic compound.

In China, a tea made from the flowering plant is used for treating conjunctivitis, boils and liver ailments. The infusion is also used as an aid in circulation, diuretic for kidney ailments and an anti-mutagenic. The Chinese consider self-heal a panacea for almost every illness, including tumors. Recent Chinese studies indicate immune-boosting potential. A recent discovery shows that *Prunella* is the best source of the antioxidant rosmarinic acid. Self-heal is currently being studied as an anti-AIDS agent.

Seneca Snakeroot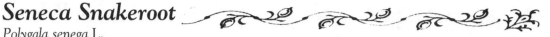
Polygala senega L.

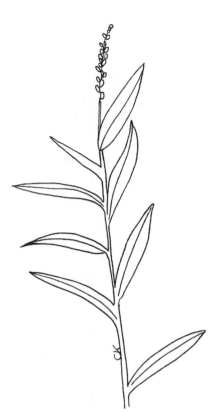

Common names
Mountain flax, rattlesnake root, Senega root.

Habitat
Prairies and dry woods from Michigan to Georgia, Arkansas to South Dakota.

Description
Seneca snakeroot is a member of the Polygalaceae (milkwort) family.

Seneca snakeroot is a perennial with slightly hairy stems, a stout root and alternate, stalkless leaves. Small white flowers in dense spikes at the ends of the stems bloom in July and August. Hairy seeds have white appendages.

Medicinal Uses
Many Indian tribes, including the Cherokee, Chippewa, Fox and Huron, used Seneca snakeroot root as a diaphoretic, expectorant, vulnerary, stimulant, anti-coagulant and tonic. They used a decoction to treat headaches, eczema, cramps, dropsy, asthma, rheumatism, nasal congestion, colds, pleurisy, syphilis, malignant sore throats and snakebites.

Around 1735, the Seneca Indians introduced the use of the root for curing rattlesnake bites (hence its name) to Dr. John Tennent. Dr. Tennent experimented with the root for treating pleurisy and pleuropneumonia (the symptoms were similar to those of the snakebite) with excellent results. His remedy is still used by herbalists for treating respiratory ailments.

In 1943, *The Dispensatory of the United States* tested snakeroot for treating bronchitis and asthma since the root contains saponins and methyl salicylate.

Seneca snakeroot contains the active components polygalic, virgineic and tannic acids, senagrin, resin, saponins and methyl salicylate. Herbalists recommend using a root decoction as an alterative, cathartic, diuretic, emmenagogue, emetic, expectorant, purgative, sudorific and tonic. The decoction is a beneficial remedy for chronic rheumatism, asthma in elderly people, dropsy and respiratory ailments

Senna

Cassia marilandica L. and *C. fasciculata* Michx.

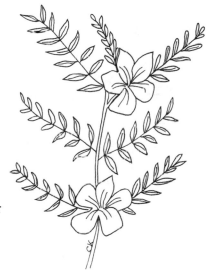

Common names
America senna, cassia, locust plant, partridge pea, wild senna.

Habitat
Dry roadsides and thickets from Ohio to Florida and Arkansas to Iowa.

Description
Senna is a member of the Fabaceae (pea) family. Wild senna (*C. marilandica*) is named after the Old World species, *C. senna*, which it resembles. Note: some botanists prefer to call the genus *Senna*, rather than *Cassia*, except for Partridge Pea, which they call *Chamaecrista fasciculata*. Partridge pea was named by the French botanist Andre Michaux, the first trained botanist to explore Illinois. His discoveries were published in 1803 in *Flora Boreali-American*, which named over three hundred new species.

Senna is an erect perennial or annual. Compound leaves have four to eight pairs of elliptical leaflets. The yellow flowers are in loose clusters at the leaf axils and blooms in July and August. The fruits are jointed seed pods.

Medicinal Uses
The Cherokee and settlers used a root decoction of senna for treating fevers, cramps, heart ailments and as a mild laxative. The bruised root was used in a poultice for treating wounds and sores.

Senna contains the active components saponin, cyanogenic glycosides, the anthraquinones sennosides A and B, aloe-emodin, cathartic and tartaric acid, catharlin, catharkaempferol, crysophonic acid, salicylic acid, mucilage, sennacrol and sennapicrin. Herbalists recommend using a leaf and/or pod infusion as a powerful laxative (*Cassia senna* and *C. augustifolia* are the source of commercial senna, an important laxative). Sennosides act chiefly on the lower bowel to stimulate and increase peristaltic movements of the colon. A paste made from powdered leaves and vinegar can be used for skin ailments and removing pimples. Research has shown that aloe-emodin and beta-sitosterol are useful in the treatment of certain cancers.

All cassia species contain cyanogenic glycosides that are toxic to sheep and other animals. Nursing mothers should not use senna because the laxative agent can be passed to the infant. Prolonged use of cassia species may lead to colon problems. The leaves may cause severe and painful dermatitis on contact.

231

Shepherd's Purse
Capsella bursa pastoris (L.) Medic

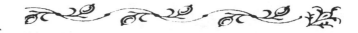

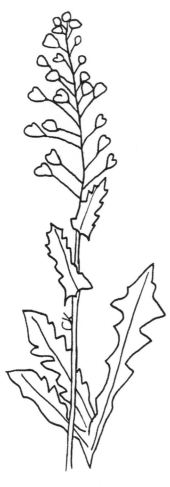

Common names
Mothers heart, Poor man's pharmacy, witches pouches.

Habitat
Roadsides, open fields and waste areas throughout the Heartland.

Description
Shepherd's purse is a member of the Brassicaceae (mustard) family.

Shepherd's purse is an annual or biennial herb. Entire or pinnately lobed basal leaves are arranged in a rosette. The small, lanceolate stem leaves are clasping and sagitate at the base. Small, white flowers are in terminal racemes and bloom from January through April. The fruit is a triangular silicula that looks like an old-fashioned leather purse.

Medicinal Uses
The common name, shepherd's purse, comes from its association with the shape of the purse carried by the shepherds of Bethlehem. Poor man's pharmacy, refers to its past medicinal uses and inexpensive availability. Shepherd's purse has been traditionally used to check hemorrhaging of the stomach, lungs, ulcers, kidneys, open wounds and during childbirth. Many children all over the world have had a pleasant snack by eating the leaves.

Culpeper said that shepherd's purse helps bleeding from wounds, inward or outward, and "if bound to the wrists, or the soles of the feet, it helps the jaundice. The herb made into poultices, helps inflammation and St. Anthony's Fire... A good ointment may be made of it for all wounds, especially wounds in the head."

Herbalists have traditionally recommended using a dried leaf tea to stop internal bleeding of the stomach, lungs and kidneys. Juice from the plant, applied to a cottonball, was inserted in the nostrils to soothe the membranes of the nose, and to stop nosebleeds. The juice was also used in a tea to treat hemorrhoids, diarrhea and dysentery.

Shepherd's purse was introduced into the United States early in the eighteenth century, reaching the Heartland between 1826 and 1859. Indians, pioneers, frontiersmen, settlers

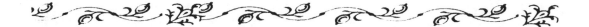

and colonists valued the herb for its astringent properties. It was used to prevent scurvy and to stop internal and external bleeding. The Indians used it as a pot herb (it tastes somewhat like cabbage), and to stop internal bleeding. The Chippewa used shepherd's purse in an infusion for treating diarrhea, dysentery and stomach cramps. The Mohegan used the seed pods for relieving stomachaches and expelling worms.

Shepherd's purse contains the active components saponin, mustard oil, the alkaloid bursine, the flavonoid glycoside diasmium, organic acids, tannin, large quantities of vitamin C and K and the amines choline, acetylcholine and tyramine. Herbalists recommend using an infusion (the herb must be free of the parasitic fungus *Cystopus candidins*) as an astringent, diuretic and hemostat. The infusion is used to stop profuse menstrual, uterine, gastric and pulmonary bleeding. It is also used for gastritis, enteritis, diarrhea, urinary and kidney disorders and children's bedwetting problems. Externally, the infusion is used to bathe wounds, eczema and other skin disorders.

Shepherd's purse is one of the most important anti-coagulant herbs due to the presence of vitamin K and the amines choline, acetylcholine and tyramine.

Any internal use of shepherd's purse should be in moderation as large doses may be poisonous. Always consult a qualified medical or herbal practitioner before using.

Skunk Cabbage

Symplocarpus foetidus (L.) Nutt.

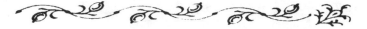

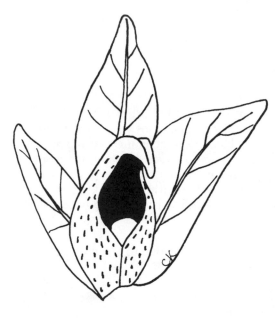

Common names
Meadow cabbage, polecat weed, skunk weed.

Habitat
Swamps and wet areas in woods and along stream banks from Michigan to Georgia, Arkansas to Iowa.

Description
Skunk cabbage is a member of the Araceae (arum or calla) family.

Skunk cabbage is a perennial herb with large upright rhizomes. Massive heart-shaped leaves have smooth margins and thick pale ribs; six to eight leaves stand in tight a cluster beside the spathe (a petal-like sheath enclosing the flowers). The fleshy, distinctive mottled brown and yellow-green spathe emerges tightly closed with a slit-like opening. Within the spathe stands a knobby spadix covered with bright yellow anthers. It blooms from mid-February through April.

Medicinal Uses

The roots and young leaves of skunk cabbage served as food for many Indian tribes, including the Iroquois and Seneca. The Meskquakie applied the rhizome directly on an inflamed tooth to ease the pain. They also crushed the leaf as a dressing for severe bruises, sores, and to help draw out thorns and splinters. The Menomini used a root tea in a poultice to reduce swellings, stop external bleeding and as an underarm deodorant. The Winnebago and Dakota used a root tea to treat asthma, hysteria, coughs, epilepsy, cramps, convulsions and to increase menstrual flow.

Skunk cabbage contains the active components tannin, a volatile oil, iron, silica, manganese and resin. Herbalists recommend using a root decoction as an antispasmodic, diaphoretic, emetic, emmenagogue, expectorant, narcotic, sedative and stimulant. The decoction is used for asthma, cancer, chorea, convulsions, coughs, dropsy, epilepsy, headaches, parturition, rheumatism, sores, toothaches, wounds and to expel worms. Skunk cabbage is an ingredient in many herbal ointments and powders.

In large doses, skunk cabbage may cause nausea, vomiting, headache, vertigo and dimness of vision. Skin contact may cause itching and inflammation.

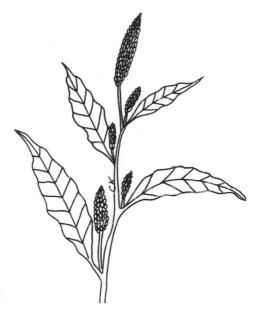

Smartweed
Polygonum sp.

Common names
Marshpepper, pale persicaria, pale smartweed,
Pennsylvania smartweed, swamp smartweed.

Habitat
Open fields, roadsides and wet ground throughout
the Heartland.

Description
Smartweed is a member of the Chenopodiaceae
(goosefoot) family.

Smartweed varieties (*Polygonum coccineum,*
P. hydropiper, P. lapathifolium, P. pennsylvanicum,
P. punctatum) are annual herbs (*P. coccineum* is a
perennial) with ascending or prostrate branched
stems. Alternate, broadly ovate to lanceolate,
leaves with undulate margins, and usually a brown
half-moon shaped spot and whitish dots on upper
surface. Small pinkish or green-white flowers are in long, dense, terminal erect spikes.
Perianth segments, peduncles and leaves are glandular. It blooms from June to frost.
The fruit is a three-sided achene.

Medicinal Uses
In Europe, smartweeds were used interchangeably as a hemostat to control internal- and
hemorrhoidal-bleeding. The Cherokee, Chippewa, Fox, Menomini, Ojibwa and
Potawatomi Indians used a herbal infusion for treating fevers, stomachs, colds, diarrhea, and
for pediatric flux. Externally, the infusion was used as a wash for treating hemorrhoids,
mouth sores or wounds. The pungent-tasting leaves were rubbed on a child's thumb to stop
thumb sucking. The Meskquakie used smartweed as an emetic for poisons and an antidote
for peyote poisoning.

Smartweeds contain the active components tannin, a bitter compound, an essential oil, a
glycoside and large amounts of vitamin C. Herbalists recommend using a flowering stem
infusion as an anti-coagulant, anti-inflammatory, strong astringent and diuretic for internal
and external bleeding, diarrhea, dropsy, various urinary aliments and hemorrhoids. Fresh,
bruised or powdered leaves are applied to bleeding or slow-healing wounds.

Large doses of smartweed may cause gastrointestinal irritation. The fresh juice may also irritate the
skin. Always consult a qualified medical or herbal practitioner before using for self medication.

Soapwort

Saponaria officinalis L.

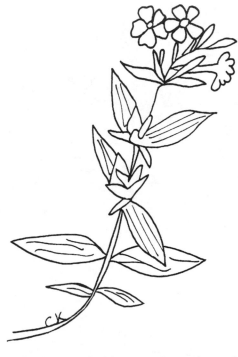

Common names
Bouncing bet, bruisewort, wild sweet William, wood-phlox.

Habitat
Along railroads, waste area and roadsides throughout the Heartland.

Description
Soapwort is a member of the Caryophyllaceae (pink) family.

Soapwort is a perennial herb with erect or ascending stems that branch at the top. Opposite, sessile, ovate to elliptic leaves are three-veined. Pink tubular flowers are in terminal panicles and bloom in July and August. The fruit is a ovoid capsule with small black seeds.

Medicinal Uses
The use of soapwort as a natural cleanser (due to the presence of a saponin which produces a soapy lather) to wash fabrics and tapestries dates back to ancient Greece. Later, soapwort was also used for producing a "head" on beer.

Soapwort contains the active components triterpenoid saponins, flavonoids and sugar. Herbalists recommend using a rhizome decoction as a cholagogic, diuretic, diaphoretic, expectorant and laxative for asthma, jaundice, gout, syphilis, rheumatism, coughs and bronchitis. A poultice is used for acne, eczema, boils, psoriasis and poison-ivy rash.

Soapwort contains saponins which can cause hemolysis, a break down of the red blood corpuscles that results in severe irritation to the gastrointestinal tract. It is dangerous if taken in large doses or over a prolonged period of time. Take internally only under the supervision of a qualified medical or herbal practitioner.

Solomon's Seal

Polygonatum biflorum (Walt) Ell., *P. commulatum* Schult A. Dietr.

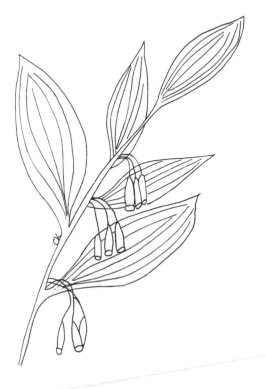

Common name
Great Solomon's seal.

Habitat
Moist woodlands and roadsides from Michigan to Florida, Texas to Nebraska.

Description
Solomon's seal is a member of the Liliaceae (lily) family.

Solomon's seal is a perennial with arched, angled, slender, smooth, stems and thick, white creeping rhizomes. The upper surface of the thick, horizontal, coarse root bears the scars of previous growth that resemble the ancient seal of King Solomon, thus the common name, Solomon's seal. It has alternate, ovate to elliptic leaves with prominent linear veins and smooth margins. Yellow-green, drooping tubular flowers are on a slender stalk and bloom from April to June. It produces blue-black, pea-sized berries.

Medicinal Uses
American Indians used the rhizome of Solomon's seal in a tea for treating internal pains and female ailments. It was also used externally as a wash for poison ivy, erysipelas, skin irritations and hemorrhoids. Fresh bruised leaves were applied directly onto bruises and poison ivy. A poultice was used to treat external inflammations and wounds. Settlers used Solomon's seal as a substitute for digitalis in the treatment of heart problems, kidney ailments, back pain, arthritis, lung congestion and to accelerate the healing of broken bones.

Solomon's seal contains the active components convallarin, asparagin, starch, saponins, mucilage, tannin, sugar and organic pigments. Herbalists recommend using a root decoction as an astringent, demulcent, diuretic, expectorant, hypoglycemic, mucilaginous and vulnerary for neuralgia, inflammation of the stomach and bowels, and diarrhea. Externally, a decoction is used in compresses and bath preparations for treating rheumatism, bruises, eczema, and other skin disorders. The decoction is also used as a douche for menstrual irregularities, and to soothe and tone female reproductive organs.

All parts of Solomon's seal are poisonous and should be taken internally only under supervision of qualified medical or herbal practitioner.

Spikenard
Aralia racemosa L.

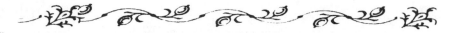

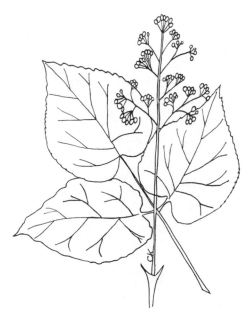

Common names
American sarsaparilla, old man's root, pigeon weed.

Habitat
Rich woods throughout the Heartland.

Description
Spikenard is a member of the Araliceae (ivy) family.

Spikenard is a perennial. Compound serrated leaves consist of three branching stems with five leaflets. Green-white flowers bloom from June through September. It produces small, dark red berries.

Medicinal Uses
The Chippewa and Potawatomi Indians used spikenard roots in a decoction for treating coughs, breast pains, menstrual irregularities, lung ailments and headaches. A hot poultice was used to treat sores and inflammations. The berry juice and oil of the seeds was used to cure earaches. In Appalachia, the rhizomes were used to treat colds, coughs, gout, skin diseases, fevers, asthma and blood poisoning.

Spikenard has been used as a folk remedy in a root tea or tincture as a diuretic, "blood purifier," febrifuge and astringent in the treatment of stomachaches, fevers, coughs, asthma, rheumatism, syphilis and kidney ailments. A root poultice was applied to wounds, ulcers, boils, carbuncles, rheumatic swellings and infections.

Millspaugh suggested mixing spikenard with the root of elecampane (*Inula helenium*) as a remedy for chronic coughs, asthma and rheumatism. He also recommended a tincture of the roots and fruit for treating stomachs.

Spikenard contains the active components resin, the saponin-like glucoside aralin and tannin. Herbalists recommend using an infusion as an alterative, diaphoretic and stimulant for syphilis, rheumatism, pulmonary disorders and skin diseases. A syrup made with spikenard flavored with peppermint is a good remedy for coughs and colds.

Stinging Nettle
Urtica dioica L.

Common names
Ground nettle, forest nettle.

Habitat
Rich woods, moist waste grounds throughout the Heartland.

Description
Stinging nettle is a member of the Urticaceae (nettle) family.

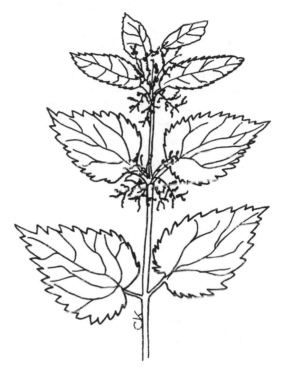

Stinging nettle is a perennial with an unbranched erect stem bearing short bristly, hollow hairs. Opposite, closely spaced leaves that are coarsely serrated and conspicuously veined are covered with bristly hairs that are broad at the base and tapered to a pointed tip. Small, green flowers are in branched clusters from leaf axils and bloom from June through September. Each tiny hair on the stems and leaves is hollow with a jagged point at the tip and a bulb at its base. A bump against the hair squeezes the bulb, forcing the release of an irritating chemical. The venom stings like bee venom and produces a red rash.

Medicinal Uses
Archaeologists found nettle fabric wrapped around a body in a Bronze Age burial site in Denmark. A tenth century Anglo-Saxon herbalist said it was one of nine powerful herbs assigned the job of combating "evils." During the sixteenth century, Gerard, herbalist to King James I of England, used nettles as an antidote to the poisonous herb henbane (*Hyoseyamus niger*). Europeans traditionally used stinging nettle leaves in a tea as a "blood purifier," diuretic and astringent to treat enlargement of the spleen, mucus discharges of the lungs, internal bleeding (they affect the action of white blood corpuscles, aiding coagulation and formation of hemoglobin in the red blood corpuscles), diarrhea and dysentery. One old herbalist contended that nettles were useful in weight-reduction diets. During World War I, the Germans used stinging nettle as a cotton substitute.

Shoshone, Cherokee, Potawatomi and Paiute Indians used the roots in a decoction for treating diarrhea, anemia, rheumatism, ague, dyspepsia, intermittent fevers and urine retention. A leaf decoction was used to treat colds. In a sweat bath, the fumes were inhaled for

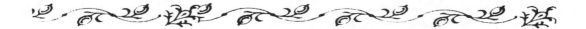

relieving the symptoms of flu or pneumonia. The seeds were used as an antidote for venomous bites, stings and poisonous plants such as henbane (*Hyoscyamus niger*), hemlock (*Conium maculatum*) and deadly nightshade (*Solanum dulcamara*).

Stinging nettle contains the active components tannin, formic acid, acetylcholine, glucoquinones, organic acids, histamine, 5-hydroxytryptamine, vitamin C, beta carotene, provitamin A and mineral salts. Herbalists recommend using a flowering stem and/or leaf infusion as an anti-coagulant, anti-rheumatic, astringent, "blood-purifier," diuretic and galactagogic for rheumatism, gastritis, enteritis urinary, liver, respiratory and skin disorders. The young leaves and shoots, rich in vitamin A, can be added to salads or cooked like spinach to improve the skin's complexion. Since the virulent qualities of nettle are destroyed by cooking or drying, simply boiling or steaming the foliage which is rich in iron, can produce a satisfying vegetable. Stinging nettle seeds have also been used to treat consumption and goiters.

Nettle tea combined with honey is used as an expectorant and general tonic for treating asthma, cystitis and nephritis, mucous conditions of the lungs, chronic coughs, anemia (vitamin C assures proper absorption of iron), diarrhea, dysentery, gout (increases excretion of uric acid), glandular diseases, and to expel worms.

Externally, the fresh leaves are used as a rubefacient for treating wounds, cuts, stings and burns. Commercial hair and skin-care products often contain stinging nettle as an antiseptic and cleansing agent. The stems can be used for fishing line or clothing.

Studies suggest that stinging nettle is a central nervous system depressant, antibacterial and mitogenic that inhibits the effects of adrenaline. Recently, Germans have been using the roots in the treatment of prostate cancer. The Russians use a leaf tincture for treating cholecystitis (inflammation of gall bladder) and hepatitis.

Handle with great care as the hypodermic needle-like tips of the plant hairs can inject formic acid, a histamine, acetylcholine and hydroxytryptamine as a stinging venom into the skin. The British recommend using the various Rumex species to get rid of those nasty nettle hairs: "Nettles in, dock out."

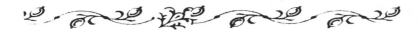

St. Johnswort
Hypericum perforatum L.

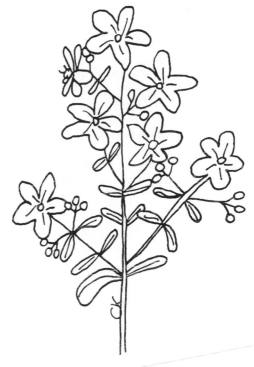

Common name
Common St. John's wort.

Habitat
Roadsides, dry pastures and fields throughout the Heartland.

Description
St. Johnswort is a member of the Hypericaceae (St. John's wort) family. The generic name, *Hypericum*, is derived from the Greek meaning "over an apparition," referring to the belief that the herb was so obnoxious to evil spirits that a whiff of it would cause them to fly.

St. Johnswort is a perennial herb with clumps of erect, branched stems (woody at the base and with two raised longitudinal lines) and stout creeping rhizomes. Opposite, ovate to oblong, sessile leaves have several reddish translucent granular dots. Yellow flowers with black-dotted sepals and petals are in terminal cymes and bloom from June through September. The fruit is a capsule.

Medicinal Uses
For centuries it was thought that St. Johnswort had the power to drive out devils. It was believed that hanging the plant in windows on St. John's birthday (June 24, also called Midsummer Day) would keep away ghosts, devils and familiars for a year. According to early Christians, St. Johnswort bloomed on St. John the Baptist's birthday and bled red oil from the leaf glands on the day in August when he was beheaded. It was also believed that if a young maiden picked the plant on the eve of St. John's Day and hung in on her bedroom wall, she would dream of her future husband. During the Middle Ages it was used to heal deep sword wounds.

Herbalists believed that St. Johnswort was more potent medicinally if it was harvested on St. John's Day. In the seventeenth century, St. Johnswort was used for treating nervous disorders, anemia, bedwetting, uterine cramping and to expel intestinal parasites. At one time, the leaves, soaked in wine or brandy, were drunk to counter melancholy and madness.

St. Johnswort contains the active components tannin, an essential oil, catechol, the red-pigmented flavonoid glycoside hypericin, the flavonoid glycosides rutin and hyperin.

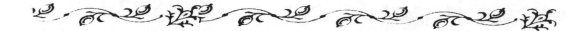

Herbalists recommend using a flowering stem infusion as an analgesic, anti-inflammatory, antiseptic, aromatic, astringent, cholagogic, diuretic, expectorant and mild sedative. Infusions are used for chronic infections, gynecological disorders, respiratory disorders, dysentery, hysteria, hemorrhages, ulcers, gastritis, jaundice, diarrhea and to soothe the digestive system. Infusions are also used externally for bruises, mastitis and hemorrhoids. An infusion given to children before retiring will relieve bedwetting.

German research has confirmed that St. Johnswort has anti-bacterial properties. Studies have shown that hypericin acts as an anti-depressant.

Excessive or prolonged usage of St. Johnswort may cause photodermatitis, a skin allergy which becomes aggravated by exposure to the sun.

Stoneroot
Collinsonia canadensis L.

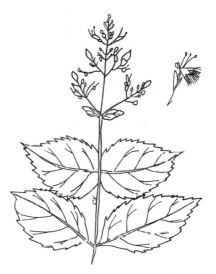

Common names
Citronella, horsebalm, horseweed, knotroot, pile wort.

Habitat
Rich, moist woods from Ohio to Florida, Tennessee to Wisconsin.

Description
Stoneroot is a member of the Laminaceae (mint) family.

Stoneroot is a perennial with branching square stems and thick, woody rhizomes. Opposite, ovate leaves are serrated. Lemon-yellow flowers bloom from July through September.

Medicinal Uses
The Cherokee Indians used stoneroot leaves in a tea for treating mastitis in nursing mothers. They used the bruised flowers and leaves as an underarm deodorant. A root tea was used by the settlers for treating laryngitis, indigestion, diarrhea, dysentery, dropsy, kidney and bladder ailments. The tea was used externally as a wash for hemorrhoids, and in a poultice for treating burns, bruises, wounds, sores and sprains.

The American Dispensatory considered stoneroot an "alterative, tonic, stimulant. Valuable in laryngitis... 'minister' sore throat... in diseases of stomach and intestines... improves appetite, promotes flow of gastric juice; tonic effect upon organs involved. A good remedy in indigestion, dyspepsia, chronic gastritis, increasing the secretion from kidneys and skin."

Physicians in the nineteenth century considered stoneroot an excellent remedy for urinary disorders, a cardiac tonic, and for relieving painful hemorrhoids, particularly those experienced by pregnant women. Stoneroot was used, with or without goldenseal (*Hydrastis canadensis*), for catarrh and gastritis when circulation was defective.

Stoneroot contains the active components saponin, glucosides, tannin and resin. Herbalists recommend using a root decoction as an antispasmodic, astringent, diaphoretic, diuretic, sedative and tonic for hemorrhoids, diarrhea and spasmodic pains of the colon. The decoction is also used to strengthen the structure and function of varicose veins. The decoction is used externally in a poultice for treating bruises, wounds, sores and cuts, in a douche for leucorrhea, or as a gargle for sore throats.

The fresh leaves may cause vomiting when taken in large doses or for prolonged periods of time.

Sweet Ciceley

Osmorhiza claytoni (Michx.) Clarke

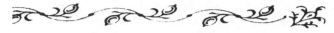

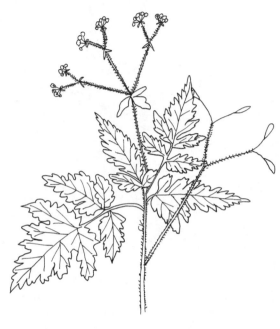

Common names

Sweet anise, sweet jervil, wild anise, wild licorice.

Habitat

Rich moist, shady woods from Michigan to Alabama, Arkansas to Wisconsin.

Description

Sweet ciceley is a member of the Apiaceae (parsley) family.

Sweet ciceley is a perennial with erect, smooth green stems that have five hairs at the nodes. The large, compound leaves are subdivided into three parts or are deeply serrated, appearing somewhat fern-like. The fleshy, carrot-shaped taproot has a distinct anise or licorice odor. Tiny white flowers are in loose umbel-like sprays and bloom from April through June. The fruits are small, sticky, two-part capsules.

Medicinal Uses

The Chippewa, Omaha, Painte, Shoshone and Winnebago Indians applied the mashed root of sweet ciceley to boils, cuts, sores and wounds. The Ojibwa used a root decoction for parturition and sore throats. Illinois-Miami Indians used sweet ciceley to treat eye ailments. Western Indians chewed the roots for relieving sore throats. They used a warm decoction to cure colds, fevers, diarrhea, influenza, pulmonary disorders, and to regulate menstrual irregularities. Sweet ciceley was highly important in the fight against venereal diseases (dose - one-half cup daily for two to three weeks).

Pioneers used sweet ciceley to relieve colic, gas, indigestion and to improve the appetite. They used a warm poultice as a wet dressing for treating cuts, sores, swellings, skin rashes, lice and snakebite. They chewed the raw root for relieving toothaches.

Many mistake sweet ciceley for the poisonous water hemlock (Cicuta maculata). Sweet ciceley smells like anise, whereas, water hemlock has an odor similar to parsnips.

244

Tansy

Tanacetum vulgare L.; also known as *Chrysanthemum vulgare*

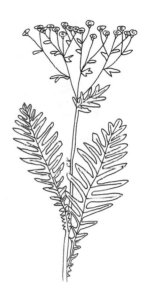

Common names
Bachelor's button, ginger plant, golden buttons.

Habitat
Fields and waste grounds throughout the Heartland.

Description
Tansy is a member of the Asteraceae (sunflower) family. The generic name, *Tanacetum*, and tansy are both thought to derive from the Greek word *athanatos*, meaning immortality, referring to the belief that the plant had powers to prolong life.

Tansy is a perennial herb with an erect, angled, almost hairless, reddish stem that is branched at the top. Alternate, dark-green leaves are pinnately lobed and serrated. Terminal rayless, button-like flowerheads with short tubular, bright-yellow florets are in dense, flat-topped corymbs and bloom from July through September. It produces greenish-white, ribbed achene. All parts smell like camphor.

Medicinal Uses
In ancient Rome and Greece, tansy was used for preserving the dead. According to legend, tansy was given to Ganymide to make him immortal. In the Middle Ages, tansy was strewn on the floor to deter fleas and other insects. In the sixteenth century, tansy cakes (called tansies) were eaten on Easter Day as a remembrance of the bitter herbs eaten by the Jews at Passover. Gerard prescribed tansy as a spring tonic and gout remedy. He also recommended chewing the seeds to rid one of worms. Culpeper mentioned tansy as an aid in treating freckles, sunburn and pimples. Millspaugh recommended an infusion of the flowers to treat those convalescing from a chronic illness.

Tansy contains the active components thujone, the bitter glycosides tanacetin, sesquiterpene lactones, the terpenoid pyrethrins, vitamin C, oxalic acid and tannin. Herbalists recommend using a flowerhead and/or leaf infusion as an anthelmintic, diuretic, emmenagogue, sedative and tonic. In small doses, the infusion is used to strengthen the digestive system, promote menstruation, quiet hysteria, aid kidney ailments and expel intestinal worms in children. Externally, the infusion is applied to swellings, bruises, sprains, sore muscles and varicose veins. The infusion is also used as a wash for feverish patients. Tanacetin oil, distilled from tansy, is used as an insect repellent.

Tansy, rich in thujone, is potentially damaging to the central nervous system and may cause dermatitis if taken in large doses or for a prolonged time. Tansy should be used internally only under strict supervision of a qualified medical or herbal practitioner.

Toadflax
Linaria vulgaris Mill

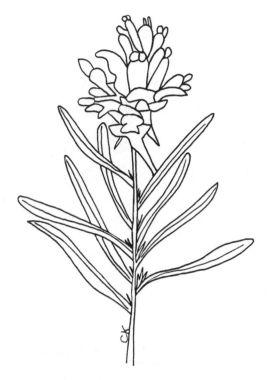

Common name
Butter and eggs.

Habitat
Waste areas and occasionally cultivated throughout the Heartland.

Description
Toadflax is a member of the Scrophulariaceae (flax) family. The genus name, *Linaria*, is from the Latin word *linum*, for flax.

Toadflax is a perennial herb with an erect, leafy branched stem, creeping rhizomes and alternate, linear, gray-green leaves. Yellow flowers in a dense, elongated spike. The corolla is a two-lipped tube that is extended at the base into a long pointed spur. A bright orange spot at the throat of the tube acts as a honey-guide for bees. It blooms from May through November and produces an ovoid capsule with winged seeds.

Medicinal Uses
Toadflax has long been used in folk remedies as a laxative, strong diuretic and tonic used to treat dropsy, jaundice, enteritis, skin diseases and hemorrhoids. The smoked plant was inhaled to relieve bronchitis. A leaf infusion was used as a spring tonic for winter weary children. A "tea" made in milk was used as an insecticide.

Toadflax contains the active components pectin, phytosterine, citric and tannic acids, vitamin C and the flavonoid glycosides linarin and pectolinarin. Herbalists recommend using a flowering stem infusion as an anti-inflammatory, diaphoretic, diuretic and mild laxative for constipation, dropsy, inflamed kidneys and disorders of the liver and spleen. The infusion is used externally in compresses or bath preparation for skin rashes, varicose veins and hemorrhoids. The juice of the herb is considered by herbalists to be a good remedy for inflammation of the eyes and for cleansing ulcerated sores. In Sweden, toadflax flowers, boiled in milk, are considered an excellent, old country fly poison.

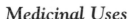

Trillium

Trillium flexipes Raf., *T. recurvatum* Beck.

Common names

Birthwort, papoose root, red trillium, squawroot, white trillium, wake robin.

Habitat

Moist woods in Michigan, Ohio, Indiana, Tennessee and Illinois.

Description

Trillium is a member of the Liliaceae (lily) family. The generic word, *Trillium*, comes from two Latin words, *tres* (three) and *lilium* (lily).

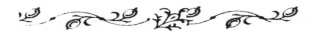

Trillium is a perennial with three triangular or ovate leaves. Flowers have three colored sepals and three green, shorter petals and bloom in April and May. It produces a red, many-seeded berry.

Medicinal Uses

Various Indian tribes including the Chippewa, Menomoni and Potawatomi, used trillium to treat open wounds and sores, menstrual disorders, menopause, internal bleeding, to induce childbirth, and as an aphrodisiac.

Trillium was also used by pioneers to induce labor, to stop post-partum hemorrhage and for other child birthing problems. Traditionally, physicians used a root tea for the same treatments as the Indians used. The tea was also used for treating hemorrhages, asthma, difficult breathing and chronic lung disorders. A poultice was also used to treat snakebites, stings and skin irritations.

Trillium contains the active components trillin, tannic acid, the saponin diosgenin, resin, and a glycoside resembling convallamarin. Herbalists recommend using an infusion as an antiseptic, astringent, expectorant and tonic for gastro-intestinal bleeding, diarrhea, dysentery and to promote parturition. Externally, a poultice is used for tumors, inflammations and ulcers.

Research has shown that diosgenin has a close relationship to human sex hormones, cortisone, vitamin D and cardiac glycosides.

Turtlehead

Chelone glabra L.

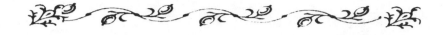

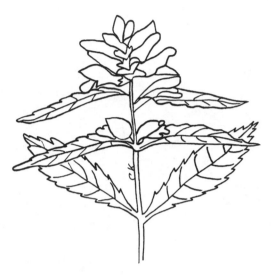

Common names
Balmony, true snakehead, turtlebloom.

Habitat
Low lands, stream borders and moist woodlands from Ohio to Georgia, Missouri to Minnesota.

Description
Turtlehead is a member of the Scrophulariaceae (flax) family. The genus name, *Chelone*, is from the Greek meaning "tortoise," and the species name, *glabra*, is from the Latin meaning "smooth."

Turtlehead is a perennial herb with a single smooth, square stem and creeping roots. Dark green, opposite, long, narrow, leaves have short winged petioles and sharply, serrated margins. Whitish to yellow-green flowers are shaped like a turtle's head with its mouth open, are in dense terminal spikes. They bloom from July through September. The fruit is an oval capsule with small winged seeds.

Medicinal Uses
The Cherokee used turtlehead in an infusion to treat fevers, skin eruptions and sores, to stimulate the appetite and to expel intestinal parasites. Malecite Indians used the infusion as a contraceptive, anti-inflammatory, anthelmintic and tonic. The Potawatomi used an ointment to treat tumors. Turtlehead was a valuable folk remedy for stimulating the appetite and to treat fevers, jaundice, constipation and expel intestinal parasites. An ointment was used to treat inflamed breasts, hemorrhoids, painful ulcers and herpes.

Herbalists use turtlehead as an anthelmintic, anti-inflammatory, cholagogue, laxative, purgative and bitter tonic. An infusion is used as an appetite and digestive stimulant, to regulate the liver and gallbladder, to treat gallstones and gallbladder infections, and to rid the body of round worms (it is especially gentle for treating children). A poultice was used externally for mastitis, ulcers and hemorrhoids.

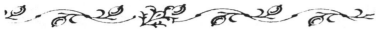

Twinleaf
Jeffersonia diphylla (L.) Pers.

Common names
Helmet pod, rheumatism root, squirrel pea.

Habitat
Rich, damp, shaded woods in Indiana, Kentucky, Tennessee, Illinois and Wisconsin.

Description
Twinleaf is a member of the Berberidaceae (barberry) family. The generic name, *Jeffersonia*, is in honor of Thomas Jefferson; the species name, *diphylla*, is from the Latin meaning "two-leafed," referring to the distinct leaves divided into two wing-like segments.

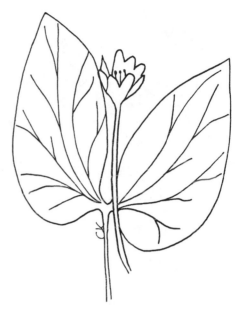

Twinleaf is a perennial herb with a dense fibrous mat of wavy rootlets. The distinctive leaf with smooth margins is divided into two leaflets that resemble a butterfly. Resembling bloodroot, the delicate white flower has eight flat petals and four green sepals and blooms in April and May. The fruit is an upside-down, pear shaped capsule with several rows of small brown seeds.

Medicinal Uses
Both Indians and settlers used twinleaf roots in a tea for treating rheumatic pain, syphilis, cramps, ulcers, mild cases of scarlet fever, muscle spasms, kidney stones, dropsy, diarrhea, sore throats, and as an emetic to induce vomiting. A wash was used externally for treating rheumatism, sores, ulcers, inflammations and cancerous sores.

Twinleaf contains the active components a bitter principle, an acid similar to polygalic acid and the alkaloid berberine. Herbalists recommend using a root infusion as an alterative, antispasmodic, diaphoretic, diuretic, emetic and expectorant for chronic rheumatism, muscle spasms, dropsy, syphilis, cramps and ulcers. In small doses the infusion is an expectorant, and in large doses, it is an emetic. Externally the infusion is used as a gargle for sore throats.

Virginia Snakeroot
Aristolochia serpentaria L

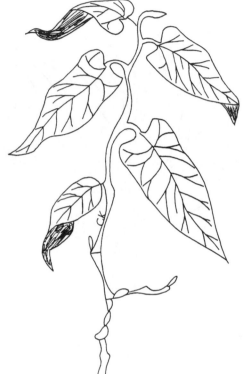

Common names
Serpentaria, snakeroot, snakeweed.

Habitat
Rich woodlands throughout the Heartland.

Description
Virginia snakeroot is a member of the
Aristolochiaceae (birthwort) family.

Virginia snakeroot is a perennial with elongate,
arrow-shaped leaves. Purplish-brown flowers are
calabash melon or pipe-shaped and bloom from
May through July.

Medicinal Uses
The Cherokee often used Virginia snakeroot for
treating ague, chest pains, colds, coughs, dyspepsia,
fever, headaches, pain, pleurisy, rheumatism, sore
throats, typhus and vertigo. They applied the root
directly to relieve toothaches. Other Indian tribes
used a root tea for treating Bright's disease
(nephritis), prostate disorders, renitis and to expel
worms.

Virginia snakeroot was boiled with rum in Virginia as a cure for leukemia and skin cancers.
A root infusion was gargled for malignant sore throats. In small doses, Virginia snakeroot
was said to promote the appetite, tone up digestive organs and act as a cardiac stimulant.
The Blacks of South Carolina used the powdered root to treat low stages of pneumonia.
Until recently, Virginia snakeroot was listed as an official drug in *The United States
Pharmacopoeia.*

Virginia snakeroot contains the active components borneal, serpentarin, aristolactone, aris-
tolochine and an essential oil. Herbalists recommend using an infusion as an alterative,
antispasmodic, diaphoretic, dyspeptic, emmenagogue, expectorant, gastric stimulant, stomachic, sudorific and vermifuge. The infusion is used for amenorrhea, dyspepsia, pneumonia,
sore throat, fevers, stomachaches, indigestion, suppressed menses and snakebites. In large
doses, it promotes arterial action and diaphoresis.

Watercress
Nasturtium officinale L.

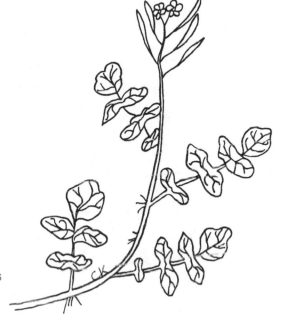

Common names
Nasturtium, scurvy grass.

Habitat
Ditches, slow streams, brooks and ponds throughout the Heartland.

Description
Watercress is a member of the Brassicaceae (mustard) family.

Watercress is a perennial, semi-aquatic herb with creeping or ascending, hollow, angled, hairless stems and roots at the stem nodes. Alternate, odd-pinnate leaves have one to four pairs of oval, entire, or slightly serrated leaflets and a large terminal leaflet. The lowermost leaves are stalked, and the upper leaves are sessile. The leaves and stems stay green all year. Small white flowers in terminal racemes bloom from April through October. The fruit is a stalked, sickle-shape silicula with ovoid seeds

Medicinal Uses
According to Culpeper, bruised watercress leaves, or the juice, would free the face of blotches, spots and blemishes when applied in a lotion.

Watercress contains the active components nicotinamide, the glucosinalate gluconasturtium which decomposes into a pungent essential oil, provitamin A, vitamins (B complex, C, D and E), iodine, iron, manganese, sulfur, copper and calcium. Herbalists recommend using a leaf and/or stem (collected before flowering) infusion as a diuretic, stimulant, and tonic for kidney ailments, arthritis, anemia, poor digestion, high blood sugar and as a blood purifier. The diluted juice or an infusion of the dried herb is used for treating digestive, gall bladder and respiratory disorders. The fresh juice is used externally to treat some skin disorders. Watercress, chewed raw, invigorates and strengthens the gums. The leaves and tender young stems are rich in more organic minerals than spinach, without the oxalic acid.

Fresh or dried, watercress should always be used with care. Large doses may cause inflammation of the bladder and gastrointestinal tract.

Water Hemlock

Cicuta maculata L.

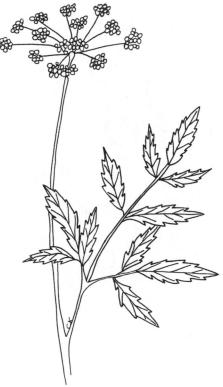

Common names
American cowbane, beaver poison, spotted cowbane, wild parsnip.

Habitat
Wet prairies, moist woods and marshes throughout the Heartland.

Description
Water hemlock is a member of the Apiaceae (parsley) family.

Water hemlock is a perennial with many branches and smooth stems with purple streaks. The reddish leaves are a two or three times feathery-compound with long, pointed leaflets. The white root smells and look like parsnips. The tiny white flowers are in erect, umbrella-like clusters and bloom from May to September.

Medicinal Uses
Children have been poisoned by using the hollow stems of water hemlock as pea shooters. A walnut-sized piece of the root is sufficient to kill a cow. The poison cicutoxis, concentrated primarily in the roots, acts on the central nervous system.

Many Indian tribes used the roots to commit suicide. The Cherokee chewed the poisonous root for four days as a contraceptive, hoping to become sterile but often ending up dead (this is definitely not recommended). The Iroquois used a root poultice for reducing sprains and inflammations.

Rafinesque stated that water hemlock was "a strong narcotic, a good substitute for *Conium maculatum*, being more powerful, and requiring a lesser dose." Powdered leaves were used by white settlers in small doses to alleviate the pain of scirrhus cancer, headaches and neuralgia.

Water hemlock, containing the volatile alkaloid cicutine found in poisonous hemlock (Conium maculatum) should never be used for self medication without strict supervision of a qualified medical or herbal practitioner.

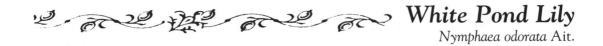

White Pond Lily

Nymphaea odorata Ait.

Common name
Sweet scented water lily.

Habitat
Ponds and lakes throughout the Heartland.

Description
White pond lily is a member of the Nyphaeceae (pond lily) family.

White pond lily is a perennial aquatic herb with stout, creeping rhizomes bearing long-stalked, round, leathery leaves that are green above and often reddish below. White flowers on long stalks have two to five showy petals; the innermost ones are longer than the sepals. They bloom from June through August. The fruit is a globose, fleshy capsule.

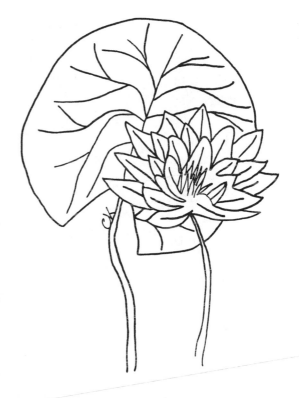

Medicinal Uses
In the Middle Ages, the root of white pond lily was used for fluxes of the blood and "reining of the reins," for venereal problems, to take away freckles, spots, sunburn and morphew of the skin. Chippewa and Marotine Indians placed the dried root in the mouth for treating sores, colds, flu and swellings. Indian squaws used a root decoction as a douche for leucorrhea.

White pond lily contains the active components tannin, the alkaloids nupharine and nuparidine, glycosides, gallic and tartaric acids. Herbalists recommend using a rhizome decoction as an antiseptic, antispasmodic, astringent, cardiotonic and demulcent.
The decoction is used as a gargle for sore throats, a vaginal douche for leucorrhea or as an eye wash. A lotion is used for smoothing the legs and treating sores.

White pond lily was long thought to be anaphrodisiac that was used to reduce the libido. Presently, white pond lily is included in some proprietary medicines used to reduce sexual drive.

White water lily is not suitable for self medication and should be used only under the supervision of a professional medical or herbal practitioner.

White Sage

Artemisia ludoviciana Nutt.

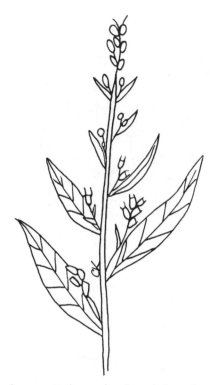

Common names
Mexican sagewort, white mugwort, wormwood.

Habitat
Dry, open areas throughout the Heartland.

Description
White sage is a member of the Asteraceae (sunflower) family. The generic name, *Artemisia*, is Latin for mugwort. Pliny stated that the name honors Artemisia, wife of Mausolus, King of Caria. After the king's death, Artemisia built the renowned mausoleum, one of the seven wonders of the world. The species name, *ludoviciana*, means "of Louisiana," referring to the Louisiana Territory.

White sage is an aromatic perennial. The lanceolate leaves are white-woolly beneath. Erect flowerheads are in dense panicles and bloom in July and August.

Medicinal Uses
The Dakota-Lakota Indians used white sage for cleansing the body in some purification rites. Short Bull, a well-known Lakota chief, said that the men used white sage, and the women used dwarf sagebush (*A. cana*), by either burning or drinking a ceremonial tea for protection against evil influences. They also used white sage for treating stomach ailments, constipation, urine retention and difficulty in childbirth. The Cheyenne Indians crushed the leaves as a snuff for sinus attacks, nosebleed and headaches. The Crow made a salve for treating sores and to use as a deodorant and antiperspirant. The Kiowa made a tonic to reduce phlegm, and to relieve pulmonary and stomach ailments. The Meskquakie used a leaf poultice to cure sores and drive mosquitoes away. They also gargled a tea to treat tonsillitis and sore throats. Pawnee women drank a bitter tea during menstrual periods.

White sage contains the active components thujone, the lactone glycosides santonin and artemisin. Herbalists recommend using an infusion as an anthelmintic, cardiac stimulant and sedative for hysterics, spasms, palpitations of the heart and to expel worms.

Recent research has shown that the lactone glycosides santonin and artemisin, found in all *Artemisia* species, account for the anthelmintic properties.

White sage, containing thujone, is poisonous in large doses and should not be used for self medication.

White Snakeroot
Eupatorium rugosum Houtt

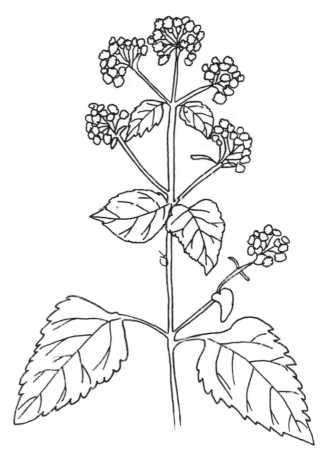

Common name
Snakeroot.

Habitat
Rich, rocky woodlands throughout the Heartland.

Description
White snakeroot is a member of the Asteraceae (sunflower) family. The genus name, *Eupatorium*, is from the Greek meaning "good father," in honor of Mithridates Eupator (132-63 B.C.); the species name, *rugosum*, is Latin meaning "wrinkled," referring to the appearance of the leaves.

White snakeroot is a perennial herb with a sticky stem and tough knotty rhizomes. Opposite, heart-shaped leaves have sharp, serrated margins and conspicuous veins that give a wrinkled appearance. Tight little buttons of tiny snow-white flowers are in loose open, flat-topped clusters and bloom from July through October. Fruits have small black seeds crowned with tuft of hairs.

Medicinal Uses
American Indians used a root tea of white snakeroot for treating ague, diarrhea, painful urination, fevers, kidney stones and in a poultice for snakebites. The smoke of the burning herb was used to revive unconscious patients.

In 1818, Abraham Lincoln's mother, Nancy Hanks Lincoln, died from a brief, agonizing illness caused by a disease known as milk sickness. "Milk sickness," was one of the most dreaded diseases in early America. In the Heartland, it was the leading cause of death. Dr. Anna Pierce Hobbs of Rock Creek, located in the southeastern part of Illinois, discovered the cause of "milk sickness" in the fall of 1834. Dr. Anna realized that "milk sickness" must be caused by something that the cows ate. One day while following a herd to collect specimens

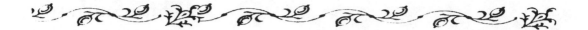

of what they ate, she met a Shawnee medicine woman who showed her that white snake-root was the cause of the trembles and milk sickness. After learning this, Dr. Anna reproduced milk sickness in cows, and carried out the first thorough white snakeroot eradication program. In 1925, J. F. Couch identified trematol (an alcohol), which accumulates in the milk of lactating animals to produce "the trembles."

White snakeroot contains the active components the flavonoid eupatorin, trematol, a volatile oil and resin. Herbalists recommend using a root decoction as an antiseptic, diaphoretic, diuretic and emmenagogue for kidney and urinary disorders, prostate and pelvic inflammatory disorders, painful periods, rheumatism and gout. Research has shown that eupatorin may have anti-cancer properties.

Wild Coffee
Triosteum perfoliatum L.

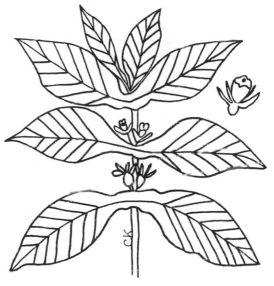

Common names
Horse gentian, horse ginseng, feverwort, white ginseng.

Habitat
Moist woods, thickets from Michigan to Georgia, Oklahoma to Minnesota.

Description
Wild coffee is a member of the Caprifoliaceae (honeysuckle) family.

Wild coffee is a perennial with hairy stems. Joined green leaves taper at the base, meeting and encircling the stems. Bell-shaped blossoms, with petals and five green, yellow and brown-purple sepals, arise from the leaf and stem axil. They bloom from May through July. It produces orange to red, egg-like berries with three hard seeds.

Medicinal Uses
American Indians used a root tea of wild coffee for treating irregular to profuse menses, constipation and urinary disorders. A root poultice was used to treat snakebites and sores. Cherokee Indians made a tea for treating fevers. They used a root bark infusion for treating constipation. The Onondaga used a root poultice for soothing and healing painful swellings and as a general tonic. The Meskquakie used a root infusion for washing the sore head of a newborn infant.

Historically, wild coffee has been used by physicians and herbalists for treating headaches, colic, vomiting, diarrhea and indigestion. A poultice was used to relieve the pain and swelling of painful wounds, a remedy derived from the Onondaga Indians. The seeds, dried, roasted and ground, were used as a coffee substitute by the Pennsylvania Dutch, and for controlling intestinal parasites and bladder problems.

Wild Garlic
Allium canadense L.

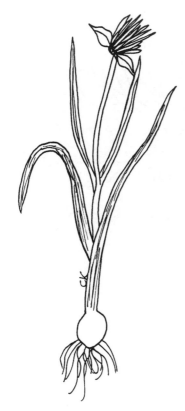

Common names
Meadow garlic, wild onion.

Habitat
Open woods and thickets throughout the Heartland.

Description
Wild garlic is a member of the Liliaceae (lily) family.

Wild garlic is a perennial with narrow, grass-like linear leaves that are flattened on one surface and slightly convex on the other, rather than hollow. Leaves arise from a shallow, small bulb. The flower stalk is topped with a spherical cluster of numerous aerial bulblets. Slender flowers have six white to pinkish petals, colored sepals and two or three broad bracts enclosing the base. The fruit is a small capsule with one or two black seeds.

Medicinal Uses
Similar to cultivated garlic, *Allium sativum*, the antiseptic properties of wild garlic were known to both Indians and early settlers. They mixed the smoked, sliced bulb juice and maple sugar for a cough syrup. The juice was often applied directly to heal wounds, burns and hives. The Cheyenne, Dakota and Winnebago crushed the bulb and stem to make a poultice for boils and bee stings. Pioneers and early explorers used wild garlic in an infusion to treat scurvy, fevers, blood disorders, lung troubles, internal parasites, skin problems, hemorrhoids, earache, rheumatism and arthritis. Wild garlic was listed in *The United States Pharmacopoeia* from 1820 to 1903 and *The National Formulary* from 1916 to 1936.

Wild garlic contains the active components folic acid, the pungent volatile oil ajoene and the sulphuric compound allilin. Herbalists recommend using a bulb infusion as an anti-bacterial, anti-fungal, diaphoretic, expectorant and weak anthelmintic for intestinal infections, fevers, earaches, respiratory disorders and to expel worms.

Recent research has shown that high levels of folic acid may play a major role in preventing heart attacks by lowering cholesterol levels.

 ## Wild Geranium
Geranium maculatum L.

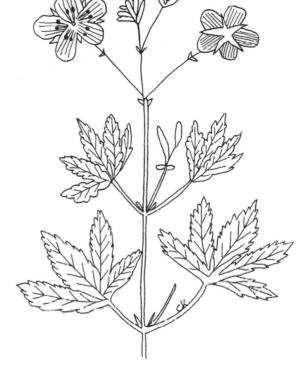

Common names
Alumroot, American cranebill, storksbill.

Habitat
Rich moist open woodlands. Michigan to Georgia, Arkansas, Kansas to North Dakota.

Description
Wild geranium is a member of the Geraniaceae (geranium) family. The generic name, *Geranium*, is from the Greek for "heron" or "crane," probably because seed capsule resembles the beak of a bird. The species name, *maculatum*, is from Latin for "spotted."

Wild geranium is a perennial with an erect, hairy, branched stem. The plant's thick, coarse, rootstock has knobby rhizomes. Large, round leaves have three to five lobes and margins with prominent teeth. Basal leaves have large petioles. Opposite, stem leaves have brown and white spots. Rose-lavender, saucer-shaped flowers with five rounded petals, five green small, narrow, pointed petals and delicate veining are in loose, open clusters at end of weak hairy flower stalks. They bloom from April through June. The fruit is an erect capsule with five parts, each with one seed.

Medicinal Uses
Wild geranium, a very powerful astringent, is mixed with yarrow (*Achillea millefolium*) and plantain (*Plantago major*) as a douche. It is also mixed with sage (*Salvia* sp.) to heal canker sores. Boiled in water and mixed with sugar and milk, wild geranium is easily administered to children as an astringent without bitterness or bad taste.

Meskquakie, Ottawa, Chippewa, Cherokee and Huron Indians used the dried, powdered roots in a tea to heal bleeding, neuralgia, pyorrhea, dysentery, diarrhea, hemorrhoids and for birth control. The Blackfeet Indians steeped wild geranium in water for an eyewash. They also applied a root paste to sores and swellings. Cherokee Indians used a root decoction mixed with wild grape as a mouth wash for children with thrush.

259

In 1795, at Fort Massac in Southern Illinois, wild geranium was used to treat a chronic disease called Racine a Becquet. Pioneers used it as an astringent for diarrhea, especially for children and people with delicate stomachs. The leaves and roots, high in tannin, were used by early settlers for tanning hides.

Wild geranium contains the active components tannic and gallic acids, gum and resin. Herbalists recommend using an infusion as an astringent, styptic and tonic for diarrhea, gum problems, children's cholera, chronic dysentery, sore throats and to stop hemorrhage of the digestive tract. Externally, the infusion can also be used as a body or face wash to awaken lazy skin, as a douche for leucorrhea, a soothing wash for hemorrhoids and in an herbal bath to give the bather aphrodisiac thoughts. The leaves of the scented geranium are used in potpourris along with almond, lime, rose balm, lemon, pineapple, village oak, and other scents, and in deodorants, cosmetics, perfumery and as a mordant in dyeing.

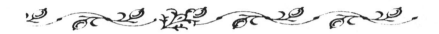

Wild Ginger
Asarum canadense L.

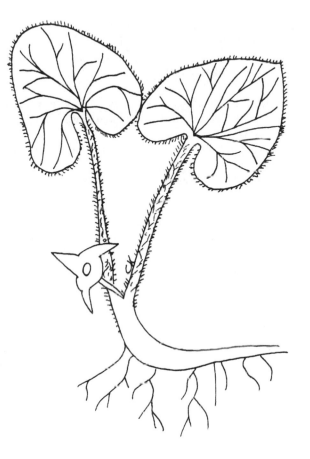

Common names
Catsfoot, chocolate flower, ginger root, Indian ginger, Canada snakeroot.

Habitat
Rich woodlands throughout the Heartland.

Description
Wild ginger is a member of the Aristolochiaceae (birthwort) family.

Wild ginger is a perennial with an unusual root stock that grows horizontally and is branched and shows prominent scars of previous leaf growth. The root has a sweet, spicy, ginger aroma. The leaf petioles arise directly from rootstock. Two large, dark green leaves are deeply indented to form a crude heart or kidney shape with smooth margins and prominent veining. A single flower droops on a hairy stalk in the notch of the two leaf petioles. The maroon to rich brown, bell-shaped flower is dull and covered with stiff white hairs. The flower with three pointed, rather thick, fleshly sepals joined together at the base to form a cup, does not have petals. It blooms in April and May. The fruit is a fleshly, six-celled capsule.

Medicinal Uses
Galen (130-200 A.D.) used wild ginger as one of eight ingredients in a cure-all medicine called "sacraed bitters." Settlers used the roots, boiled with sugar, to make a natural candied spice, as a substitute for Jamaica ginger. Wild ginger was regarded highly as a remedy for whooping cough, nausea, respiratory ailments, fevers, heart palpitations and to control nervous disorders. Powered wild ginger was also inhaled as a snuff to relieve headaches and sinus congestion.

American Indians including the Chippewa and Meskquakie, used wild ginger in an infusion for treating nausea, coughs, cramps and fevers. They applied the crushed rhizomes to wounds, fractures and skin inflammations. A root tea was "dropped" into the ear to cure ear

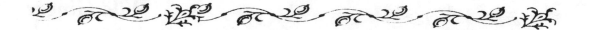

infections. Warriors mixed wild ginger with dried fruits and meats to keep them fresh on long journeys, and to ward off evil. The Catawbas used an infusion to relieve heart arrhythmia and pains. The Illinois-Miami used the powdered root in a tea to relieve birthing pains, promote menstruation and as a contraceptive.

Wild ginger contains the active component aristolachic acid. Herbalists recommend using an infusion as a carminative, diaphoretic, diuretic and stimulant for chronic chest complaints, dropsy and painful spasms of the stomach and bowels. Wild ginger is included in many herbal formulas to increase their effectiveness as a circulatory stimulant.

Research has shown that wild ginger does have anti-bacterial, anti-fungal and anti-tumor properties.

Wild Hyssop
Verbena hastata L.

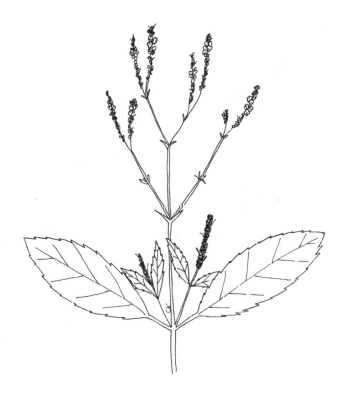

Common names
Blue vervain, Indian hyssop, ironweed.

Habitat
Dry, hard soils, roadsides and fields throughout the Heartland.

Description
Wild hyssop is a member of the Verbenaceae (vervain) family. The generic name, *Verbena*, is from the Latin word *verberi* meaning "stick," referring to the prominent stems with few leaves.

Wild hyssop is a perennial with erect, branched, angled stems. Opposite, lanceolate leaves are doubly serrate, strongly veined and gray-pubescent beneath. The small, blue flowers are in dense slender spikes and blooms from July through September.

Medicinal Uses
The Cherokee, Dakota, Delaware and Menomini Indians used wild hyssop to treat mastitis, kidney ailments, colds, coughs, dysmenorrhea, dropsy, dysentery, fever, flux, stomachaches and to expel afterbirth. The Chippewa used the dried flowers in a snuff to stop nosebleeds.

During the American Revolution, doctors used wild hyssop to induce vomiting and to clear respiratory tracts of mucus. Settlers used a leaf tea as a spring tonic known as Simpler's Joy. It was listed in *The National Formulary* from 1916 to 1926 as a diaphoretic and expectorant.

Wild hyssop contains the active components tannin, a bitter principle, the glucosides verbenalin and verbenin. Herbalists recommend using an infusion as an anthelmintic, anti-rheumatic, anti-periodic, antispasmodic, emetic, expectorant, sedative, and tonic for treating intermittent fevers, diseases of the spleen and liver, epilepsy, stones, gravel, to restore blood circulation and as an antidote to poke (*Phytolacca americana*) poisoning.

Research shows that verbenalin increases the flow of mother's milk and promotes menstruation.

263

Wild Indigo

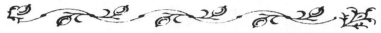

Baptisia tinctoria (L.) R. Br.

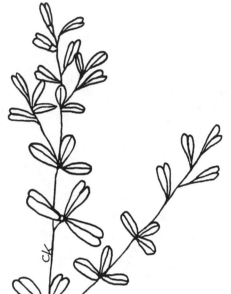

Common names
American indigo, rattlebush, yellow broom.

Habitat
Dry woods and open fields throughout the Heartland.

Description
Wild indigo is a member of the Fabaceae (pea) family. The generic name, *Baptisia*, is from the Greek word *bapto* (to dye).

Wild indigo is a perennial with smooth, blue-glaucous stems and small, alternate, palmate, trifoliate leaves. Yellow flowers on numerous racemes bloom from May through September. It produces legumes with short, bluish-black seeds.

Medicinal Uses
American Indians used a root infusion as an emetic and purgative to treat mucous colitis and amoebic dysentery. The infusion was used externally as a wash for inflammations, cuts, wounds, bruises and sprains and in a compress for relieving toothaches.

Wild indigo contains the active components resin, the glucoside baptisin, the alkaloids cytisin and baptoxin. Herbalists recommend using a root decoction as an antiseptic, astringent, cathartic, emetic, febrifuge and tonic for prolonged fevers, scarlatina, typhus, sepsis and inflammations of the lymph glands. Strong doses may be purgative or emetic. An ointment or poultice is good for treating gangrenous ulcers, sores or ulcerated nipples.

Wild indigo was listed in *The United States Pharmacopoeia* from 1831 to 1842 and in *The National Formulary* from 1916 to 1936.

German research indicates that Baptisia species are potential stimulants to the immune system.

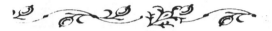

Wild Lettuce

Lactuca biennis (Moech) Fern., *L. canadensis* L.

Common names
Tall blue lettuce, wild opium.

Habitat
Moist open woods and waste grounds throughout the Heartland.

Description
Wild lettuce is a member of the Asteraceae (sunflower) family.

Wild lettuce is a biennial. The leaves are irregularly divided and coarsely serrated. Bluish to creamy-white flowers bloom from July through September.

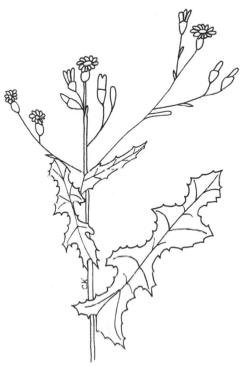

Medicinal Uses
Legend has it that after Emperor Augustus of Rome was cured of a dangerous illness by wild lettuce, he built an altar and erected a statue in its honor.

American Indians used a root tea for treating diarrhea, heart and lung ailments, hemorrhaging, nausea and to relieve pain. The milky sap from the stems was used for treating skin eruptions. The bruised leaves were applied directly to insect stings. Cherokee Indians used wild lettuce as a nervine and sedative. They drank a tea for curing milk sickness caused by white snakeroot, *Eupatorium rugosum*. Chippewa, Lumbee, and Menomoni Indians rubbed the milky sap on warts, poison ivy or poison oak. The Meskquakie used the juice for various infantile diseases. The Bella Coola used a root decoction as an analgesic, anti-diarrheal, anti-emetic and hemostat for heart and lung ailments. Both Indians and pioneers used a leaf tea to hasten milk flow after childbirth and as a spring tonic.

Wild lettuce contains the active component lactucarium (lettuce opium, chemically similar to opium). Herbalists recommend using the latex in cough mixtures to replace opium as an anodyne, expectorant, slight narcotic and sedative to soothe nervous, dry irritating coughs, especially whooping cough. Wild lettuce can be eaten before bedtime as a sleep aid. The latex, warmed with oil of rose, can be used in a compress for relieving headaches.

Wild Pansy
Viola tricolor L.

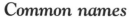

Common names
Heartsease, Johnny-jump-up, love-lies-bleeding.

Habitat
Open fields, waste areas and cultivated throughout the Heartland.

Description
Wild pansy is a member of the Violaceae (violet) family.

Wild pansy is an annual with angled stems. Serrated leaves, with large, leaf-like stipules, are strongly divided. Purple, white and yellow flowers are pansy-like and bloom from May through September.

Medicinal Uses
Gerard stated about pansy: "It is good... as are sick of ague, especially children and infants, whose convulsions and fits of the falling sickness it is thought to cure. It is commended against inflammations of the lungs and chest, and against scabs and itching of the whole body and healeth ulcers."

Wild pansy gets the common name "heartsease," from the belief that an infusion of wild pansy would ease a broken heart. In Europe, a leaf tea was used as a diuretic, expectorant, mild sedative and "blood purifier" for treating fevers, asthma and heart palpitations. The tea was also used as a gargle for sore throats.

Wild pansy contains the active components violine, salicylates, saponin, alkaloids, tannin, the flavonoid rutin and mucilage. Herbalists recommend using an infusion as an anti-inflammatory, diaphoretic, diuretic and expectorant for painful and frequent urination, skin diseases, arthritis, gout and respiratory ailments. The infusion is also used to prevent bruising and broken capillaries, prevent edema, reduce arteriosclerosis and lower high blood pressure.

Wild pansy is an excellent remedy for treating skin diseases, both internally and externally. A compress or ointment applied to affected areas is excellent for treating eczema, psoriasis, acne and skullcap in babies.

266

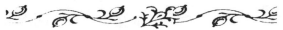

Wild Strawberry
Fragaria virginiana Duchesne and *F. vesca* L.

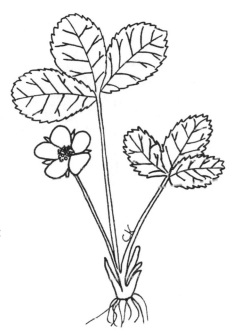

Common names
Virginia strawberry, wood strawberry.

Habitat
Woodlands, prairies and fields throughout the Heartland.

Description
Wild strawberry is a member of the Rosaceae (rose) family.

Wild strawberry is a perennial herb with a short rhizome, long stolons rooting at the nodes, and a rosette of trifoliate basal leaves. Long-stalked leaves are bright green above and white felted below. White flowers with the sepals curving backwards are in a terminal loose raceme and bloom from May through August. The fruits have achenes spread over the surface of the fleshy, juicy, usually red receptacle.

Medicinal Uses
Wild strawberries were described in the first book on American plants by Thomas Harriot in 1588. Many Indian tribes made a tea-like drink of the leaves, and used the strawberries in bread. The Virginia strawberry was first taken to Europe in 1629, crossed in cultivation with the Chilean strawberry and hybridized to produce the large edible strawberry. Linnaeus believed that eating wild strawberries cured his gout. A root infusion was also used at one time in England to treat gonorrhea.

Wild strawberry contains the active components tannin, an essential oil with a lemon-scented component and vitamin C. Herbalists recommend using the dried, leaf tea that has a bitter, aromatic taste as an astringent, diuretic and tonic. The tea is used to treat diarrhea especially for children, dysentery, anemia, nervousness, kidney and urinary diseases, gastrointestinal disorders, gout and to heal spongy gums. The leaves are used in herbal baths for relieving pains and aches of the hips and thighs.

The fruit contains the active components magnesium, potassium, beta carotene, iron, malic and citric acids. Herbalists recommend eating the raw fruit or in an infusion as an astringent, diuretic and laxative to whiten the teeth and treat diarrhea. The infusion is also used to break up calcareous kidney, gallbladder or bladder stones. The juice is used in cosmetics and soaps for the complexion.

Wintergreen
Gaultheria procumbens L.

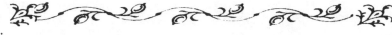

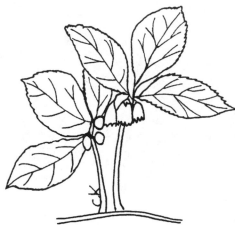

Common names
Boxberry, checkerberry, teaberry.

Habitat
Dry, wooded areas from Michigan to Georgia, Alabama to Wisconsin.

Description
Wintergreen is a member of the Ericaceae (heath) family.

Wintergreen is a perennial with creeping stems and a flowering, upright stem and alternate, leathery, shining green leaves. White, bell-shaped, drooping flowers bloom in June and July. It produces red, waxy berries.

Medicinal Uses
According to Lenope Indian legend, the mastodons were put on earth for people to use. However, they became too destructive and unruly. All the other animals fought the mastodons in a great, bloody battle in a bog. The mastodons lost. The Great Spirit compensated for the loss of meat by transforming the spots of blood into winterberry berries which dot the bogs with red to this day.

Wintergreen contains the active components tannin, the glucoside gaultherin, methyl salicylate, the crystalline principles arbutin, ericolin and ursone. Herbalists recommend using a fresh or dried leaf tea as an antiseptic, aromatic, carminative, diuretic, emmenagogue, galactagogue, rubefacient, sedative and stimulant for delayed, irregular or painful menstruation, to ease the pain of childbirth, to relieve the pain of rheumatism and childbirth and to promote the milk flow of nursing mothers. The tea is also used as a gargle for sore throats and as a douche for treating leucorrhea.

Gaultherin, upon hydrolysis, yields the volatile oil gaultheria (wintergreen oil consists mostly of methyl salicylate). The oil is used as an anodyne, antiseptic, and counter-irritant in treating rheumatic fever, rheumatism, lumbago, sciatica, hives, swellings, arthritis and sore nipples. Oil of wintergreen is a flavoring agent in candies, soft drinks and dental preparations.

Large doses or prolonged internal usage may cause stomach ulcers and external usage may cause skin ulcers. Do not use wintergreen for self medication without the supervision of a qualified practitioner or herbalist.

Wood Sorrel
Oxalis sp.

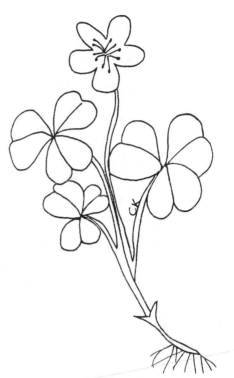

Common names
Creeping wood sorrel, purple oxalis, yellow wood sorrel.

Habitat
Woods, fields, prairies, roadsides and bluffs throughout the Heartland.

Description
Wood sorrel is a member of the Oxalidaceae (wood sorrel) family. The generic name, *Oxalis*, is from the Greek word *oxys* (sour or acid).

Oxalis species (O. *violacea* L., O. *stricta* L. and O. *dillenii*) perennial herbs with slender, creeping scaly rhizomes bearing long-stalked leaves (aerial stem at root head). Bright yellow-green, clover-like compound leaves with three obcordate leaflets that fold along the midrib and droop at night. O. *violacca* has white to purple flowers; both O. *dillenii* and O. *stricta* have yellow flowers which bloom April through October. The flowers have five spreading petals, each with a conspicuous notch. The fruit is a five-angled capsule.

Medicinal Uses
Culpeper recommended wool sorrel to strengthen a weak stomach, stop vomiting, to quench thirst and as an excellent remedy for fevers. A leaf infusion was used as an ointment for skin infections. The juice was used as an excellent gargle for mouth ulcers, a wash to heal wounds and to stop bleeding.

Wood sorrel contains the active components oxalic acid, potassium oxalate, mucilage and vitamin C. Herbalists recommend using a flowering stem infusion as an anti-scorbutic, diuretic and weak antipyretic for scurvy, urine retention and infected gums. The fresh herb or juice can be used as a tonic to treat scurvy. The juice, in a syrup, may be used as effectively as the infusion. Compresses from the macerated leaves are safe to apply to skin infections and swellings. Fresh leaves improve the flavor of spring salads and soups.

Fresh leaves should be used with caution and never by those with kidney or urinary disorders. Oxalic acid and potassium oxalate are irritants and in large doses can cause poisoning resulting in hemorrhage, diarrhea and even kidney failure.

Wormwood

Artemisia absinthium L.

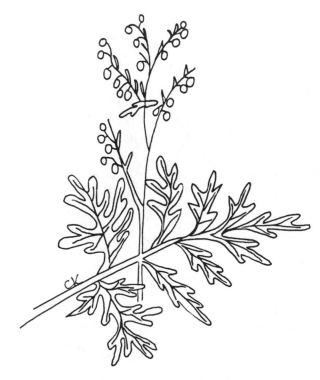

Common name
Absinthium.

Habitat
Roadsides and open fields throughout the Heartland.

Description
Wormwood is a member of the Asteraceae (sunflower) family.

Wormwood is a perennial herb with tall, erect, furrowed angled stems. Alternate, narrow, silvery-green leaves are finely divided. Yellow, rayless flowerheads are in drooping, long racemose panicles and bloom in July and August. The fruit is a cylindrical, slightly flatten achene. All parts of the plant are covered with silvery-white down.

Medicinal Uses
Dioscorides and Pliny considered wormwood as a stomachic, tonic and anthelmintic. In the sixteenth century, wormwood was used to repel fleas, moths and insects. It was also used as an antidote to hemlock (*Conium maculatum*) and toadstool poisoning, and the bite of the seadragon. Linnaeus considered wormwood good for treating intermittent fevers, gout, scurvy, calculus, hepatic and spleenic obstructions. According to Rafinesque, the dark green essential oil of wormwood is a powerful stimulant, antispasmodic and vermifuge. Wormwood wine is an excellent tonic. Some wines, ales and beers are medicated by wormwood.

Wormwood was the principal ingredient in the liqueur Absinthe until 1915 when it was banned in France. Millspaugh relates that the effects of too much Absinthe are: derangement of digestive organs, intense thirst, vertigo, tingling in the ears, trembles, numbness of the extremities, delirium, general paralysis and death.

Wormwood contains the active components tannin, the bitter glycosides absinthin, absinthic acid and succinic acid, an essential oil with thujone, chamazulene, azulene and camphene. Herbalists recommend using a flowering stem infusion as an anthelmintic, antiseptic, carminative, choleretic, anti-diarrheal, diuretic, emmenagogue, febrifuge, lactagogue, stomachic, tonic and vermifuge for arthritis, diarrhea, dropsy, dysmenorrhea, gout, gravel,

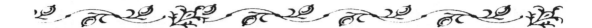

hepatitis, jaundice, malaria, neuralgia, rheumatism and spleenosis. The infusion is used externally as a gargle, and in a compress for treating bruises and sprains. Wormwood, crushed in vinegar and applied to the body, repels flies and fleas. The twigs repel moths. The leaves and twigs can be stuffed into pillows as a flea repellent for cats and dogs. Oil of absinthin, used in medical and veterinary liniments, is reported to be an abortifacient, antiseptic and narcotic. The FDA classifies this as an unsafe herb because it contains thujone, a known narcotic poison. Thujone-free derivatives have been approved for use in foods by the FDA.

Habitual use or large doses can cause convulsions, insomnia, nausea, nightmares, restlessness, tremors and vertigo. Taken over a long period, wormwood leaves become habit forming and will eventually cause serious brain damage. It is advisable to take wormwood internally only under the supervision of a qualified medical or herbal practitioner.

Yarrow

Achillea millefolium L.

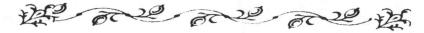

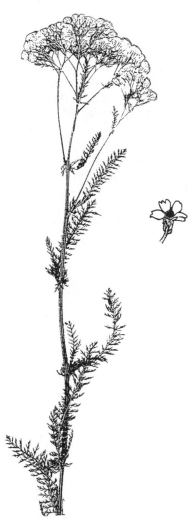

Common names

Milfoil, sneezewort, achillea.

Habitat

Open fields, thickets, roadsides and waste areas throughout the Heartland.

Description

Yarrow is a member of the Asteraceae (sunflower) family. The generic name, *Achillea*, is named after Achilles, the Greek legendary hero of the Trojan war, who used yarrow to heal his soldiers' wounds.

Yarrow is a perennial with erect, furrowed, hairy stems and creeping rhizomes. Dark green, lanceolate, finely-divided basal and stem leaves. Small flowerheads with white ray florets and occasionally pink disc florets are clustered in dense, flat corymbs. They bloom from May through August. The fruit is a strongly-compressed, slightly winged achene.

Medicinal Uses

Fossil records reveal yarrow pollen in Neanderthal burial caves. The Greek physician Dioscorides smeared yarrow on ulcers to prevent inflammation. In 1500, the British herbalist Gerard recommended yarrow for "swelling of those secret parts." Nicholas Culpeper, the seventeenth century herbalist, recommended it for wounds. Anglo-Saxons used a tonic tea to break the fever of a severe cold, to heal burns, and to treat insect bites and venomous snakebites. During the Middle Ages, yarrow was thought to be a witches' herb and was brought to weddings to ensure seven years of love. Linnaeus prescribed freshly bruised yarrow as a vulnerary and styptic for rheumatism.

Yarrow was used in a wide variety of medicinal treatments by at least fifty eight Indian tribes as a stimulant, laxative, analgesic, diuretic, hemostat, antiseptic, cholagogue, emmenagogue and tonic. Algonquin, Blackfoot, Cherokee, Illinois-Miami, Lakota, Micimac and Ute Indians applied yarrow leaves to injuries, sores, blisters, burns, and hemorrhoids to soothe, heal and curb bleeding. The Aberaki smoked the leaves for asthma. The Cheyenne used a tea for colds, coughs, sore throats and nausea. The Chippewa inhaled the steam from

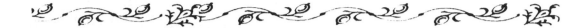

a hot infusion for headaches. Mohawk and Mohegan Indians drank an infusion for cramps, diarrhea, nausea and stomach ailments. Cahuilla and Crow Indians made a tea to soothe toothaches and sore gums.

Shakers used yarrow as an alterative, aromatic, aid for indigestion, cathartic, detergent, diuretic, stimulant and tonic and stomachic in treatments ranging from hemorrhages to flatulence.

Yarrow contains the active components rutin, coumarin, saponin, the bitter glycoalkaloid achilleine, salicylic acid, cyanidin, tannin, sterols, triterpenes, the alkaloids achilletin, aquiline and strachydrine, a volatile oil with azulene, boreal, cineol, menthol and camphor. Herbalists recommend using a leaf and/or flower infusion as an astringent, antiseptic, antispasmodic, diaphoretic, stimulant and stomachic for nausea, diarrhea, flatulence, menstrual disorders, venereal diseases, colds, fevers, bronchitis and as a tonic for the heart and circulatory system. The infusion can be used externally as a douche for leucorrhea, and in a poultice for treating severe wounds, slow-healing wounds, skin rashes, eczema, chapped skin and boils.

Research has demonstrated that achilleine is an effective anti-coagulant, suppresses menstruation and lowers blood pressure. Cyanidin affects the vagus nerve, slowing the heart beat. Achillatin is an anti-coagulant. The tannins are anti-bacterial. Both cyanidin and aquline are anti-inflammatories.

The dried leaves and flowering tips of yarrow were officially listed in *The United States Pharmacopoeia* from 1863 to 1882 as a tonic, stimulant and emmenagogue. It is still listed in some pharmacopoeias in Europe. In China, yarrow is used fresh as a poultice for healing wounds. An infusion of the whole herb is prescribed for stomach ulcers, amenorrhea and abscesses. In Norway, yarrow has been used as a cure for rheumatism. In Sweden, yarrow (field hips) has been used in brewing a very intoxicating beer.

Yarrow should always be taken in moderation and for short periods because it may cause skin irritation.

Cultivated
Herbs

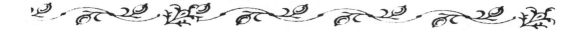

Alfalfa
Medicago sativa L.

The first recorded mention of alfalfa is in a book on plants by the Emperor of China written in 2939 B.C. The Chinese used alfalfa to treat ulcers, stimulate the appetite and strengthen the digestive tract. Alfalfa was brought to the United States in 1852 and was quickly accepted by the Indians for its nutritive and medicinal qualities. The Great Plains Indians called alfalfa "buffalo grass." Many of the tribes made an alfalfa infusion for relieving rheumatism and arthritis.

Alfalfa, grown for fodder, contains unusually high amounts of vitamins A, D, E and K and phosphorous. It also contains eight important digestive enzymes: lipase is a fat splitter; amylase breaks down starch; coagulase coagulates milk and clots blood; emulsin breaks down sugar; invertase changes cane sugar to dextrose; peroxidase oxidizes the blood; pectinase forms vegetable jelly from pectin; and protease breaks down proteins.

A nutritious fresh or dried leaf tea has traditionally been used as a diuretic, hemostat and appetite stimulant. Drunk daily, the tea will improve the appetite, aid in the cure of peptic ulcers, act as a mild diuretic and aid in bowel regulation. Alfalfa can also relieve dropsy, help narcotics and alcoholics kick their habit, and stimulate the supportive connective cells (excellent for relieving rheumatic and arthritic pain).

Alfalfa sprouts are delicious and contain more protein than wheat or corn. If eaten often, they help rebuild decayed teeth.

Studies have shown that alfalfa has anti-fungal and estrogenic properties. Alfalfa is an excellent commercial source for chlorophyll and carotene used in the manufacture of many staple foods.

Consuming large quantities of alfalfa may cause the breakdown of red blood corpuscles. Recent reports suggest that alfalfa sprouts or seeds containing caravarine may be associated with stimulating the re-occurrence of lupus in patients in which the disease has become dormant.

Asparagus
Asparagus officinalis L.

Asparagus shoots, a most delicious food and diuretic, have been grown and used by epicurians since the earliest times. In medieval times it was believed that a decoction of asparagus roots, boiled in wine and drunk while fasting from other foods, would stir up bodily lust in man or woman. According to Gerard, a decoction of asparagus roots "boiled in wine, clears the sight."

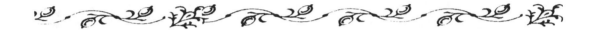

Culpeper wrote that asparagus is "good against the strangury or difficulty of making water. It expelleth the gravel and stone out of kidneys ...the decoction of the roots (Asparagus) boiled in wine, and taken, is good to clear the sight and being held in the mouth easeth the toothache." American Indians used asparagus as a diuretic for treating kidney and bladder disorders. In 1889, the settlers of Wyoming were reminded in their local paper that "asparagus purifies the blood and especially acts on the kidneys."

Asparagus contains the active components vitamin A and B, asparagin, beta-sitosterol, choline, betaine, rumatakenin, saponins, flavonoids, volatile oil, glucosides, resin, tannin and mineral salts. Herbalists recommend using an infusion or the cooking water as a diaphoretic, diuretic, laxative and sedative for fevers, constipation, rheumatism, and as a diuretic for edema caused by heart failure (since the mineral salts act to stimulate the bladder).

The Japanese report that green asparagus aids protein conversion into amino acids. The Chinese report that the roots lower blood pressure. Studies have shown that the seeds possess antibiotic activity.

Basil
Ocimum basilicum - sweet basil; *O. minimum* - bush basil

In ancient Italy, basil signified love; but in ancient Greece, basil signified hate. In India, basil was sacred to Krishiva and Vishnu, gods of the Hindus. They also used basil as an antidote for snake venom. In Europe, pots of basil were placed outside the house to repel fleas. Culpeper called basil "basilicon" because it was the herb of Mars and under Scorpion. According to Culpeper, basilicon "applied to the place bitten by the venomous beasts, or stung by a wasp or hornet, it speedily draws the venom to it. Every like draws its like." He also recommended using basil mixed with honey and nutmeg for diarrhea, easing childbirth and to expel the afterbirth.

Basil contains the active components tannin, glycosides, saponin, an essential oil with eugenol, estrogal, lineol, linalool, thymol and basil camphor. Herbalists recommend using a flowering stem infusion as an antispasmodic, galactagogue, carminative, expectorant, mild sedative and stomachic for chronic gastritis, stomachache, flatulence, constipation, respiratory disorders such as coughs and whooping cough, and urinary infections. Basil tea is excellent for the prevention of motion sickness and for pregnant women suffering from morning sickness. Externally, the infusion is used in invigorating baths, in compresses for slow-healing wounds and in gargles for sore throats. Oil of basil massaged into the temples relieves nervous tension and headaches.

The essential oil, obtained by steam distillation from fresh basil, is widely used in the perfumery and food industries. In cooking, basil leaves are used to flavor soups, salads, meat and fish dishes.

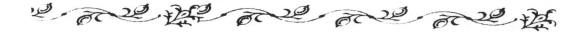

Borage
Borago officinalis L.

Fresh borage leaves, with a cucumber-like flavor, are a cooling accent to salads, pickles, iced beverages and herb teas. The flowers are excellent for floating in wine punches, fruit juice and gin with sugar. The flowers may also be candied or included in jams, jellies and syrups.

The leaves and/or the flowers were traditionally used in folk remedies for treating breast or facial cancers and tumors. An infusion was used as an anti-inflammatory, demulcent, diaphoretic, emollient, expectorant, febrifuge, lactagogue, laxative and tonic for treating kidney stones, bronchitis, coughs, cramps, fevers, sore throats, jaundice and urogenital ailments.

Borage leaves and flowers contain the active components saponins, silic and malic acid, mucilage, tannin, potassium, calcium, vitamin C, allantoin, and high levels of gamma linolecic acid, particularly in the seeds. Herbalists recommend using an infusion as an anti-inflammatory, mild diuretic, diaphoretic, demulcent and tonic for urinary infections, colds, bronchitis and rheumatism. The infusion can be used externally in a compress for treating skin rashes.

Caraway
Carum carni L.

Evidence of caraway seeds have been found among Mesolithic food remains. Caraway was mentioned in Ebers Papyrus, a medicinal manuscript dating to 1500 B.C, and in a twelfth century German medical work. Caraway seeds were used as a culinary herb and medicinally to relieve flatulence, indigestion, colic in babies and to promote milk flow in nursing mothers.

Caraway contains the active components tannin, an essential oil with carvone and linosine, proteins, starch, sugar and fatty oil. Herbalists recommend using the seeds as an anthelmintic, antiseptic, antispasmodic, carminative, galactagogue and stomachic. The powdered seeds taken in hot milk is an excellent remedy for warding off colds. Caraway seeds are ideal for use in children's medicines for flatulence and upset stomachs. The powdered seeds are also used in a poultice to dissolve bruises. Distilled caraway oil is an effective anesthetic for toothache (place a cotton ball soaked in the oil into the cavity).

Caraway seeds or oil are an ingredient in the alcoholic beverages Kummel and gin. The fleshy root, with a better taste than parsnips, can be eaten as a vegetable. The young leaves are added to salads and soups. The seeds are also widely used as a culinary herb.

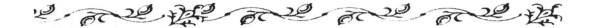

Castor Bean
Ricinus communis L. - Palma Christi

Castor bean has been cultivated in India and tropical Africa since ancient times for its oily seeds. In ancient Egypt and the Orient, the seed oil was used to beautify the hair and complexion. The seeds have been found in numerous ancient tombs. Dioscorides described the plant and gave a detailed description of extracting the oil from the seeds. He recommended that the oil be used only as an external medicine because the seeds were an extreme purgative.

Castor bean contains the active components ricin, glycerin, palmitic and ricinoleic acid. Herbalists recommend using the seed oil as an anti-fungal, anthelmintic, antiseptic, cathartic, emollient and purgative. Castor oil, in small doses, is regarded as the most valuable laxative for relieving constipation, especially in children, convalescents and the elderly. Currently, castor oil is used as a laxative in cases of food poisoning and as a purgative before X-ray diagnostic exams. Larger doses can be used as a purgative for chronic constipation and for expelling intestinal parasites.

Externally, the oil is used for treating ringworm, hemorrhoids, rashes and abscesses. The oil is also used in hair tonics for treating dandruff and in industrial lubricants, varnishes, plastics and other products.

Edgar Cayce, the "psychic doctor," recommended the external use of castor oil packs for treating at least fifty different illness including the removal of warts, healing skin ulcers, soothing irritated eyes and stimulating the liver, kidneys or stomach.

The seeds should never be eaten whole as ricin is extremely poisonous. One seed may be fatal to a child and two or three may be fatal for an adult. The nauseating taste of the oil may induce vomiting. Large doses may cause vomiting and severe diarrhea. Prolonged use may cause dermatitis.

Celery
Apium graveolens L

Celery seeds were used medicinally by the ancient Greeks and Romans, and by Europeans up until the seventeenth century. In medieval times it was said that witches ate the seeds to keep from getting a cramp or falling off their brooms while flying.

Celery contains the active component apiol. Herbalists recommend eating the stalks or seeds as a diuretic, sedative and stimulant for hysteria, bronchitis, swollen glands, rheumatism and

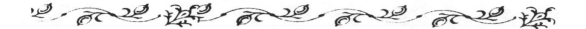

insomnia. Celery stalks containing organic sodium are used as a neutralizer and diuretic. Eating the stalks is an excellent aid in the treatment and prevention of arthritis as the sodium keeps insoluble inorganic calcium in solution until the body eliminates it. In general, celery seeds promote a healthy muscular condition. Because celery sodium is a neutralizer in the body, it is also a helpful antidote to alcoholism. A celery stalk with tomato juice is particularly helpful after a heavy night of alcohol consumption.

Chamomile
Anthemis nobilis L. - Roman chamomile

The medicinal properties of Roman chamomile (similar to scented mayweed, commonly called German chamomile) were known by the ancient Egyptians who dedicated the herb to the sun because it cured agues. In herbal medicine, an infusion was used for treating fevers, dyspepsia, nausea, migraine headaches, painful menstruation and insomnia. A tincture was given to children for summer diarrhea, to lower nervous excitability, neuralgia, and to relieve tooth- and ear-aches. Cherokee Indians used the flowerheads of this introduced species for treating bowel complaints, colic, delayed menstrual periods, hysteria, nausea, rheumatism and ulcers.

Chamomile contains the active components bitter compounds, an essential oil with azulone, the flavonoids quercitrin and choline. Herbalists recommend using a flowerhead tea as an anti-inflammatory, antiseptic, antispasmodic, diaphoretic, diuretic, emmenagogue, mild sedative and stomachic. Chamomile tea is used to relax restless or hyperactive children and in small amounts for teething babies. It is also used for indigestion, flatulence, edema, heartburn, diarrhea and painful menstrual periods. Externally, a strong infusion of chamomile flowers is used for ulcers, eczema and wounds.

Chamomile is used in bath herbs and in facial lotions to firm the tissues for young-looking skin, to brighten the eyes and to relieve weariness. Blondes can use an infusion in a hair rinse to maintain their hair color. Distillation of fresh flowering stems yields the oil used by the pharmaceutical industry.

Coriander
Coriandrum sativum L.

Cultivated over three thousand years, coriander seeds have been found among funeral offerings in ancient Egyptian tombs. Ancient Hebrews used coriander as one of the bitter herbs in the

280

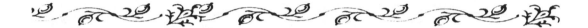

ritual of Passover. There are several Old Testament references to coriander as the herb that God showered upon the Israelites during their trek out of Egypt (Exodus 16:31). The fruit is similar to the mysterious food manna. Both Greek and Roman physicians made medicines from coriander. Hippocrates also used it as a spice. The Chinese used coriander as far back as the Han dynasty, 207 to 220 A.D. In the Arabian fantasy tales *One Thousand and One Nights*, coriander is mentioned as an aphrodisiac. Indeed the seeds can be narcotic if consumed in excessive amounts.

All parts of coriander smell strongly like bed bugs. However, the fruits lose their disagreeable scent when ripe, becoming pleasantly spicy and aromatic. Coriander (also called cilantro) fruits and fresh leaves are an important culinary herb widely used for flavoring food and gin. The cooked root is an excellent addition to any meal.

Coriander contains the active components tannin, an essential oil with coriandrol and pinene, fatty oil, protein, pectin, sugars and vitamin C. Herbalists recommend using the dried fruits by themselves or in tea mixtures as an aromatic, carminative, emmenagogue, mild sedative, stimulant and tonic to relieve migraine headaches, regulate menstrual periods, as a digestive tonic, and as a mild sedative. Coriander tea is a good general tonic for children. The fruits or coriander oil are included in ointments for painful rheumatic and sore muscles. Chewing the seeds will soothe and relieve stomachaches and toothaches.

Dill
Anethum graveolens L.

In the Middle Ages, dill was used by magicians in their spells and charms against witchcraft. Culpeper says of dill: "Mercury has the dominion of this plant, and therefore to be sure it strengthens the brain ...it stays the hiccough, being boiled in wine and but smedded unto being tied in a clothe ...and is used in medicines that serve to expel wind."

Dill was once an important medicinal herb for treating coughs, headaches and as an astringent in ointments. Dill is still used by herbalists but is chiefly known as a vegetable and seasoning herb.

Dill contains the active components tannin, an essential oil (dill-seed oil) with carone, limonene, fatty oil, proteins and mucilage. Herbalists recommend using a fruit and/or flowering stem infusion as a carminative, diuretic, galactagogue, laxative, stimulant, stomachic and tranquilizer. Dill water (gripe), made from the fruits, is given to babies for hiccups, colic and to induce sleep. The essential oil is used in the manufacture of liqueurs and in cosmetic preparations. Dill is used as a flavoring agent by the food industry.

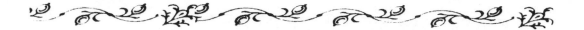

European and American herbalists use both the seeds and leaves to dispel flatulence, increase mother's milk, treat breast congestion resulting from nursing, stimulate the appetite, and relieve colic in babies. Oil of dill is used in many over-the-counter medicines for digestive problems.

Fennel
Foeniculum vulgare Mill

Fennel was known to the ancient civilizations of China, India and Egypt. Hippocrates and Dioscorides both recommended fennel for increasing milk flow in nursing mothers. Pliny prescribed at least twenty-two remedies using fennel. In Medieval times, people nibbled on fennel seeds during church and on fast days to suppress the appetite. Bunches of fennel, with or without St. John's wort, were hung over doors on Midsummer's Eve to ward off witches and were thrown on carpetless floors to keep homes sweet smelling and free from infection.

Culpeper wrote that all parts of the fennel plant "are much used in drink or broth to make people lean that are too fat." Culpeper believed that fennel helped to break kidney stones, quiet hiccups, prevent nausea and gout, clear the liver and lungs, and was an antidote to poisonous mushrooms. Fennel tea (the famous "gripe water") was used to cure colic in babies. Teas were gargled as a breath freshener, applied as an eyewash and drank to expel intestinal worms. A poultice was used to relieve breast swelling in nursing mothers. An infusion of ground seeds was used to make a steam facial.

The young fresh leaves and seeds are excellent for flavoring food, especially fish. The roots and swollen leaf bases can be eaten as a vegetable.

Fennel contains the active components proteins, fatty oils, a fixed oil with petroselenic-, oleic-, and linoleic acid, calcium, sugars, mucilage, an essential oil with anethole, estragole, limonene, camphene, pinine and fenchone. Herbalists recommend using a seed tea as an antispasmodic, aromatic, carminative, galactagogue, stomachic, and depending on dosage, as a weak diuretic for both long-term constipation and diarrhea, to ease flatulence, colic pain, urinary disorders, coughs, bronchitis and to stimulate milk flow in nursing mothers. The oil of fennel is used in tinctures as a gargle and eyewash. The oil is used also for scenting soaps and perfumes.

The volatile oil of the seeds can be irritating or even dangerous to those with allergies or sensitive skin.

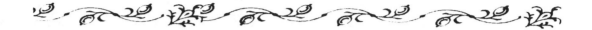

Fenugreek
Trigonella foenum-graecum L.

Fenugreek seeds have been used as a spice and medicine since the days of the Babylonian and Egyptian empires. Arabians roasted the seeds as a "coffee" substitute. The seeds, which taste like celery, were used in spice combinations for curries and in preserves. They have been used in folk medicine as an aphrodisiac and for increasing lactation in nursing mothers. The seeds were also used as a substitute for cod-liver oil in the treatment of scrofula, rickets, anemia and debility following infectious diseases.

Fenugreek contains the active components the steroidal saponin diosgenin, flavonoids, mucilage, proteins, vitamins A, B and C, calcium, iron, the alkaloids trigonelline, choline, gentianine and carpaine. Herbalists recommend using a seed infusion as an antibiotic, astringent and emmenagogue for reproductive disorders (the therapeutic steroidal saponins closely resemble the body's own sex hormones) and as a soothing remedy for bronchitis. The powdered seeds make an excellent poultice for treating rheumatic pains, ulcers, *Staphylococcus* infections and boils. In China, fenugreek is prescribed for male impotence, menopausal depression and recurring hot flashes.

Fenugreek should never be used as a medication during pregnancy because of its stimulatory effect on the uterus.

Foxglove
Digitalis purpurea L.

Various foxglove species have been cultivated for herbal medicines as far back as 1000 A.D. Its action against dropsy, discovered by William Withering in the 1770s, led to the wide use of the plant in medical practice. English herbalists used foxglove as a cough medicine, a treatment for epilepsy and a cure for swollen glands.

Foxglove contains the active components tannin, saponins, several cardiac glycosides (including digitoxin, digitalin, digitonin, and purpurea glycosides A and B in various concentrations), organic acids and mucilage. Herbalists recommend using a dried leaf infusion as a cardiac stimulant. The dried leaf is listed as an official drug in the British Pharmacopoeia. A beautiful decorative garden plant, foxglove should be picked in its second year when it is flowering and the alkaloid digitalis is the most concentrated.

Digitalis is a powerful cardiac stimulant that increases the force of systolic contractions in congestive heart failure, lowers venous pressure in hypertensive heart failure and elevates low

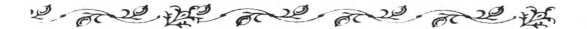

arterial blood pressure. This, in turn, alleviates water retention and reduces edema by acting as a strong diuretic. Digitalis is also used in the treatment of internal hemorrhages, inflammatory diseases, epilepsy, delirium tremors and acute mania. It is an excellent antidote to aconite poisoning.

Digitalis is cumulative and even relatively small doses, taken often, induce the symptoms of poisoning. Symptoms of poisoning include abdominal pain, irritation of the stomach and bowel, nausea, abnormal heart action and perhaps tremors and convulsions. Death can result. All parts of foxglove species are extremely poisonous and should never be collected and used for self medication without the supervision of a qualified medical or herbal practitioner.

Garlic
Allium sativum L.

Medicinally, garlic has been prescribed since prebiblical times in the Far East. Garlic has been cultivated in the Middle East since 3000 B.C. Ancient herbalists used it to treat high blood pressure and respiratory problems. Garlic is mentioned in the Calendar of Hsai, which dates back to 2000 B.C. Garlic is mentioned in the Bible as one of herbs used in embalming. Garlic was used with hyssop to treat leprosy.

Theophratus relates that the ancient Greeks placed garlic on piles of stones at cross-roads as a supper for Hecate. The poet Homer related that Odysseus used garlic to prevent the sorceress Circe from turning him into a pig. Egyptians swore on a clove of garlic when they took a solemn oath. An Egyptian medical listing of 1550 B.C. recommended using garlic for treating headaches, bites, worms, tumors and heart ailments. It is said that garlic was eaten by laborers who built the pyramids of Egypt, Roman solders on long marches and in battle (they believed that it was the herb of Mars, the Roman God of War), and the Israelites before their escape from Egypt in order to keep up their strength. In India, garlic was used to wash wounds and ulcers.

Pliny the Elder (484-475 B.C.) stated: "Garlic has powerful properties, and is of great benefit against changes in water and residence." He recommended garlic for poisonous snakebites, intestinal parasites, asthma and as a cough suppressant.

In Marseilles during the plagues of 1772, garlic was the main ingredient of "Four Thieves Vinegar" used for protection against the plague. It is said that four thieves confessed that they were protected by a liberal use of the "vinegar" when plundering the dead victims of the plague. European legend says that if a man chews a garlic bulb during a foot race, no one will be able to pass him. Long considered to have power to ward off evil, garlic is still used today by the Chinese, Arabs and Egyptians for that purpose.

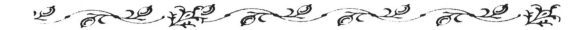

In 1858, Louis Pasteur experimentally confirmed the anti-bacterial activity of garlic. During World War I and II, many doctors daubed garlic juice on sterilized sphagnum moss and applied it to infected wounds to prevent septic poisoning and gangrene.

Garlic is a perennial plant, native to Asia west of the Himalayas, that has been used for eons as a stimulant, carminative, diuretic, expectorant for bronchitis, antiseptic, diaphoretic, cold syrup, for infantile catarrh, abscesses, earaches, insect and serpent wounds, intestinal complaints, diarrhea, hysteria, pimples and many others. Garlic has also been used, internally and externally, to prevent and arrest tumors, to kill intestinal worms, to cure sinus infections, as an arthritic painkiller, to normalize blood pressure, to stimulate the growth of healthy bacteria in the system, for toothaches, to prevent or cure colds and when hung about the house, to keep out vampires.

Garlic contains the active components calcium, iron, vitamins A, C and B-complex, folic acid, iodine, potassium, a pungent volatile oil with ajoene and the sulfuric compounds diallyl disulfide, diallyltrisulfide and allilin. Herbalists recommend using fresh or dried bulbs eaten or made into a tea, syrup or tincture, as a diaphoretic, anti-bacterial, anti-fungal, diuretic, expectorant, weak anthelmintic, chloretic and stimulant for intestinal infections, hypertension, colds, flu, fever, earache, respiratory disorders and sinus congestion. Garlic is also excellent for stimulating bile secretion, therapeutic prevention of arteriosclerosis, lowering blood lipid and cholesterol levels, to increase arterial blood flow, catarrh and rhinitis. To make the syrup, simmer ten garlic cloves in one pint of milk, add honey to taste. Take the syrup in one tablespoon doses as needed. It is especially good for coughs.

Studies have shown that garlic is an excellent diuretic and does lower blood pressure and serum cholesterol. Research has also shown that ajoene (formed by combining allicin and diallyl-disulfide) and allilin (which breaks down into the pungent allicin and diallyldisulphides when the cell tissue is damaged and is responsible for garlic's characteristic odor) are natural antibiotic and anti-fungal agents. They destroy or inhibit *Staphlococcus* and *Streptococcus* bacteria, the organisms responsible for cholera, typhus, dysentery, enteritis and yeast.

In China, garlic is used for treating digestive difficulties, diarrhea, dysentery, colds, whooping cough, pinworms, old ulcers, swellings and snakebites.

Excessive use of fresh garlic may dull the sight, cause flatulence, injure the stomach and induce thirst.

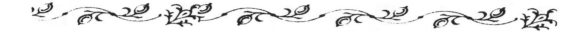

Henbane
Hyoscyamus niger L.

Henbane was mentioned in the Arabian tale *One Thousand and One Nights*. The guards were drugged by someone who cast henbane leaves into the fire. Henbane was recommended by Dioscorides as a sleep aid and to allay pains. Henbane was smoked by the magician of a black mass during the Middle Ages in order to work up his fury and his magicianship.

Henbane contains the active components the choline, mucilage, calcium oxalate, alkaloids scopolamine, hyoscyamine, atropine and hyoscine, the bitter glucoside hyoscytricin and potassium nitrate. Herbalists recommend using an infusion as an antispasmodic, hypnotic and mild diuretic. Applied to the eyes, the infusion dilates the pupils and aids in curing internal inflammation. The oil of henbane is often included in anti-rheumatic ointments and liniments. It has also been used in the treatment of Parkinson's disease.

Scopolamine, extracted in alcohol, is used as a tincture to kill pain, to treat asthma, relieve muscle spasms and nervous, irritable conditions, and to relieve the griping caused by excessive vomiting. It is also substituted for opium in bath herbs to cause sleep. Hyoscamine which affects the central nervous system, tends to check secretion and to relax spasms of the involuntary muscles. The narcotic effect of hyoscine has a slight somnifacient action, and lessens spasm pains in unstriated muscles, lead colic and cystitis.

Henbane is a narcotic and a slight stimulant that is poisonous to pigs and chickens but seems to be tolerated by cows, horses, dogs and goats. It was listed as an official medicine in the British Pharmacopoeia as a sedative and analgesic for depressing the brain and producing drowsiness.

Henbane is a strong narcotic and should never be used for self-medication without supervision from a qualified medical or herbal practitioner.

Lavender
Lavandula sp.

In the Middle Ages, lavender was considered to be a herb of love, both as an aphrodisiac and for chastity. Perfume of lavender was used by the Romans in their baths and to fumigate a room in preparation for childbirth, serving to promote the menses and expel the afterbirth. Lavender oil was used as a powerful antiseptic to dress wounds in World War II when commercial sterilizers were in short supply.

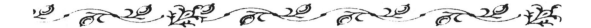

Lavender contains the active components tannin, the coumarins coumarin, hemiarin, pinene, limonene and umbelliferone, flavonoids, a volatile oil with laveneulyl acetate, triterpenoids, camphor, borneol, linalyl acetate, linabool, terpinenol and cineole. Herbalists recommend using a flower or flowering stem infusion as an antispasmodic, carminative, rubefacient, mild sedative, and tonic for headaches, flatulence, nausea, nervous disorders, insomnia and coughs. Externally, the infusion is an excellent wash for acne to normalize the sebaceous glands, to soothe painful sore feet and as douche to treat leucorrhea.

Oil of lavender, obtained by steam distillation, has aromatic, sedative, stimulant, antiseptic, anti-bacterial and carminative properties. Herbalists have traditionally used the oil to suppress and kill the bacterium that cause diphtheria and typhoid. Lavender oil is one of the best reme dies for eczema and psoriasis, burns, stings and cuts due to its strong antibacterial action. It is also used to treat rheumatism, respiratory ailments and as a sedative to treat nervous headaches, stomachaches and high blood pressure. The essential oil is used in therapeutic baths to reduce nervousness. A few drops of the oil is an effective insect repellent. The oil is used commercially in fine perfumes, soaps, toilet articles, cosmetics and to mask unpleasant odors in medicines.

Maize - Corn
Stigmata mirdis or *Zea mays* L.

Native to tropical Central America, the Mayan Indians used maize (corn), soaked in water, for treating bloody urine. The Zuni Indians of New Mexico used corn pollen for treating heart palpitations and dried corn for treating pneumonia. They also used corn smut (*Ustilago zeae*, a fungus that grows on corn cobs) in a tea to ease labor, parturition and post-partum hemorrhage and in a compress to treat sore throats.

Maize contains the active components saponin, a fatty oil, a volatile oil, glycosides, alkaloids, vitamin C and K, allantoin, potassium, calcium, tannins, sugars and resin. Herbalists recommend using an infusion of corn silks collected before pollination, or seed oil as a cardiotonic, cholagogic and diuretic. An infusion made with the silks is used for many urinary problems including bedwetting in the elderly and young, urinary tract infections, the passage of urinary stones, treatment of gonorrhea, and as a soothing enema. French herbalists use corn silk to thin bile and to promote its flow.

The seed oil (corn oil) also contains allantoin and is an excellent health food for treating arteriosclerosis and high blood pressure.

Studies have confirmed that corn extracts do have diuretic and cardiotonic properties. Chinese research indicates that corn silks do increase bile output.

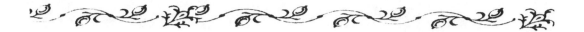

Onion
Allium cepa L.

Onion was cultivated as a vegetable and medicinal plant in Mesopotamia, India and Egypt. It was depicted on Egyptian tomb paintings. The Greeks and Romans praised its healing properties but damned its odor. Alexander the Great fed onions to his troops to give them strength in battle. A southern Black slave used the juice of red onions and horsemint to dissolve his master's kidney stone. For this deed, he was given his freedom.

Onions contain the active components sugar, vitamins, mineral, organic sulfur-containing compounds which are excellent antiseptics, and essential oils. Herbalists recommend using the fresh bulbs as an anthelmintic, choleric, diuretic, expectorant, hypoglycemic, hypotensive and stomachic. Onions have been a popular remedy for treating coughs, bronchitis, common colds and other infections of the respiratory passages and the digestive system. An onion diet seems to reduce cholesterol and increase the production of high-density lipoprotein which clears the arteries of fatty deposits.

Crushed fresh onion can be applied to insect bites and boils. A paste made from fresh onions is used to prevent infections in wounds and burns, and to inhibit blood clotting.

Oregano
Origanum vulgare L.

The Romans and Greeks used wild oregano as a tonic to strengthen the brain, and to cleanse and revive the system. A powder mixed with honey was used to remove bruises. An ointment made from the oil was used to relieve the pains of sore joints and arthritis. The ancient Roman scholar Pliny recommended using a poultice of oregano for treating scorpion and spider bites. Culpeper recommended oregano for relieving appetite loss, coughs and consumption, urine retention, delayed menstruation, dropsy, scurvy and yellow jaundice. He also recommended using the essential oil on a cotton ball to relieve toothaches and earaches.

In early America, oregano was used in a tea as a stimulant and carminative for chronic coughs and asthma. Doctors used oil of oregano for treating toothaches, rheumatic limbs and sprains.

Oregano contains the active components, tannin, an essential oil with thymol, origanene, carvacrol and bitter compounds. Herbalists recommend using a flower and/or leaf infusion as an antiseptic, antispasmodic, astringent, carminative, diaphoretic, expectorant, stomachic

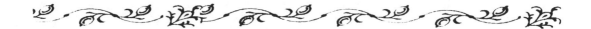

and mild tonic for stomach and gall bladder disorders, diarrhea, coughs, asthma, nervous headache, general exhaustion, flatulence and menstrual pain.

Externally, oregano is used in gargles, bath preparations, liniments and inhalants. A strong infusion will ease the discomfort of earaches. Oregano oil aids aching teeth and the surrounding gums (in an emergency, try chewing some fresh leaves). For glossy hair, try massaging the scalp after shampooing with a strong infusion. A muslin bag of oregano leaves in a steaming bath is recommended for relieving aches and stiff joints.

Oregano is a culinary herb that is used in soups, salads, sauces and many meat dishes throughout the world. Marjoram (*O. onites*) and sweet marjoram (*O. marjorama*) have a scent and flavor similar to oregano. They are both used for the same culinary and medicinal purposes as is oregano.

Parsley
Petroselinum crispum (Mill.) Nym.

The Romans seem to have been the first to use parsley as a food. The Romans used it at orgies to cover the smell of alcohol on the breath and to aid digestion. The use of parsley as a medicinal and sacred plant dates from ancient Greek times. In ancient Greece, parsley was used in funeral ceremonies, probably to cover the odor. Parsley was placed in wreaths given to winning athletes because the Greeks believed that Hercules had chosen parsley for his garlands. In Greek mythology, parsley was a sacred herb that sprang up where the blood of Archemorus the Hero was spilled when he was eaten by serpents.

By the Middle Ages, parsley made its appearance into herbal medicine. It was said to be a key to comfort and cleanse the stomach, liver, kidneys, spleen and intestines. It was also used for treating asthma, dropsy, jaundice and female problems.

Parsley contains the active components iron, iodine, manganese, copper, the flavonoid glycosides myristicin and apin, large quantities of vitamins A, B and C, an essential oil with apiolin, apiol and pinene. Herbalists recommend using an infusion as a carminative, strong diuretic, emmenagogue and stomachic to stimulate the appetite, aid indigestion, regulate menstrual flow, and alleviate kidney and bladder disorders. Doctors still continue to prescribe parsley tea for young females with bladder problems.

Crushed leaves or juice from the roots heals or reduces the swelling of wounds and sprains and relieves itching insect bites. A cup of parsley tea sipped regularly will help ease the discomfort of hemorrhoids. A cold infusion of freshly-picked and crushed parsley leaves applied to the eyes,

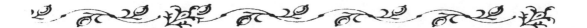

will help clear bloodshot eyes. Parsley oil is used in cosmetics, shampoo, perfumes, soap, creams and skin lotions.

Parsley oil in large amounts may be toxic, causing a decrease in blood pressure and pulse rate, followed by muscle weakness and paralysis, lung congestion and swelling of the liver. Pregnant women should avoid parsley oil and refrain from eating large quantities of parsley. Very strong doses can be toxic, causing hemorrhage and nervous disorders. The essential oil obtained by steam distillation from ripe fruits (parsley seed oil) should be used only under strict medical supervision.

Peony
Paeonia officinalis L.

Named after Paion, a physician of ancient Greece, peony has a long history of medical use. There are many superstitions connected with the plant. In ancient times, it was thought to be of divine origin. Later, the seeds were believed to ward off evil spirits. In the Middle Ages, peony was thought to guard the home against storms and devils. The peony seeds were ground to a powder and taken in the morning and at night to ward off nightmares and melancholy dreams. It was also a custom to wear a chain of beads cut from peony roots as a protection against all sorts of illness and injury, to assist children in teething and as a remedy for insanity.

The American Indians used a tea of the root for lung troubles, for cleansing the uterus and as a general tonic.

Peony contains the active components tannin, glycosides, the alkaloid peragrinine, asparagin, sugars, mucilage and the anthocyanidin pigment paeonidin (found only in the flowers). Herbalists recommend using an infusion as an antispasmodic, diuretic, emmenagogue, sedative and vasoconstrictive. Peony was once used internally to relieve spasms of the smooth muscles, asthmatic attacks, epileptic seizures, gout, kidney stones, hemorrhoids and as an abortifacient. Peony is now rarely used by western herbalist, but remains popular in Chinese medicine.

All parts of the plant are poisonous, especially the flowers, and should be used only under strict medical supervision.

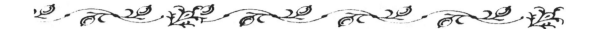

Pepper
Capsicum sp.

The American Indians began cultivating the various pepper species long before the settlers came to America. They used peppers medicinally and as an excellent source of nutrition. The Spaniards, in the sixteenth century, introduced peppers to Europe.

The fruits of the mild sweet pepper varieties are green when young and turn red or yellow when ripe. An excellent source of vitamin C, sweet peppers are used in salads or eaten raw (perhaps accompanied by a sour cream dip). The dried, powdered red berries of this plant produce the spice known as paprika. Chili powder comes from ground berries of another variety.

Cayenne peppers (*Capsicum frutescens*) with its long, hot, pungent red fruits, are preferred for medicinal preparations. The dried fruits containing the oily, irritant capsaicin (used in "self-defense" pepper sprays), carotenoids, vitamins B_1, B_2, C and E and fats, are used as an astringent, digestive stimulant and a major circulatory stimulant. The peppers, eaten raw or cooked, ease flatulence and relieve stomach and intestinal pains. Cayenne peppers, eaten raw or powdered, are an excellent remedy for warding-off chills, particularly at the onset of a cold, by causing profuse sweating. They also support the body's defense system, due in part to their anti-bacterial properties and large quantities of vitamin C. Cayenne powder is a powerful local stimulant that is used externally in extracts, tinctures, ointments and plasters as a counter-irritant to improve blood flow in the skin and mucosa in the treatment of muscle pains, arthritis, sciatica, unbroken chilblains, pleurisy, neuralgia and lumbago. A pill prepared from cayenne powder stimulates circulation by influencing the heart action first, followed by the arteries and capillaries and finally the nerves. Equal parts of tincture of capsicum (obtainable from a herbalist) and glycerin, shaken together, is excellent for relieving the pain of arthritic joints.

Excessive consumption of cayenne peppers may cause digestive, liver or kidney disorders.

Peppermint-Spearmint
Mentha piperita and M. *spicata*

The Romans used mints as a specific scent for the arms (deodorant) and as crowns during various ceremonies. The Roman scholar Pliny thought that mint was the loveliest of herbs. The Greeks used mints in herbal treatments and temple rites, while the Pharisees paid their tithes with mint.

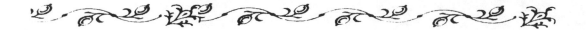

American Indians used a leaf tea for treating cholera, colds, colic, cramps, dyspepsia, fever, gravel, headaches, hysteria, upset stomachs and pneumonia.

Mentha species contain the active components tannin, rosmarinic acid, carotenoids, betaine, choline, flavonoids, vitamins (B, C and E), bitter compounds, a volatile oil with menthol, menthone, limonene, pulegone, cinole, bisabole, isomenthol, neomenthol and azulene. Herbalists recommend using a leaf (free of mint rust, *Puccina menthiae*) infusion as an anti-bacterial, anti-parasitic, carminative, chologogue, mild antispasmodic, expectorant, local anesthetic and stomachic. An infusion is used to treat respiratory infections, digestive and gall bladder disorders, diarrhea, flatulence and abdominal spasms and stimulate the appetite. Peppermint is the mint of choice for dyspeptic adults, good for nausea and diarrhea; spearmint is milder and more beneficial for children. Peppermint-spearmint leaves are used in proprietary medicines.

Studies have shown that menthol, an antibacterial and antiparasitic agent, is an effective agent against *Herpes simplex* and other viruses. Menthol also has an antispasmodic affect on the smooth muscles of the digestive system, which makes it an effective remedy for colic and flatulence. The flavenoids stimulate the liver and gallbladder, increasing bile flow. Azulene has anti-inflammatory and ulcer healing effects.

Fresh leaves make a refreshing tea substitute and addition to various foods for flavoring. They are also used in potpourris and bath herbs. Mint oils have a characteristic agreeable odor and powerful taste that leave a sensation of coolness when air is drawn in. The oils also have antibacterial properties and are used in dental creams, mouth washes, toothpaste, cough drops, chewing gum, pharmaceutical preparations, liqueurs and confectionery and rheumatic ointments.

Inhalation of the herb or oil is effective against excessive respiratory mucous. *However, prolonged usage of the inhalant may damage the nasal and sinus mucous membranes, and should never be used for babies or very young children. The mint oils are toxic if taken internally and prolonged external usage may cause dermatitis.*

Pot Marigold
Calendula officinalis L.

Pot marigold is an annual herb that has been grown in gardens since the Middle Ages for their bright orange or yellow flowers; some have sweetly scented foliage while others have a strong rank scent. Gypsies used the flowers in ointments for treating sprains, wounds and skin problems. Pot marigold, believed to have many magical properties, was one of the necessary ingredients in

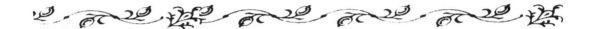

potions used to see the fairies. Pot marigold was also used for treating fevers, ear inflammations, chronic ulcers, varicose veins and as an emetic. The flowers were used in bath-herb mixtures as a diaphoretic to induce fevers and as a hair rinse to bring out highlights for blondes and brunettes. During the Civil War, the petals were often used in compresses to staunch wounds.

Pot marigold contains the active components mucilage, an essential oil, carotenoids, saponins, flavonoid glycosides and resin. Herbalists recommend using the deep orange flowers in an infusion as an anti-bacterial, anti-fungal, diaphoretic, emmenagogue and stimulant to relieve painful menstruation and to bring on delayed periods. The infusion is excellent as a gargle after tooth extraction and to cure thrush (*Candida albicans*). It is also used externally in extracts, tinctures, ointments, complexion creams and lotions to cleanse, soothe and heal stubborn wounds, inflamed or ulcerated sores, bed sores, persistent ulcers, varicose veins, bruises, skin rashes, burns, scalds, stings and impetigo.

Studies have shown that a pot marigold tincture is as effective as bleach in killing germs, without being as harsh or irritating to the skin.

Pot marigold should be avoided during pregnancy due to its emmenagogic properties.

Pumpkin
Cucurbita pepo L.

Pumpkin is native to Central America, where it has been cultivated for over a thousand years. Pumpkin seeds have been a popular folk remedy for expelling worms and treating urinary complaints. Gypsies ate the seeds daily to prevent a decrease in masculine vigor and to preserve male potency.

Pumpkin contains the active components resin, fatty oils, proteins, the glycoside cucurbitin, vitamins and minerals. Herbalists recommend using the seeds or the juice as a catarrh, demulcent and anthelmintic. Pumpkin juice, a mild diuretic, is recommended for urinary complaints.

Recent research has shown that pumpkin seeds have anti-tumor properties, in particular, for treating an enlarged prostate.

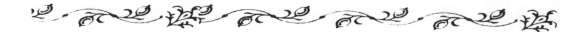

Rose
Rosa sp.

In the Middle Ages, a preparation of roses was eaten for treating respiratory ailments, gonorrhea, soreness of the bladder and to purge the body of toxins. Roger Bacon, the thirteenth century English philosopher, used this same preparation as a soothing, refreshing drink. The preparation was also used as a vaginal douche for menstrual complaints, a wash for ulcers and sores of the mouth, ears and anus, and as an ointment for chapped hands and lips.

American Indians used roses for ornaments and for health care long before the settlers arrived. They also combined the powdered petals with bear grease to cure mouth sores and blisters. They bathed sore eyes with rainwater-soaked flowers. The inner bark of the roots was applied to boils. Young Indian braves gathered roses for their brides.

The fruits, rosehips, are rich in vitamin A, B, C (richer than oranges), E and K, organic acids, pectin, carotenes, sugars, tannins, malic and citric acids, nicotinamide and fatty oils. Herbalists recommend using a rosehip infusion as a mild laxative, astringent and diuretic. An infusion is used for scurvy, infections, chest congestion, bladder ailments, to combat stress and diarrhea. Attar of rose or Rose Otto (*Rosa damascena*) is used for rejuvenating and regulating the menstrual cycle. In Britain, a syrup made from the rosehips of the Wild of Dog Rose (*Rosa canina*) is an excellent remedy for treating sore throats, colds and coughs. Rose petals are used in tonics and gargles to cure catarrhs, sore throats, mouth sores and stomach disorders. Rose flower wash is used as a hydrating agent for young-looking skin. Soothing, cooling rose oil is inhaled as a sleep aid and rubbed on the temples to relieve headache and mental stress. The roots of rose bushes are also used in teas for their astringent properties. Chinese herbalists use rose flowers to regulate vital energy and to treat poor circulation, liver pains, stomachaches, mastitis, dysentery and vaginal infections.

Rosemary
Rosmarinus officinalis L

Native to the Mediterranean, rosemary has been used as a culinary and medicinal herb since ancient Greek and Roman times. Rosemary, considered the herb of remembrance and fidelity, was used to strengthen the memory. At exam time, students intertwined rosemary in their hair or rubbed rosemary oils onto the forehead or temples in order to insure good marks.

In 1525, *Branches' Herbal* (the first book devoted exclusively to herbs) stated that rosemary teas were greatly valued against all manner of evils in the body. The famous "Hungary Water" made

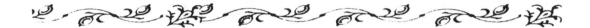

from rosemary oil and alcohol was concocted by a hermit for Queen Elizabeth of Hungary. He supposedly cured her paralysis of the joints by rubbing the concoction on them. During the fourteenth and fifteenth centuries, rosemary branches were burned in homes to keep away black death. During World War II, a mixture of rosemary leaves and juniper berries were burned in the hospitals of France to kill germs.

Herbal physicians prescribed an infusion of rosemary leaves for the treatment of depression, headaches and muscle spasms. Externally, an ointment made from oil of rosemary was reputed to benefit rheumatism, sores, eczema, bruises and wounds.

Rosemary contains the active components tannin, monoterpene hydrocarbon, saponin, the flavonoids diosnin and rosmanicine phenolic acids, carnoesic acid, triterpenic acid and a volatile oil with cincole, linalool, verbenol camphore and borneal. Herbalists recommend using a leaf and/or young shoot tea as an antiseptic, antispasmodic, aromatic, cholagogue, diuretic, rubefacient, sedative and tonic. A rosemary tea aids the stomach, liver and gallbladder, improves circulation, and at bedtime calms the nerves and induces sleep. Externally, the dried herb and rosemary oil are components of anti-rheumatic liniments, skin tonics, hair conditioners, herbal bath preparations, disinfectants and are used extensively in perfumes.

Studies have shown that as rosmanicine breaks down in the body it stimulates the smooth muscles of the digestive tract and gallbladder. The flavonoid diosnin improves circulation by strengthening fragile blood vessels.

Rosemary oil should never be taken internally. Very strong doses can irritate the stomach, intestine and kidneys.

Saffron
Crocus sativus L.

Saffron has been cultivated and highly valued in the Middle East for at least four thousand years as an aromatic flavoring, perfume, dye, medicine and aphrodisiac. It has been so prized that at times it has been worth its weight in gold. Saffron was mentioned in the Bible in the Song of Solomon. It was used as a royal dye, in scented salves and thrown about early Greek halls and courts and in the Roman baths. It became so popular that it was appropriated by the hetaerae (professional female entertainers of that time). It takes about seventy-five thousand flowers to make one pound of saffron. Because it was so expensive, its use was usually limited to flavoring certain dishes. It was also used medicinally as a carminative, diaphoretic, anodyne and to treat women's menstrual complaints.

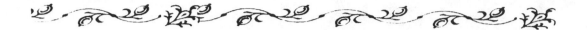

Saffron contains the active components the bitter glycoside picrocrocine, a series of crocine glycosides, an essential oil containing colchicum and trepenes. Herbalists recommend using the stigma in an infusion as an antispasmodic, carminative, diaphoretic, emmenagogue and stomachic. An infusion is used to stimulate menstruation, ease painful periods, treat gout and arthritis.

Research has shown that colchicum has anti-cancer properties. Drugs derived from colchicum were the first to be used effectively against leukemia.

Saffron is a powerful medicine not suitable for self medication; large doses can cause hemorrhage, vomiting, diarrhea and vertigo. Use only under the strict supervision of a qualified medical or herbal practitioner.

Sage
Salvia officinalis L.

The Romans used sage in their baths as a specific to ease aching muscles and sore, tired feet. Since the early eighteenth century, sage has been used to disguise the flavor of slightly putrefying meat when there was no other way of keeping food. Sage tea was drank for treating running of the reins (a nice medieval term for discharge from the penis), to bring on a menstrual cycle and to expel the afterbirth.

Sage contains the active components tannin, oestrogenic substances, carnoesic acid, phenolic acid, the bitter compounds salvin and picroslavin, resin, terpene, a volatile oil with thujone, borneol, cineole, linalool, pinine and camphor. Herbalists recommend using a leaf infusion as an anti-bacterial, anti-diaphoretic, anti-fungal, antiseptic, antispasmodic, astringent, carminative and diuretic for stomach and intestinal ailments, hot flashes during menopause, painful periods, and to dry the flow of breast milk in nursing mothers. It is also excellent for lowering blood sugar in diabetics and as a general tonic for promoting a long and healthy life.

A bunch of fresh sage leaves tied together and held under hot running tap water, washes healing oils into the water giving relief to rheumatic suffers and soothing dry, itchy skin. A few sage leaves rubbed gently on the teeth will remove plaque, help clear stains and stimulate the gums. An infusion of sage and Chinese tea will help restore the natural color to graying hair. Sage tea, with small amounts of cider vinegar, is an excellent gargle for sore throats, laryngitis and tonsillitis. The essential oil is used by the pharmaceutical, perfumery, liquor and food industries.

Research has shown that phenolic acid is anti-bacterial, especially against *Staphlococcus aureus*, and that thujone is a strong antiseptic.

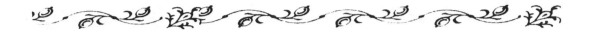

Sage should not be taken in large doses for a long period because of the thujone it contains. Thujone is potentially damaging to the central nervous system and may cause dermatitis if taken in large doses or for a prolonged period of time.

Scented Mayweed
Matricaria chamomile L. - German chamomile

Scented mayweed is often confused with Roman chamomile, but botanically it is not a true chamomile, and scented mayweed is the preferred name. It is one of the most widely used herbal medicines, particularly for children's ailments. In herbal medicine, an infusion is used for colds influenza, insomnia and "nerves." Externally, scented mayweed is used in compresses, bath preparations and for eye and mouth washes.

Scented mayweed contains the active components fatty acids, the coumarin umbeliferone, salicylate derivatives, choline, polysaccharides, tannin, the flavonoids rutin, mertrin and quercimetrin, cyanogenic and coumarin glycosides, valerianic acid mucilage, an essential oil with chamazulene, bisabolol and farnescene. Herbalists recommend using a flowerhead tea as an anti-inflammatory, antiseptic, antispasmodic, carminative, diaphoretic and sedative. The tea is excellent for relaxing restless or hyperactive children and in small amounts for teething babies. It is a traditional remedy for treating upset stomachs, flatulence, heartburn and diarrhea.

German chamomile oil, derived from the wild plants, is used externally to treat dental caries, in the ear canal for pain, as a rub for hard swellings and pains in the joints. According to the Egyptians, a simple way to make chamomile oil is to take fresh (preferably) or dried flowers and beat them up with pure olive oil, steep the flowers in the oil for twenty-four hours and then strain. This oil can be used to rub over the body of a person afflicted with ague or rheumatism or for massaging overstrained or cramped muscles. The person should then be put to bed, covered very warmly, and left to sweat the soreness away in a manner similar to steaming in a sweat or sauna bath.

Studies have shown that chamazulene, a component of azulene, is a powerful antibiotic and antiseptic. Chamazulene, an anti-inflammatory and anti-spasmodic, encourages wound healing, acts on the smooth muscles of the intestine and uterus to relax spasms, and is effective against *Staphlococcus aureus*. Bisabolol, an anti-microbial, speeds up the healing of ulcers and prevents them from occurring. Belliferone (an anti-fungal) plus chamazulene is effective against thrush, *Candida albicans*.

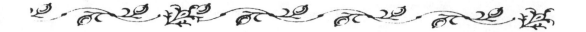

Scotch Pine
Pinus sylvestris L.

Scotch pine contains the active components fatty acids, resin, an essential oil with bornyl acetate and large amounts of vitamin C. Herbalists recommend using the young, fresh shoots in an infusion as an antiseptic, diuretic, expectorant and rubefacient for dropsy, rheumatic afflictions, liver and kidney ailments. Externally, the infusion is used in inhalant mixtures for treating coughs, bronchitis, asthma and other respiratory disorders. The infusion is also used in bath preparations, and in poultices for treating rheumatism, rashes and ulcerous conditions. Resin extracts of Scotch pine (spirits of turpentine) are used in liniments and plasters for treating rheumatic and arthritic pain, strained muscles and frostbite.

Large doses or prolonged usage are potentially harmful and may irritate the kidneys.

Sunflower
Helianthus sp.

Sunflower is a native of North America, where it was first cultivated by American Indians some time before 1000 B.C. Spanish conquerors of Central and South American civilizations found the plant was holy to the sun worshippers of Peru and used in religious ceremonies. Reproduc-tions of sunflowers, sculpted in pure gold, were placed in many temples. The priestesses in the temples of the sun were crowned with sunflowers and carried them in their hands.

The Spaniards took the seeds to Old World in the sixteenth century and from there sunflowers spread across Europe. However, it did not become a regular food plant until it reached Russia. Some Russians are said to eat the seeds daily to preserve male potency

The Indians of North America used the sunflower seeds for food and as source of oil.
The Indians used the oil as a hair grease and as a warm rub for rheumatic parts. They used the flowerheads as a diuretic, carminative, anti-inflammatory and anti-diarrheal in an infusion or tea. Dakota, Meskquakie and Potawatomi Indians used the roots baked or in a tea for respiratory ailments, rheumatism, bruises, contusions, snakebites and for malaria. The astringent leaves were used in herbal tobaccos, powdered or in an ointment to treat sores, blisters and swellings.

High in vitamin B and a high-quality protein, the seeds are eaten as a food, and yield an oil containing glycerides of unsaturated linolenic and oleic acids, saturated palmitic and arachic acids. The oil contains about eighty percent polyunsaturates, which reduce the cholesterol

298

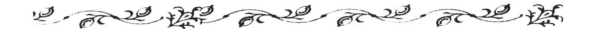

level in the blood. The oil is used in salves, plasters, and liniments for rheumatic pain. The leaves are used for fodder, the flowers for their yellow dye. In homeopathy, a tincture from the seeds is used internally to relieve constipation, and externally on cuts and bruises.

Sweet Violet
Viola odorata L.

Violets were used by ancient Athenians "to moderate anger," to induce sleep and to strengthen the heart. Pliny prescribed a liniment of violet and vinegar for gout and disorders of the spleen. He also recommended that a garland of violets worn about the head would dispel the fumes of wine, preventing headache and dizziness.

The Cherokee used the roots of various violet species as a poultice for boils. They used a decoction for treating coughs, dysentery, constipation and general debility. The decoction was sprayed in the nostrils for catarrh. The leaves were bound to the head to relieve headaches.

Syrup of violet (the flowers in honey or sugar) is a mild laxative and is used as a coloring or flavoring agent in other medicines. The syrup was also used to treat epilepsy, inflammation of the eyes, pleurisy and jaundice. Gerard stated that "it has the power to ease inflammation, roughness of the throat and comforteth the heart, assuageth the pains of the head and causeth sleep."

Sweet violet contains the active components saponin, mucilage, the aromatic essential oil myrosin, the glycoside violarutin, methyl salicylate, vitamin A and C and in the flowers, anthocyanin. Herbalists recommend using a leaf, flower and/or rhizome infusion as an antiseptic, diuretic, expectorant and mild sedative for bronchitis, whooping cough, head colds and rheumatic pain. Fresh leaves infused in fresh water for twelve hours and drank daily or applied in a poultice over a period of time is reported to be an old folk remedy for curing cancer. A strong infusion of the rhizomes is used as an emetic and purgative. Externally, sweet violets are included in mouth washes and gargles, and in compresses for swellings, slow-healing wounds, ulcers and rashes. When fresh flowers are inhaled, it is said that the smell eases the pains of a headache caused by lack of sleep. The many garden varieties of violet with their large, unscented flowers are not used medicinally.

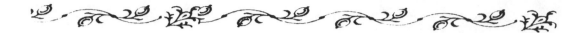

Tarragon
Artemisia dracunculus L.

Tarragon was named after Artemis, the Greek goddess of hunting and of virginity, although some forms were used to induce abortions. The species name, dracunculus, means "small dragon." The long thin leaves were seen as tiny dragons' tongues.

Tarragon contains the active components rutin, an essential oil with estragale and phelladrene, a bitter compound and tannins. Herbalists recommend using a flowering stem infusion as an anthelmintic, anti-inflammatory, carminative, diuretic, emmenagogue, a general tonic, mild sedative, stimulant and vermifuge. Tarragon vinegar (fresh leaves infused in white vinegar overnight and strained for use) stimulates the appetite and digestive processes. This mild medicinal is also used as an herb to flavor food and to aid digestion. The distilled essential oil is used in the manufacture of some toilet preparations.

Studies have shown that rutin is a cancer-preventive, diuretic and anti-inflammatory that also decreases capillary permeability, fragility and hypertension.

Thyme
Thymus vulgaris L.

The antiseptic and preservative properties of thyme were known to the ancient Egyptians who used the oil for embalming. The Romans valued the oil for its antiseptic properties, using it as an antidote for headaches and depression. They also burned it as incense in their temples. In the Middle Ages, knights wore a sprig of thyme as a symbol of strength and courage, believing it to be a source of strength. Thyme was also used in the Middle Ages to treat women's problems: to induce the menses, increase and soothe urination and to provoke abortion. The leaves were slept on or inhaled for melancholy diseases and for epileptics.

This low-growing bush with small, bright, glossy green leaves is easily grown in an apartment as a potted plant. It is also an excellent plant outdoors as bees love it and the honey produced is particularly healthful.

Thyme contains the active components saponin, tannins, bitter components, organic acid, an essential oil with thymol, terpinene, linalool, phenol and carvacrol. Herbalists recommend using a flower tea as an anthelmintic, antiseptic, antispasmodic, carminative, deodorant and expectorant for headaches and respiratory ailments. The tea is also an excellent remedy for treating sore throats and infected gums. The hot tea is sweat-inducing and very effective against the common

300

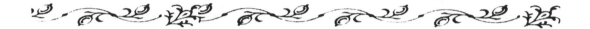

cold. The volatile oil is partially excreted through the lungs, and therefore, is an excellent remedy for bronchitis and whooping cough.

Externally, an infusion is used as a wash for scabies, gout, rheumatism, insect bites, eczema and as soothing skin tonic. An ointment made from thyme is used to treat shingles (*Herpes zoster*). The dried leaves and flowers are an excellent addition to potpourris or a herb cushion. Tied in a muslin bag, sprigs of thyme, fresh or dried, are added to bath water for a refreshing perfumed bath.

Thyme oil, with its powerful anti-bacterial and anti-fungal properties, is used as an antiseptic, antipyretic, deodorant, disinfectant, parasiticide, rubefacient, stimulant and vermifuge for treating muscular aches and congested mucous membranes. The distilled essential oil is used in pharmaceutical, cosmetic and food industries in dentifrices, mouth washes, hair tonics, cough drops, ointments to remove warts and relieve swollen testicles and as a specific for hookworm.

The herb tea is safe to consume, except during pregnancy. The isolated volatile oil is toxic in any quantity and should be used internally only under the strict supervision of a qualified medical or herbal practitioner.

Valerian
Valeriana officinilis L.

According to Culpeper, valerian was an important remedy that was effective as a nervine tonic. The dried, powdered roots in an infusion or tincture, were used to induce sleep, ease pain and as a tranquilizer without any side effects. Culpeper recommended using valerian in all cases of neuralgia.

Presently, valerian is a leading over-the-counter tranquilizer throughout Europe. The rhizomes and roots of second year plants are used in an infusion as a sedative, hypnotic and antispasmodic. They are included in pharmaceutical preparations prescribed for nervous heart disorders, convulsions, nervous dyspepsia, depression and chronic insomnia. Cats are said to be as attracted to the root as they are to catmint. Some people also use the roots as a rat poison.

Valerian contains the active components choline, tannins, resins, the valepotriate valtrate, the glycoside valerosidatum, a volatile oil with limonene, sesquiterpene, valerian camphor, chatinine, valerianine, actinidine, valerian and esters of acetic-, butyric, and isovaleranic acids, which upon drying yield isovaleranic acid. Isovaleranic acid gives valerian its characteristic smell. Herbalists recommend using a root infusion as an antispasmodic, calmative and nerve tonic for hypochondria, nervous headaches, irritability, depression and insomnia.

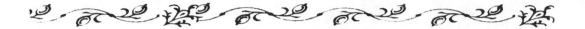

Research has shown that valerian tea, tincture and/or extracts are central nervous system depressants. Valerian acts as an antispasmodic and sedative when agitation is present. It also acts as an anti-bacterial, anti-diuretic, a stimulant when fatigued and is a liver protectant. Valerian does not interfere with the sleep cycle when taken for insomnia.

Valerian may be addictive in large doses or when taken for a prolonged period. Headaches, muscle spasms, palpitations, visual illusions, giddiness and restlessness may also occur. Always consult a qualified medical or herbal practitioner before using valerian.

Wild Plum
Prunus americana Marsh.

The Cherokee, Chippewa, Fox, Omaha, Meskquakie, Mohegan and Omaha Indians used the bark of wild plum in a decoction for treating intestinal parasites, bladder and kidney ailments, upset stomachs, diarrhea and asthma. The decoction was also used as a wash to treat wounds and canker sores.

Wild plum contains the active components phloretin, beta carotene, potassium, phosphorus, B-complex and vitamin C. Herbalists recommend using wild plum as an antiseptic, laxative and astringent. Fresh or dried plums (prunes), eaten raw or cooked, are an excellent laxative. The inner bark and twigs in a decoction is an excellent folk remedy for treating mouth sores and sore throats.

Research has shown that phloretin is an active anti-bacterial agent against both gram positive and negative bacteria.

Appendix I:
Active Medicinal Components

Component	Action	Plant
Acetylcholine	Anticoagulant	Shepherd's Purse
Achillatin	Anticoagulant	Yarrow
Achilleine	Emmenogogue, hemostat, heart tonic	Yarrow
Actin	Inhibits granular secretion	Jimsonweed
Agropyrone	Broad antibiotic	Quack grass
Ajoene	Anti-bacterial	Garlic, wild garlic
Alantolactone	Anti-bacterial, anti-fungal, antitumor, anthelmintic, hyperglycemic	Elecampane
Allantoin	Cell proliferant of connective tissue, bone and cartilage	Bearberry, borage, comfrey, maize
Allilin	Anti-bacterial, anti-fungal	Garlic, onion, wild garlic
Allylisothiocynate	Counterirritant	Horseradish, shepherd's purse
Apiol	Diuretic, emmenagogue	Celery, parsley
Apocymarin	Antitumor, cardiac tonic	Indian hemp
Arbutin	Diuretic, toxic antiseptic	Bearberry, cramp bark
Aristolochine	Anti-bacterial, anti-cancer, anti-fungal	Virginia snakeroot, wild ginger
Artemisin	Anthelmintic	Mugwort, white sage, wormwood
Asparagin	Diuretic	Asparagus, dandelion, hops, horseradish, Lily-of-the-Valley, peony, Solomon's seal
Atropine	Analgesic, antispasmodic	Jimsonweed
Aucubin	Anti-bacterial	Mullein, plantain, self-heal
Azulene	Anti-bacterial, anti-fungal anti-inflammatory, anti-spasmodic	Bearberry, elecampane, peppermint-spearmint, chamomile, sweet may weed, wormwood, yarrow
Berberine	Anti-bacterial, anti-convulscent, astringent, carminative, choloretic, hemostat, lowers blood pressure	Barberry, bloodroot, blue flag, goldenseal, moonseed, twinleaf

Component	Action	Plant
Betulinol	Anti-cancer (melanoma)	Birch
Bisabolal	Anti-bacterial, anti-fungal, anti-inflammatory	Balm of Gilead, sweet mayweed, peppermint-spearmint
Camphor	Anodyne, antiseptic, carminative, diaphoretic, stimulant	Basil, lavender, rosemary, sage, sassafras
Caryophylene	Anti-inflammatory, anti-viral, immunostimulant	Coneflower
Caulosaponin	Cardiac tonic, uterine stimulant	Blue cohosh
Cedarwood oil	Antiseptic	Red cedar
Chamazulene	Anti-bacterial, anti-fungal, anti-inflammatory, anti-spasmodic	Bearberry, elecampane, peppermint-spearmint, chamomile, sweet mayweed, wormwood, yarrow
Choline	Anticoagulant	Asparagus, chamomile, chickweed, dandelion, fennel, henbane, peppermint-spearmint, scented mayweed, shepherd's purse, valerian, willow
Cimcifugin	Cardiac tonic	Black cohosh
Cineole	Expectorant	Mugwort, peppermint-spearmint, rosemary, sage, spicebush, yarrow
Citronellol	Antiseptic, anthelmintic	Catmint
Colchicum	Anti-cancer (leukemia)	Saffron
Convarallin	Cardiac tonic	Lily-of-the-valley, Solomon's seal
Cymarin	Antitumor	Indian hemp
Digitalis	Cardiac tonic	Foxglove
Diogenin	Estrogenic	Fenugreek, trillium, wild yam
Diosmin	Estrogenic	Rosemary
Echinacin	Anti-inflammatory, anti-viral, immunostimulant	Coneflower
Emodin	Cathartic	Rumex, senna
Eugenol	Analgesic, anti-fungal, antiseptic	Basil
Eupatorin	Anti-cancer	Boneset, Joe-Pye weed, white snakeweed
Fragarine	Oxytecic	Blackberry-raspberry
Ginsenin	Lowers blood sugar	American ginseng
GLA	Cerebral tonic, heart tonic, immunostimulant	Borage, hops, evening primrose

Component	Action	Plant
Humulone	Anti-bacterial, anti-inflammatory, for gastric and duodenal ulcers	Balm of Gilead, coneflower, hops
Inulin	Anti-diabetic	Buckbean, burdock, chicory, coneflower, dandelion, elecampane
Isoquercitrin	Anti-inflammatory	Witch hazel
Isoquinoline	Central nervous system depressant	Dutchman's breeches, moonseed
Juglone	Antiseptic, antitumor, anthelmintic	Butternut, walnut
Kaempferol	Anti-cancer, anti-inflammatory, diuretic	Boneset, clover
Lobeline	Diuretic, expectorant	Indian tobacco
Lobelenin	Expectorant, diuretic, expectorant to resuscitate newborn infants	Indian tobacco
Lupulone	Anti-bacterial, anti-inflammatory for gastric and duodenal ulcers	Hops
Marrubiin	Chloretic, expectorant, heart tonic	Horehound
Menthol	Anti-bacterial, anti-viral (herpes) anthelmintic, antispasmodic	Passion flower, peppermint-spearmint, yarrow
Methylcytine	Expectorant, carminative, raises blood pressure	Blue cohosh
Methyl salicylate and its derivatives	Analgesic, anti-inflammatory, cardiac tonic	Birch, black cohosh, blue flag, clover, honeysuckle, passion flower, pennyroyal, plantain, scented mayweed, Seneca snakeroot, senna, sweet violet, wild pansy, willow, wintergreen, yarrow
Menispine	Central nervous system depressant	Moonseed
Myricetin	Anti-bacterial, chloretic	Barberry, parsley, witch hazel
Naphtholoquinone	Anti-fungal	Jewelweed
Nepatalactone	Insecticide, non-addictive sedative	Catmint
Panacen	Analgesic, central nervous system stimulant	American ginseng
Panaquilin	Cathartic	American ginseng
Panaxin	Cardiac stimulant, tonic	American ginseng
Phytolaccogenin	Powerful molluskcide, paracide	Poke
Pinene	Anti-bacterial, anti-inflammatory expectorant	Angelica, coriander, fennel, parsley, pennyroyal, poke, Queen Anne's lace, sage, sassafras

Component	Action	Plant
Procyanidin	Cardiac tonic	Hawthorn
Protopine	Analgesic, cardiac tonic	Bloodroot
Prussic acid	Expectorant, sedative	Wild black cherry
Queretrin	Anti-cancer, anti-inflammatory	Boneset, chamomile, elderberry, goldenrod, gum plant, hops, New Jersey tea, scented mayweed
Ranunculin	Central nervous system depressant	Black cohosh, buttercup
Resperpine	Anti-cancer	Periwinkle
Rosmarin	Antioxidant	Rosemary
Rotenone	Anti-cancer (lymphocytic leukemia)	Devil's shoe string
Rumicin	Chloretic, rubefacient	Rumex
Rutin	Anti-cancer, diuretic, anti-inflammatory	Boneset, chickweed, elderberry, ground ivy, hawthorn, hops, New Jersey tea, scented mayweed, St. Johnswort, tarragon, wild pansy, yarrow
Sanquinarine	Anodyne, anti-fungal, antiseptic, plaque-inhibitive	Bloodroot
Saponiogenin	Central nervous system stimulant	American ginseng
Scopalamine	Analgesic, anti-inflammatory, narcotic sedative	Jimsonweed, henbane
Scopoletin	Muscle relaxant	Cramp bark
Sesquiterpenes	Anti-cancer, immunostimulatory	Birch, boneset, cone-flower, feverfew, hore-hound, Joe-Pye weed, passion flower, sweet flag, tansy, valerian, willow
Silylin	Liver tonic	Milk thistle
Solamine	Cardiac and respiratory tonic, Central nervous system depressant	Bittersweet nightshade, horsenettle
Thymol	Antiseptic, anthelmintic	Basil, catmint, horsemint, onion, oregano, thyme
Tropane	Antiseptic, central nervous system depressant	Mugwort, tansy, white sage, wormwood
Tyramine	Anti-coagulant	Shepherd's purse, stinging nettle
Umbelliferone	Anti-fungal	Angelica
Verbenalin	Emmenagogue, coagulant	Wild hyssop
Viburnin	Sedative	Cramp bark
Vincarmine	Adrenalin depressant, sedative	Periwinkle

Appendix II: Disorders, Medicinal Functions and Herbal Treatments

Ague
(see Fever - Febrifuge)

Alcoholism
Alfalfa
Celery
Evening primrose
Goldenrod

Alterative - Tonic
(Blood purifiers)
Alfalfa
Asparagus
Barberry
Bittersweet
Blackberry-Raspberry
Black cohosh
Blessed thistle
Blue flag
Boneset
Borage
Bracken fern
Buckbean
Burdock
Bush clover
Butternut
Catmint
Celery
Chicory
Clover
Compass plant
Coriander
Cornflower
Culver's root
Dandelion
Devil's shoe string
Dutchman's breaches
Elderberry
Elecampane
False Solomon's seal
Fennel
Feverfew
Ginseng
Goldenseal
Ground ivy
Hawthorn
Hepatica
Hercules' club
Indian hemp
Jewelweed
Lavender
Pot marigold

Milk thistle
Moonseed
Motherwort
Mugwort
New Jersey tea
Oregano
Ox-eye daisy
Passion flower
Peony
Prickly ash
Queen Anne's lace
Red cedar
Rose
Rosemary
Rumex
Sage
Sarsaparilla
Sassafras
Seneca snakeroot
Spicebush
Spikenard
Stoneroot
Stinging nettle
St. Johnswort
Sumac
Sweet flag
Tansy
Tarragon
Thyme
Toadflax
Virginia snakeroot
Watercress
Wild black cherry
Wild coffee
Wild geranium
Wild ginger
Wild hyssop
Wild indigo
Wild lettuce
Wild pansy
Willow
Wintergreen
Witch hazel
Wood sorrel
Wormwood
Yarrow

Amenorrhea
(See Dysmenorrhea-
Emmenorrhea)

Analgesic - Anodyne
Angelica
Balm of Gilead
Burdock
Black cohosh
Bloodroot
Blue flag
Buttercup
Catmint
Cup-plant
Dandelion
Dogwood
Evening primrose
Hemlock
Henbane
Hops
Horsenettle
Horseradish
Jimsonweed
Lavender
Marijuana
Mexican tea
Motherwort
Mullein
Oak
Passion flower
Pennyroyal
Peppermint-Spearmint
Plantain
Saffron
Sarsaparilla
Solomon's seal
Spicebush
St. Johnswort
Thyme
Virginia snakeroot
Wild lettuce
Wild ginger
Wintergreen
Witch hazel
Yarrow

Anemia
Angelica
Chickweed
Chicory
Elecampane
Horsetail
Spicebush
Stinging nettle
St. Johnswort

Watercress
Wild strawberry

Anodyne
(See Analgesic)

Anthelmintic - Vermifuge
Alumroot
Angelica
Balm of Gilead
Bittersweet nightshade
Blackberry-Raspberry
Blessed thistle
Bloodroot
Blue flag
Bracken fern
Buckbean
Caraway
Catmint
Cattail
Compass plant
Devil's shoe string
Dogwood
Elecampane
Fennel
Feverfew
Garlic
Hercules' club
Hollyhock
Honeysuckle
Horehound
Horsemint
Horseradish
Indian hemp
Indian nettle
Indian physic
Indian tobacco
Lavender
Pot marigold
Mayapple
Mexican tea
Milkweed
Motherwort
Mugwort
Onion
Pennyroyal
Peppermint-Spearmint
Pumpkin
Queen Anne's lace
Rose
Sage
Shepherd's purse
Skunk cabbage
Spicebush
Stinging nettle
St. Johnswort
Sumac
Tansy
Tarragon
Thyme
Turtlehead
Virginia snakeroot

Walnut
White sage
Wild black cherry
Wild coffee
Wild garlic
Wild hyssop
Wild plum
Wormwood

Anti-bacterial
(See Antiseptic)

Antibiotic
(See Antiseptic)

Anti-coagulant
(Hemorrhage, Hemostat)
Alfalfa
Alumroot
Amaranth
Butternut
Ginseng
Balm of Gilead
Bearberry
Bloodroot
Buckbean
Blue cohosh
Chickweed
Clover
Dogwood
Evening primrose
False Solomon's seal
Fleabane
Foxglove
Goldenrod
Goldenseal
Horsetail
Indian hemp
Indian physic
Kentucky coffee tree
Melilot
New Jersey tea
Oak
Onion
Peppermint-Spearmint
Periwinkle
Plantain
Prickly ash
Rumex
Sage
Self-heal
Seneca snakeroot
Senecio
Shepherd's purse
Skunk cabbage
Slippery elm
Smartweed
Stinging nettle
St. Johnswort
Sumac
Sweet flag
Trillium
Walnut

White pond lily
Wild geranium
Wild lettuce
Wild strawberry
Willow
Witch hazel
Yarrow

Anti-fungal
(Ringworm, thrush)
Bittersweet
Bittersweet nightshade
Blackberry-Raspberry
Bloodroot
Elecampane
Garlic
Ginseng
Hepatica
Horsemint
Jewelweed
Jack-in-the-pulpit
Pot marigold
Mugwort
Mullein
Mustard
Plantain
Rosemary
Rumex
Sage
Scented mayweed
Walnut
Wild geranium
Wild ginger

Anti-inflammatory
(Erysipelas)
Barberry
Black cohosh
Black snakeroot
Blue cohosh
Blue flag
Borage
Butternut
Cattail
Chamomile
Chickweed
Chicory
Comfrey
Coneflower
Elderberry
Evening primrose
Feverfew
Foxglove
Garlic
Goldenseal
Ground ivy
Hemlock
Henbane
Hepatica
Hercules' club
Hops
Horseradish

Horsetail
Jewelweed
Jimsonweed
Joe-Pye weed
Kentucky coffee weed
Mallow
Marijuana
Melilot
Milkweed
Mullein
Oak
Passion flower
Periwinkle
Plantain
Prickly pear
Rattlesnake master
Rose
Scented mayweed
Shepherd's purse
Slippery elm
Smartweed
Solomon's seal
Spikenard
St. Johnswort
Sunflower
Tarragon
Thyme
Toadflax
Trillium
Twinleaf
Walnut
Water hemlock
Wild ginger
Wild indigo
Wild pansy
Wild strawberry
Willow
Witch hazel
Yarrow

Antiperiodic
(See Scurvy)
Antiscorbic
(See Scurvy)
Antiseptic - Vulnerary
(Anti-bacterial, antibiotic)
Alumroot
Basil
Barberry
Bearberry
Birch
Blackberry-Raspberry
Blessed thistle
Bloodroot
Bittersweet nightshade
Boneset
Bracken fern
Burdock
Buttercup
Chamomile
Chickweed

Clover
Comfrey
Coneflower
Culver's root
Dogwood
Elecampane
Garlic
Goldenseal
Hemlock
Hepatica
Honeysuckle
Hops
Horsemint
Horsenettle
Horseradish
Horsetail
Indian tobacco
Kentucky coffee tree
Lavender
Mallow
Pot marigold
Mugwort
Mullein
Mustard
Oak
Onion
Oregano
Periwinkle
Plantain
Queen Anne's lace
Red cedar
Rose
Rosemary
Rumex
Sage
Sassafras
Scented mayweed
Scotch pine
Self-heal
Seneca snakeroot
Solomon's seal
Spikenard
Stinging nettle
St. Johnswort
Sumac
Sweet violet
Tansy
Thyme
Trillium
White pond lily
Wild garlic
Wild ginger
Wild hyssop
Wild indigo
Wild plum
Willow
Wintergreen
Wood sorrel
Yarrow

Antispasmodic
Basil
Black cohosh
Black haw
Catmint
Caraway
Chamomile
Clover
Compass plant
Fennel
Fenugreek
Feverfew
Gum plant
Hemlock
Henbane
Horehound
Horsenettle
Jimsonweed
Lavender
Marijuana
Mayapple
Melilot
Mexican tea
Motherwort
Mugwort
Mullein
New Jersey tea
Oregano
Ox-eye daisy
Passion flower
Pennyroyal
Peony
Prickly ash
Saffron
Sage
Scented mayweed
Skunk cabbage
Stoneroot
Thyme
Twinleaf
Valerian
Walnut
White pond lily
Wild hyssop
Wormwood
Yarrow

Anti-viral
Bracken fern
Coneflower
Honeysuckle
Oak

Aphrodisiac
Asparagus
Boneset
Celery
Compass plant
Dayflower
Dutchman's breeches
Ginseng
Indian tobacco

Jimsonweed
Marijuana
Mayapple
Ox-eye daisy
Queen Anne's lace
Parsley
Passion flower
Periwinkle
Saffron
Sarsaparilla
Sassafras
Sweet flag
Trillium
Wild geranium
Wild lettuce

Appetite depressant
(see Obesity)

Appetite stimulants
Alfalfa
Chamomile
Ginseng
Goldenseal
Hops
Oregano
Parsley
Rosemary
Stoneroot
Sweet ciceley
Sweet flag
Turtlehead
Virginia snakeroot
Watercress

Aromatic
Catmint
Coriander
Fennel
Feverfew
Goldenrod
Horsemint
Melilot
Queen Anne's lace
Rosemary
Sweet flag
Yarrow

Arthritis - Rheumatism
Alfalfa
Angelica
Arrowhead
Balm of Gilead
Birch
Bittersweet
Bittersweet nightshade
Blackberry-Raspberry
Black cohosh
Black snakeroot
Bloodroot
Blue cohosh
Blue flag
Boneset
Buckbean

Burdock
Buttercup
Butternut
Catmint
Celery
Chamomile
Chickweed
Chicory
Clover
Comfrey
Coneflower
Coriander
Couchgrass
Cup plant
Dandelion
Dutchman's breeches
Elderberry
Evening primrose
False Solomon's seal
Fenugreek
Garlic
Ginseng
Goldenrod
Gum plant
Hemlock
Henbane
Hercules' club
Honeysuckle
Hops
Horsemint
Horsenettle
Horseradish
Indian hemp
Indian physic
Indian tobacco
Jack-in-the-pulpit
Jimsonweed
Joe-Pye weed
Lavender
Maize
Mallow
Marijuana
Mayapple
Melilot
Moonseed
Mullein
Mustard
Oak
Oregano
Pepper
Peppermint-Spearmint
Plantain
Poke
Prickly ash
Prickly pear
Rattlesnake master
Red cedar
Rosemary
Saffron
Sarsaparilla

Sassafras
Scented mayweed
Scotch pine
Seneca snakeroot
Skunk cabbage
Slippery elm
Smartweed
Soapwort
Solomon's seal
Spicebush
Spikenard
Stinging nettle
Sumac
Sunflower
Trillium
Twinleaf
Virginia snakeroot
Walnut
Watercress
Wild garlic
Wild hyssop
Wild kidney bean
Wild yam
Willow
Wintergreen
Witch hazel
Wormwood

Asthma
Bittersweet nightshade
Chamomile
Chickweed
Clover
Comfrey
Elecampane
Evening primrose
Feverfew
Garlic
Goldenseal
Henbane
Hollyhock
Honeysuckle
Horehound
Horsenettle
Horseradish
Indian hemp
Indian tobacco
Jimsonweed
Marijuana
Mexican tea
Milkweed
Mugwort
Mullein
Oak
Onion
Oregano
Parsley
Plantain
Sage
Scotch pine
Seneca snakeroot

Skunk cabbage
Spikenard
Stinging nettle
Sumac
Trillium
Watercress
Wild ginger
Wild plum
Wild yam

Astringent - Styptic
Alumroot
Amaranth
Barberry
Bearberry
Bittersweet
Blackberry-Raspberry
Black cohosh
Black snakeroot
Bracken fern
Buttercup
Clover
Comfrey
Compass plant
Cornflower
Cramp bark
Dogwood
Elderberry
Evening primrose
Goldenrod
Goldenseal
Ground ivy
Hawthorn
Hepatica
Joe-Pye weed
Mallow
Melilot
Motherwort
Mullein
New Jersey tea
Oak
Oregano
Ox-eye daisy
Periwinkle
Plantain
Prickly ash
Rose
Rosemary
Rumex
Sage
Self-heal
Shepherd's purse
Smartweed
Stinging nettle
St. Johnswort
Stoneroot
Solomon's seal
Sumac
Trillium
Walnut
White pond lily

Wild geranium
Wild indigo
Wild plum
Wild strawberry
Willow
Witch hazel

Bedwetting - Incontinence
Corn
Fennel
Hollyhock
Plantain
St. Johnswort

Birth Control - Contraceptives
Balm of Gilead
Blessed thistle
Dandelion
Dogbane
False Solomon's seal
Feverfew
Hepatica
Indian hemp
Jack-in-the-pulpit
Milkweed
Queen Anne's lace
Skunk cabbage
Tansy
Turtlehead
Water hemlock
Wild geranium
Wild ginger
Wild lettuce
Wild yam

Bladder - Kidney
(See Urinary disorders)

Blood pressure
Blue cohosh
Evening primrose
Foxglove
Goldenseal
Motherwort
New Jersey tea
Parsley
Passion flower
Pepper
Sassafras
Tarragon

Blood Purifiers
(See Alterative, Tonic)

Boils
Balm of Gilead
Buttercup
Burdock
Catmint
Cattail
Chickweed
Coneflower
Dayflower
Elderberry
Fenugreek
Goldenrod

Hercules' club
Jack-in-the-pulpit
Jimsonweed
Indian tobacco
Milkweed
Mustard
Onion
Plantain
Passion flower
Poke
Rumex
Sarsaparilla
Self-heal
Slippery elm
Soapwort
Spikenard
Sumac
Sweet ciceley
Sweet violet
Wild garlic
Yarrow

Bright's Disease - Nephritis
Indian hemp
Clover
Milkweed
Oak
Virginia snakeroot
Wild black cherry

Bronchitis
(See Respiratory
Disorders)

Bruises, Cuts, Wounds
Alumroot
Amaranth
Angelica
Arrowhead
Balm of Gilead
Basil
Birch
Blackberry-Raspberry
Boneset
Blue flag
Burdock
Butternut
Caraway
Catmint
Cattail
Chickweed
Comfrey
Coneflower
Cup plant
Dandelion
Dogwood
Elderberry
Evening primrose
Fenugreek
Garlic
Ginseng
Goldenrod
Goldenseal

Ground ivy
Hepatica
Hercules' club
Hollyhock
Honeysuckle
Hops
Horehound
Horsemint
Horsetail
Indian hemp
Indian tobacco
Jack-in-the-pulpit
Jewelweed
Jimsonweed
Mallow
Pot marigold
Mayapple
Milkweed
Mullein
Mugwort
New Jersey tea
Oak
Oregano
Ox-eye daisy
Parsley
Pennyroyal
Plantain
Poke
Prickly ash
Prickly pear
Queen Anne's lace
Red cedar
Rose
Rosemary
Rumex
Sage
Sassafras
Self-heal
Senna
Shepherd's purse
Skunk cabbage
Slippery elm
Solomon's seal
Spikenard
Smartweed
Stinging nettle
St. Johnswort
Stonewort
Sumac
Sunflower
Sweet ciceley
Sweet violet
Tansy
Trillium
Turtlehead
Walnut
White pond lily
White sage
Wild coffee
Wild garlic

Wild geranium
Wild ginger
Wild indigo
Willow
Wintergreen
Witch hazel
Yarrow

Burns - Emollients
(Sunburns)
Balm of Gilead
Barberry
Birch
Bittersweet
Bloodroot
Blue flag
Boneset
Borage
Bracken fern
Burdock
Cattail
Comfrey
Compass plant
Dayflower
Elderberry
Goldenrod
Hercules' club
Hollyhock
Horsemint
Jimsonweed
Jewelweed
Lavender
Pot marigold
Milkweed
Oak
Onion
Plantain
Sarsaparilla
Self-heal
Slipper elm
Stinging nettle
Stoneroot
Sumac
Sweet flag
Tansy
White pond lily
Wild geranium
Wild garlic
Wild lettuce
Willow
Witch hazel
Yarrow

Cancer - Tumors
Balm of Gilead
Black cohosh
Bittersweet
Bittersweet nightshade
Blessed thistle
Bloodroot
Bracken fern
Burdock

Bush clover
Chickweed
Clover
Coneflower
Devil's shoe string
Dogwood
Fleabane
Garlic
Hemlock
Honeysuckle
Horehound
Horsenettle
Indian hemp
Mallow
Mayapple
Mugwort
Mullein
Oak
Parsnip
Plantain
Poke
Pumpkin
Queen Anne's lace
Rumex
Saffron
Self-heal
Skunk cabbage
Slippery elm
Solomon's seal
Stinging nettle
Sweet flag
Sweet violet
Tarragon
Trillium
Virginia snakeroot
Water hemlock
Wild ginger
Witch hazel

Canker sores - Herpes
(External Ulcers)
Alumroot
Barberry
Blackberry-Raspberry
Blue flag
Chamomile
Butternut
Chickweed
Dandelion
Dill
Elecampane
Fenugreek
Garlic
Goldenrod
Goldenseal
Hemlock
Hercules' club
Horehound
Horsemint
Horsetail
Indian tobacco

Mallow
Pot marigold
Mayapple
Melilot
Mugwort
Milkweed
New Jersey tea
Oak
Plantain
Pennyroyal
Peppermint-Spearmint
Poke
Prickly ash
Queen Anne's lace
Red cedar
Rose
Sage
Sarsaparilla
Scented mayweed
Scotch pine
Self-heal
Slippery elm
Spikenard
Sumac
Sweet ciceley
Sweet flag
Trillium
Turtlehead
Twinleaf
Walnut
Wild geranium
Wild indigo
Wild plum
Wild strawberry
Wintergreen
Witch hazel
Yarrow

Cardiac disorders
Alfalfa
Black cohosh
Bloodroot
Blue cohosh
Chicory
Dayflower
Evening primrose
Foxglove
Garlic
Hawthorn
Horehound
Indian hemp
Lily-of-the-valley
Maize
Mexican tea
Motherwort
Oak
Plantain
Pepper
Senna
Solomon's seal
Stoneroot

Virginia snakeroot
White pond lily
White sage
Wild ginger
Wild pansy
Yarrow

Carminative
(Colic, Flatulence)
Angelica
Basil
Blessed thistle
Catmint
Caraway
Celery
Chamomile
Coriander
Dill
Fennel
Feverfew
Ginger
Goldenrod
Hercules' club
Horsemint
Lavender
Milkweed
Mustard
Oregano
Passion flower
Pennyroyal
Pepper
Peppermint-Spearmint
Periwinkle
Prickly ash
Queen Anne's lace
Saffron
Sage
Sassafras
Scented mayweed
Self-heal
Sunflower
Sweet flag
Tansy
Thyme
Wild ginger
Wintergreen
Wormwood

Catarrh
(See Respiratory
Disorders)

Cathartic, Laxative, Purgative
(Constipation)
Asparagus
Balm of Gilead
Barberry
Birch
Bittersweet
Blue flag
Boneset
Borage
Buckbean

Butternut
Chickweed
Chicory
Culver's root
Dandelion
Devil's shoe string
Dill
Elderberry
Dogwood
False Solomon's seal
Fennel
Goldenrod
Goldenseal
Gum plant
Hercules' club
Hepatica
Honeysuckle
Indian hemp
Indian physic
Joe-Pye weed
Kentucky coffee tree
Mallow
Mayapple
Milkweed
Moonseed
Motherwort
Mullein
Mustard
New Jersey tea
Plantain
Red cedar
Rumex
Saffron
Sarsaparilla
Seneca snakeroot
Senna
Slippery elm
Soapwort
Spicebush
Sweet flag
Scented mayweed
Sweet violet
Toadflax
Walnut
White sage
Wild coffee
Wild lettuce
Wild indigo
Wild plum
Wild strawberry
Yarrow

Childbirth
(See Parturition)

Cholagogue - Choleretic
(Gallbladder, Gallstones)
Alfalfa
Barberry
Bearberry
Birch
Bittersweet

Blackberry-Raspberry
Black cohosh
Blessed thistle
Blue cohosh
Blue flag
Boneset
Buckbean
Burdock
Chickweed
Chicory
Comfrey
Culver's root
Cup-plant
Dandelion
Devil's shoe string
Dogbane
Evening primrose
Fleabane
Fennel
Gum plant
Hepatica
Horehound
Horseradish
Horsetail
Lavender
Mayapple
Milk thistle
Mugwort
Oak
Onion
Oregano
Parsley
Passion flower
Peony
Queen Anne's lace
Rattlesnake master
Rumex
Sage
Scotch pine
Self-heal
Shepherd's pine
Soapwort
Stinging nettle
St Johnswort
Strawberry
Sumac
Sweet flag
Sweet violet
Toadflax
Turtlehead
Watercress
Wild hyssop
Wild strawberry
Wild yam
Wormwood
Yarrow

Cholera

Blackberry-Raspberry
Elecampane
Goldenrod

Mayapple
Peppermint-Spearmint
Prickly ash
Red cedar
Skunk cabbage
Strawberry
Sweet flag
Wild black cherry
Wild geranium

Cholesterol
Bush clover
Buttercup
Honeysuckle
Onion
Plantain
Sunflower

Colds
(See Respiratory Disorders)

Colic
(See Carminative)

Colitis
(See Carminative)

Conjunctivitis
(See Eye Disorders)

Constipation
(See Cathartic)

Convulsions
(See Sedative)

Coughs
(See Respiratory Disorders)

Demulcent
(Internal Ulcers)
Borage
Chickweed
Comfrey
Cup plant
Ginseng
Hollyhock
Hops
Plantain
Pot marigold
Self-heal
Slippery elm
Solomon's seal
St. Johnswort
Sumac
White pond lily
Yarrow

Dermatitis
(See Skin Disorders)

Diabetes
Burdock
Evening primrose
Fleabane
Indian physic
Milkweed
Queen Anne's lace
Self-heal

Sage
Sumac
Watercress

Diaphoretic - Sudoforic
Angelica
Asparagus
Bittersweet
Blessed thistle
Borage
Burdock
Catmint
Chamomile
Chickweed
Compass plant
Culver's root
Cup-plant
Devil's shoe string
Dutchman's breeches
Elderberry
Feverfew
Garlic
Goldenrod
Hercules' club
Honeysuckle
Horsemint
Indian hemp
Indian tobacco
Jack-in-the-pulpit
Joe-Pye weed
Pot marigold
Mexican tea
Milkweed
Motherwort
Mugwort
Oregano
Plantain
Pennyroyal
Prickly ash
Rattlesnake master
Saffron
Scented mayweed
Sassafras
Sarsaparilla
Seneca snakeroot
Soapwort
Spicebush
Tansy
Thyme
Toadflax
Twinleaf
Virginia snakeroot
Wild black cherry
Wild hyssop
Wild yam
Yarrow

Diarrhea, Dysentery, Flux
Alumroot
Amaranth
Balm of Gilead
Barberry

Basil
Birch
Bittersweet
Blackberry-Raspberry
Blessed thistle
Blue flag
Bracken fern
Buckbean
Butternut
Cattail
Clover
Comfrey
Dayflower
Dogwood
Feverfew
Fleabane
Garlic
Hawthorn
Hepatica
Hercules' club
Hollyhock
Honeysuckle
Horsetail
Jimsonweed
Kentucky coffee tree
Mayapple
Milkweed
Mullein
New Jersey tea
Oak
Ox-eye daisy
Pennyroyal
Peppermint-Spearmint
Periwinkle
Plantain
Poke
Prickly ash
Queen Anne's lace
Rose
Rumex
Sage
Sassafras
Scented mayweed
Self-heal
Seneca snakeroot
Shepherd's purse
Slippery elm
Smartweed
Solomon's seal
Spicebush
Stinging nettle
Stoneroot
Strawberry
St. Johnswort
Sumac
Sweet ciceley
Sweet violet
Tansy
Twinleaf
Walnut

White pond lily
Wild black cherry
Wild coffee
Wild geranium
Wild hyssop
Wild indigo
Wild lettuce
Wild plum
Wild strawberry
Willow
Witch hazel
Yarrow

Diuretic

Alfalfa
Angelica
Arrowhead
Asparagus
Barberry
Bearberry
Birch
Bittersweet
Bittersweet nightshade
Blackberry-Raspberry
Black cohosh
Blessed thistle
Bloodroot
Blue flag
Burdock
Catmint
Celery
Chamomile
Chickweed
Chicory
Compass plant
Cornflower
Couchgrass
Dandelion
Elderberry
Elecampane
False Solomon's seal
Fennel
Feverfew
Foxglove
Goldenrod
Goldenseal
Hawthorn
Henbane
Hepatica
Hercules
Hollyhock
Honeysuckle
Hops
Horsemint
Horseradish
Indian hemp
Jewelweed
Joe-Pye weed
Lily-of-the-valley
Milkweed
Moonseed

Mugwort
Onion
Ox-eye daisy
Parsley
Peony
Periwinkle
Prickly pear
Pumpkin
Queen Anne's lace
Red cedar
Rose
Sage
Sassafras
Scotch pine
Self-heal
Shepherd's purse
Skunk cabbage
Slippery elm
Smartweed
Soapwort
Solomon's seal
Stinging nettle
St. Johnswort
Stoneroot
Sweet violet
Tansy
Tarragon
Thyme
Toadflax
Trillium
Twinleaf
Watercress
White sage
Wild lettuce
Wild pansy
Wild strawberry
Wintergreen
Wormwood

Dropsy
(See Edema)

Dysentery
(See Diarrhea)

Dysmenorrhea - Emmenorrhea
Alumroot
Angelica
Asparagus
Balm of Gilead
Barberry
Birch
Bittersweet
Blackberry-Raspberry
Black cohosh
Black haw
Black snakeroot
Blessed thistle
Bloodroot
Blue cohosh
Boneset
Buckbean

Catmint
Chamomile
Chickweed
Comfrey
Coriander
Cramp bark
Dandelion
Dayflower
Elderberry
False Solomon's seal
Fennel
Fenugreek
Feverfew
Fleabane
Hawthorn
Hepatica
Hercules' club
Honeysuckle
Hops
Horehound
Horseradish
Jewelweed
Joe-Pye weed
Lavender
Marijuana
Mexican tea
Milkweed
Moonseed
Motherwort
Mugwort
Mullein
New Jersey tea
Oak
Onion
Oregano
Ox-eye daisy
Parsley
Parsnip
Passion flower
Pennyroyal
Peppermint-Spearmint
Plantain
Pot marigold
Queen Anne's lace
Red cedar
Rose
Saffron
Sage
Self-heal
Seneca snakeroot
Senna
Skunk cabbage
Solomon's seal
Spicebush
Spikenard
St. Johnswort
Stoneroot
Sumac
Sweet flag
Tansy

Tarragon
Thyme
Trillium
Twinleaf
Virginia snakeroot
White sage
Wild coffee
Wild ginger
Wild hyssop
Wild lettuce
Wild strawberry
Wild yam
Wintergreen
Witch hazel
Wormwood
Yarrow

Dyspepsia
(See Gastrointestinal
Disorders)

Earache
Bloodroot
Boneset
Blue flag
Elderberry
Feverfew
Garlic
Hercules' club
Hops
Horsetail
Indian Tobacco
Pot marigold
Milkweed
Mullein
Oregano
Passion flower
Plantain
Scented mayweed
Spikenard
Sumac
Tansy
Trillium
Wild garlic
Wild ginger

Eczema
(See Skin Disorders)

Edema - Dropsy
Alfalfa
Black cohosh
Blue cohosh
Blue flag
Boneset
Chamomile
Dandelion
Elderberry
Garlic
Goldenseal
Horsemint
Horsetail
Indian hemp
Jewelweed

Lavender
Lily-of-the-valley
Mayapple
Milkweed
Mustard
Onion
Oregano
Parsley
Pennyroyal
Plantain
Queen Anne's lace
Rattlesnake master
Saffron
Sassafras
Scotch pine
Seneca snakeroot
Shepherd's purse
Skunk cabbage
Smartweed
Spicebush
Stonewort
Sumac
Sweet flag
Toadflax
Twinleaf
Wild hyssop
Wormwood

Emetic
Alumroot
Angelica
Barberry
Birch
Bittersweet
Black haw
Blessed thistle
Blue cohosh
Blueflag
Boneset
Butternut
Compass plant
Cramp bark
Culver's root
Cup-plant
Dogwood
Elderberry
Feverfew
Foxglove
Goldenrod
Hercules' club
Honeysuckle
Indian hemp
Indian physic
Pot marigold
Mayapple
Milkweed
Mustard
Ox-eye daisy
Periwinkle
Poke
Rattlesnake master

Rumex
Seneca snakeroot
Skunk cabbage
Spicebush
Sumac
Sweet violet
Tansy
Twinleaf
Walnut
Wild ginger
Wild hyssop
Wild Indigo
Wild yam
Strawberry
Twinleaf

Emmenagogue
(See Dysmenorrhea)

Emollient
(see Burns)

Enteritis
Blackberry-Raspberry
Clover
Dayflower
Garlic
Ground ivy
Hollyhock
Horsemint
Mallow
Stinging nettle
Toadflax

Epilepsy
Boneset
Chamomile
Fleabane
Foxglove
Hemlock
Horsenettle
Indian tobacco
Mullein
Passion flower
Peony
Skunk cabbage
Smartweed
Thyme

Erysipelas
(See Anti-inflammatory)

Expectorant
(See Respiratory
Disorders)

Eye Disorders
(Conjunctivitis,
Ophthalmia)
Angelica
Asparagus
Blackberry-Raspberry
Caraway
Carrot
Chamomile
Chickweed
Cornflower

Dandelion
Dayflower
Devil's shoe string
Dogwood
False Solomon's seal
Fennel
Elderberry
Goldenseal
Ground ivy
Hemlock
Henbane
Hercules' club
Horehound
Jimsonweed
Lily-of-the-valley
Melilot
Oak
Parsley
Parsnip
Pennyroyal
Plantain
Queen Anne's lace
Rose
Sassafras
Scented mayweed
Self-heal
Sweet ciceley
Thyme
Toadflax
White pond lily
Wild geranium
Wild ginger
Wild lettuce
Wild strawberry
Willow
Witch hazel

Fever - Febrifuge
(Ague)
Angelica
Arrowhead
Barberry
Birch
Blue cohosh
Bittersweet
Blackberry-Raspberry
Black snakeroot
Blessed thistle
Bloodroot
Boneset
Borage
Buckbean
Catmint
Chamomile
Clover
Culver's root
Cup-plant
Dandelion
Dayflower
Dogwood
Elderberry

Elecampane
Fenugreek
Feverfew
Fleabane
Goldenrod
Henbane
Hepatica
Hercules' club
Honeysuckle
Hops
Horehound
Horsemint
Indian hemp
Jack-in-the-pulpit
Joe-Pye weed
Jimsonweed
Pot marigold
Mexican tea
Milkweed
Motherwort
Mugwort
Mullein
Mustard
New Jersey tea
Oak
Ox-eye daisy
Parsnip
Pennyroyal
Peony
Pepper
Plantain
Poke
Prickly ash
Red cedar
Sassafras
Scented mayweed
Self-heal
Senna
Smartweed
Spicebush
Spikenard
Stinging nettle
St. Johnswort
Sumac
Sweet ciceley
Sweet flag
Virginia snakeroot
Tansy
Thymus
Turtlehead
White snakeroot
Wild black cherry
Wild coffee
Wild garlic
Wild ginger
Wild hyssop
Wild indigo
Wild pansy
Wild plum
Willow

Wood sorrel
Wormwood
Yarrow

Flatulence

(See Carminative)

Flu

Boneset
Burdock
Dayflower
Dogwood
Goldenrod
Hercules' club
Honeysuckle
Hops
Horehound
Horsemint
Horseradish
Mustard
Peppermint-Spearmint
Sassafras
Stinging nettle
Sweet ciceley
Sweet flag
White pond lily
Wintergreen
Yarrow

Flux

(See Diarrhea-Dysentery)

Gallbladder - Gallstones

(See Cholagogue)

Gargle

(Sore Throats, Tonsillitis)
Alfalfa
Alumroot
Amaranth
Angelica
Basil
Balm of Gilead
Barberry
Birch
Bittersweet nightshade
Blackberry-Raspberry
Black cohosh
Blue flag
Black snakeroot
Bloodroot
Boneset
Butternut
Chamomile
Clover
Coneflower
Cornflower
Dayflower
Dogwood
Elderberry
False Solomon's seal
Fenugreek
Goldenrod
Goldenseal
Ground ivy

Hawthorn
Hepatica
Hercules' club
Hollyhock
Honeysuckle
Horehound
Horsemint
Horsenettle
Horseradish
Horsetail
Indian hemp
Jack-in-the-pulpit
Jimsonweed
Maize
Mallow
Milkweed
Mullein
New Jersey tea
Oak
Peppermint-Spearmint
Prickly ash
Red cedar
Rose
Rumex
Sage
Self-heal
Seneca snakeroot
Senna
Slippery elm
Smartweed
Stoneroot
Sumac
Sweet ciceley
Sweet-scented mayweed
Sweet violet
Twinleaf
Virginia snakeroot
Walnut
White pond lily
White sage
Wild black cherry
Wild geranium
Wild pansy
Wild plum
Wild strawberry
Wild ginger
Wild indigo
Wild yam
Willow
Wintergreen
Witch hazel
Wood sorrel
Wormwood

Gastrointestinal Disorders

(Dyspepsia, Indigestion.
Stomachache)
Alfalfa
Alumroot
Angelica
Arrowhead

Asparagus
Balm of Gilead
Basil
Bearberry
Birch
Bittersweet
Bittersweet nightshade
Blackberry-Raspberry
Black snakeroot
Bloodroot
Blue cohosh
Blue flag
Boneset
Bracken fern
Butternut
Caraway
Catmint
Chamomile
Chickweed
Clover
Comfrey
Coriander
Coneflower
Culver's root
Cup plant
Dandelion
Dill
Dogwood
Elderberry
Elecampane
Evening primrose
False Solomon's seal
Fennel
Fenugreek
Feverfew
Fleabane
Garlic
Ginseng
Goldenrod
Goldenseal
Ground ivy
Gum plant
Hawthorn
Henbane
Hepatica
Hercules' club
Hollyhock
Hops
Horsemint
Horseradish
Indian physic
Indian tobacco
Jack-in-the-pulpit
Jewelweed
Lavender
Mallow
Marijuana
Mayapple
Melilot
Milk thistle

Mexican tea
Milkweed
Moonseed
Motherwort
Mugwort
Mullein
Mustard
New Jersey tea
Oak
Onion
Ox-eye daisy
Plantain
Parsley
Pennyroyal
Pepper
Peppermint-Spearmint
Plantain
Poke
Queen Anne's lace
Red cedar
Rose
Rosemary
Saffron
Sage
Sassafras
Scented mayweed
Self-heal
Shepherd's purse
Spicebush
Skunk cabbage
Smartweed
Solomon's seal
Spikenard
Stinging nettle
St. Johnswort
Stoneroot
Sumac
Sweet flag
Sweet ciceley
Sweet-scented mayweed
Tansy
Tarragon
Thyme
Turtlehead
Virginia snakeroot
Watercress
Walnut
White sage
Wild coffee
Wild ginger
Wild hyssop
Wild indigo
Wild lettuce
Wild strawberry
Wild jam
Willow
Wintergreen
Wood sorrel
Wormwood
Yarrow

Gonorrhea
(See Venereal Diseases)
Gout
Angelica
Asparagus
Balm of Gilead
Birch
Boneset
Burdock
Chickweed
Cornflower
Comfrey
Dandelion
Elderberry
Fennel
Fleabane
Ginseng
Hemlock
Henbane
Horseradish
Joe-Pye weed
Marijuana
Mullein
Peony
Plantain
Queen Anne's lace
Rumex
Saffron
Sarsaparilla
Sassafras
Soapwort
Spikenard
Stinging nettle
Strawberry
Sweet flag
Tansy
Thyme
Wild strawberry
Wood sorrel
Gravel - Stones
(See Urinary Disorders)
Hallucinogen
Catmint
Indian tobacco
Jimsonweed
Marijuana
Mugwort
Skunk cabbage
Sumac
Sweet flag
Wild lettuce
Headache
Basil
Balm of Gilead
Birch
Blessed thistle
Bracken fern
Buttercup
Butternut
Catmint

Chamomile
Coneflower
Coriander
Dogwood
Elderberry
Evening primrose
False Solomon's seal
Fennel
Feverfew
Fleabane
Elecampane
Garlic
Ginseng
Goldenrod
Goldenseal
Ground ivy
Hawthorn
Hercules' club
Hops
Horsemint
Indian hemp
Indian Tobacco
Jack-in-the-pulpit
Jewelweed
Kentucky coffee tree
Lavender
Lily-of-the-valley
Marijuana
Melilot
Mexican tea
Motherwort
Mullein
Mustard
Oregano
Plantain
Passion flower
Pennyroyal
Peppermint-Spearmint
Periwinkle
Prickly pear
Rose
Rosemary
Sage
Self-heal
Seneca snakeroot
Skunk cabbage
Smartweed
Solomon's seal
Spikenard
Sweet flag
Sweet violet
Sumac
Tansy
Thyme
Virginia snakeroot
Walnut
Watercress
White sage
Wild coffee
Wild ginger

319

Wild lettuce
Wild yam
Willow
Yarrow

Hemorrhoids
Alumroot
Burdock
Catmint
Chickweed
Comfrey
Coneflower
Dayflower
Dogwood
Elderberry
Evening primrose
Fleabane
Garlic
Hemlock
Hepatica
Jimsonweed
Kentucky coffee tree
Mullein
Oak
Parsley
Peony
Peppermint-Spearmint
Periwinkle
Plantain
Poke
Self-heal
Solomon's seal
Smartweed
Stonewort
Sumac
Toadflax
Turtlehead
Wild garlic
Wild geranium
Wild plum
Witch hazel
Yarrow

Hemostat
(See Anti-coagulant)

Hepatitis - Jaundice
Barberry
Chamomile
Dandelion
Dogwood
Elderberry
Fennel
Garlic
Goldenrod
Goldenseal
Hops
Horehound
Jewelweed
Lavender
Mayapple
Oregano
Parsley

Pennyroyal
Plantain
Queen Anne's lace
Rumex
Saffron
Shepherd's purse
Spikenard
Soapwort
Stinging nettle
Toadflax
Turtlehead
Wild strawberry
Wormwood

Herpes
(See Canker sores -
Herpes)

Hysteria
(See Sedative)

Impotency
Boneset
Devil's shoe string
Fenugreek
Ginseng
Wild yam

Incontinence
(See Urinary Disorders)

Indigestion
(See Gastrointestinal
Disorders)

Inflammation
(See Anti-inflammatory)

Insect Bites
Angelica
Basil
Blackberry-Raspberry
Burdock
Coneflower
Dayflower
Feverfew
Fleabane
Garlic
Honeysuckle
Jewelweed
Lavender
Mallow
Mustard
Oak
Oregano
Plantain
Rumex
Sassafras
Stinging nettle
St. Johnswort
Sunflower
Sweet flag
Sweet ciceley
Thyme
Toadflax
Trillium
Walnut

Wild garlic
Wild lettuce
Witch hazel
Wormwood

Insect repellent
Basil
Birch
Butternut
Catmint
Chamomile
Elderberry
Feverfew
Fleabane
Goldenseal
Lavender
Mugwort
Pennyroyal
Peppermint-Spearmint
Red cedar
Sassafras
Scented mayweed
Self-heal
Sweet flag
Tansy
Walnut
White sage

Insomnia
Bittersweet nightshade
Catmint
Chamomile
Dandelion
Dill
Elderberry
Feverfew
Hawthorn
Hops
Horsemint
Indian tobacco
Lavender
Marijuana
Melilot
Mugwort
Passion flower
Peppermint-Spearmint
Prickly pear
Rosemary
Scented mayweed
Sweet flag
Wild lettuce
Yarrow

Kidney - Kidney stones
(See Urinary Disorders)

Lactagogue
Basil
Bittersweet nightshade
Blackberry-raspberry
Borage
Bracken fern
Dandelion
Chicory

Compass Plant
Fenugreek
Hercules' club
Horsenettle
Hops
Lavender
Mayapple
Milkweed
New Jersey tea
Plantain
Rattlesnake master
Rose
Sage
Slippery elm
Walnut
White pond lily
Wild garlic
Wild geranium
Wild lettuce
Wild strawberry
Willow
Wintergreen

Laxative
(See Cathartic)

Leucorrhea
Amaranth
Bittersweet
Clover
Dayflower
Devil's shoe string
False Solomon's seal
Fleabane
Goldenseal
Hepatica
Oak
Self-heal
Solomon's seal
Trillium
White pond lily

Malaria
Barberry
Black cohosh
Black snakeroot
Boneset
Dayflower
Dogwood
Jack-in-the-pulpit
Oak
Plantain
Spicebush
Stinging nettle
White pond lily
Wild hyssop
Witch hazel
Wormwood

Mastitis
Boneset
Bracken fern
Chicory

Comfrey
Dill
Elderberry
Goldenrod
Henbane
Hercules' club
Hepatica
Hops
Indian physic
Mallow
Milkweed
Mugwort
Mustard
Peppermint-Spearmint
Poke
Saffron
Solomon's seal
Spikenard
Stoneroot
Trillium
Turtlehead
Wild ginger
Wild hyssop
Wild indigo
Wintergreen

Measles
Blackberry-Raspberry
Coneflower
Dogwood
Ground ivy
Goldenrod
Horsemint
Jewelweed
Sassafras
Spicebush
Wild black cherry

Migraine
(See Headache)

Miscarriage
Blackberry-Raspberry
Boneset

Mouth - Gums
(See Gargle - Sore
throat)

Muscle relaxant
Birch
Black haw
Cattail
Coneflower
Cramp bark
Dutchman's breeches
Evening primrose
Henbane
Sassafras
Scented mayweed

Narcotic
(See Hallucinogen)

Nervous disorders
(See Sedative)

Neuralgia
Black cohosh
Black haw
Chamomile
Cramp bark
Cup plant
Dogwood
Goldenrod
Melilot
Passion flower
Pepper
Rattlesnake master
St. Johnswort
Wild Geranium
Wormwood

Nicotinism
Indian Tobacco
Sumac

Obesity
(Appetite Depressant)
Chickweed
Elderberry
Evening primrose
Fennel
Peppermint-Spearmint
Sassafras
Stinging nettle

Ophthalmia
(See Eye Disorders)

Panacea
Alumroot
Birch
Bloodroot
Blue flag
Boneset
Chickweed
Coneflower
Ginseng
Goldenseal
Oak
Plantain
Rattlesnake master
Rumex
Sage
Sweet ciceley
Sweet flag
Wild ginger
Wintergreen

Painful Menstruation
(See Dysmenorrhea-
emmenorrhea)

Parturition - Childbirth
Alumroot
Basil
Bearberry
Bittersweet
Blackberry-Raspberry
Black cohosh
Bloodroot

Blue cohosh
Elderberry
Feverfew
Fleabane
Hercules' club
Horehound
Horsetail
Indian physic
Jewelweed
Lavender
Maize
Marijuana
Milkweed
Ox-eye daisy
Peony
Red cedar
Sage
Sarsaparilla
Sassafras
Shepherd's purse
Skunk cabbage
Slippery elm
St. Johnswort
Sumac
Sweet ciceley
Trillium
White sage
Wild black cherry
Wild ginger
Wild yam

Pectoral
(see Respiratory
Disorders)

Photodermatitis
Buttercup
Motherwort

Pleurisy - Pneumonia
(See Respiratory
Disorders)

Poison
Boneset
Bush clover
Hemlock
Hercules' club
Mallow
Mayapple
Milkweed
Skunk cabbage
Water hemlock
Wormwood

Poison Ivy
Bittersweet nightshade
Blue cohosh
Horsenettle
Dogwood
Goldenseal
Indian physic
Jewelweed
Oak
Poke

Sassafras
Smartweed
Shepherd's purse
Soapwort
Solomon's seal
Sumac
Wild lettuce

Prostate
Hemlock
Ginseng
Horsetail
Joe-Pye weed
Mayapple
Pumpkin
Stinging nettle
Virginia snakeroot
Wild yam

Purgative
(See Cathartic)

Respiratory Disorders -
Expectorant
(Bronchitis, Colds,
Coughs, Pectoral,
Pleurisy, Pneumonia)
Angelica
Basil
Balm of Gilead
Barberry
Bearberry
Birch
Bittersweet nightshade
Blackberry-Raspberry
Black cohosh
Bloodroot
Blue cohosh
Boneset
Borage
Burdock
Caraway
Catmint
Celery
Chickweed
Clover
Comfrey
Compass plant
Dandelion
Dayflower
Dogwood
Elecampane
Elderberry
Fennel
Feverfew
Fleabane
Garlic
Goldenrod
Goldenseal
Ground Ivy
Gum plant
Hepatica
Hercules' club

Hollyhock
Hops
Honeysuckle
Horehound
Horsemint
Horsenettle
Horseradish
Indian hemp
Indian physic
Indian tobacco
Jack-in-the-pulpit
Jimsonweed
Kentucky coffee tree
Maize
Mallow
Melilot
Milkweed
Motherwort
Mugwort
Mullein
Mustard
New Jersey tea
Oak
Onion
Oregano
Ox-eye daisy
Pennyroyal
Peony
Pepper
Peppermint-Spearmint
Plantain
Prickly ash
Queen Anne's lace
Rattlesnake master
Red cedar
Rose
Rosemary
Saffron
Sage
Sassafras
Scotch pine
Seneca snakeroot
Senna
Shepherd's purse
Skunk cabbage
Slippery elm
Smartweed
Soapwort
Solomon's seal
Spicebush
Spikenard
Stinging nettle
St. Johnswort
Sumac
Sunflower
Sweet ciceley
Sweet flag
Sweet-scented mayweed
Sweet violet
Tansy

Thyme
Toadflax
Toothwort
Trillium
Twinleaf
Virginia snakeroot
White pond lily
White sage
Wild black cherry
Wild garlic
Wild ginger
Wild hyssop
Wild lettuce
Wild pansy
Wild yam
Willow
Yarrow

Ringworm
(See Anti-fungal)

Rubefacient
Bush clover
Horseradish
Lavender
Mugwort
Pennyroyal
Red cedar
Rosemary
Scotch pine
Sumac
Thyme
Wintergreen

Scrofula
Barberry
Burdock
Blue flag
Culver's root
Ginseng
Jack-in-the-pulpit
Moonseed
Rumex
Sweet flag
Willow

Scurvy
(Anti-periodic,
Antiscorbic)
Amaranth
Arrowhead
Balm of Gilead
Barberry
Blackberry-Raspberry
Black haw
Burdock
Chickweed
Cramp bark
False Solomon's seal
Horseradish
Mexican tea
Rose
Shepherd's purse
Wild garlic

Wild strawberry
Willow
Wood sorrel

Sedative

(Convulsions, Hysteria)
Angelica
Asparagus
Birch
Bittersweet nightshade
Black cohosh
Black haw
Black snakeroot
Bloodroot
Blessed thistle
Blue cohosh
Boneset
Buttercup
Butternut
Catmint
Celery
Chamomile
Chicory
Comfrey
Compass plant
Coriander
Cramp bark
Dandelion
Dill
Dogwood
Elderberry
False Solomon's seal
Feverfew
Foxglove
Garlic
Ginseng
Goldenrod
Goldenseal
Hawthorn
Hemlock
Honeysuckle
Hops
Horehound
Horsemint
Indian hemp
Indian tobacco
Joe-Pye weed
Lavender
Marijuana
Mexican tea
Motherwort
Mugwort
Mustard
New Jersey tea
Passion flower
Peony
Pepper
Peppermint-Spearmint
Periwinkle
Poke
Red cedar

Rosemary
Saffron
Scented mayweed
Skunk cabbage
St. Johnswort
Stoneroot
Sweet flag
Sweet violet
Tansy
Tarragon
Valerian
Walnut
Water hemlock
White sage
Wild black cherry
Wild ginger
Wild lettuce
Wild pansy
Wild strawberry
Willow
Wintergreen
Witch hazel

Skin Disorders
(Dermatitis, Eczema)
Angelic
Birch
Bittersweet
Bittersweet nightshade
Blackberry-Raspberry
Burdock
Butternut
Chamomile
Chickweed
Clover
Comfrey
Compass plant
Dandelion
Dayflower
Devil's shoe string
Dutchman's breeches
Elderberry
Evening primrose
False Solomon's seal
Feverfew
Goldenrod
Goldenseal
Hemlock
Hepatica
Hollyhock
Honeysuckle
Hops
Horehound
Horsemint
Horsetail
Indian physic
Jewelweed
Lavender
Mallow
Pot marigold
Mayapple

Melilot
Moonseed
Parsley
Plantain
Peppermint-Spearmint
Periwinkle
Poke
Red cedar
Rose
Rosemary
Sage
Saffron
Sarsaparilla
Sassafras
Seneca snakeroot
Senna
Shepherd's purse
Slippery elm
Soapwort
Solomon's seal
Spikenard
Stinging nettle
St. Johnswort
Stoneroot
Sumac
Tansy
Thyme
Toadflax
Trillium
Walnut
Watercress
White pond lily
White sage
Wild garlic
Wild kidney bean
Wild lettuce
Wild pansy
Wild strawberry
Wild yam
Wintergreen
Wood sorrel
Yarrow

Snakebite

Black cohosh
Black snakeroot
Bloodroot
Boneset
Burdock
Butternut
Coneflower
Dayflower
Feverfew
Fleabane
Garlic
Goldenrod
Hercules' club
Horehound
Indian hemp
Indian physic
Jack-in-the-pulpit

Mayapple
Milkweed
New Jersey tea
Plantain
Seneca snakeroot
St. Johnswort
Sunflower
Sweet ciceley
Trillium
Virginia snakeroot
Walnut
Wild coffee
White snakeroot

Stimulant

Angelica
Bittersweet nightshade
Blessed thistle
Blue flag
Boneset
Caraway
Catmint
Celery
Compass plant
Coriander
Cup plant
Devil's shoe string
Elecampane
Fennel
Feverfew
Goldenrod
Goldenseal
Gum plant
Horehound
Horsenettle
Horseradish
Jack-in-the-pulpit
Lavender
Pot marigold
New Jersey tea
Pennyroyal
Poke
Prickly ash
Queen Anne's lace
Red cedar
Rosemary
Sassafras
Seneca snakeroot
Skunk cabbage
Spicebush
Spikenard
Stoneroot
Tarragon
Thyme
Watercress
Wintergreen
Wormwood
Yarrow

Stomachache

(See Gastrointestinal Disorders)

Styptic

(See Astringent)

Sudoforic

(See Diaphoretic)

Sunburn

(See Burns)

Swelling

Alumroot
Angelica
Balm of Gilead
Black snakeroot
Blue flag
Burdock
Caraway
Catmint
Chamomile
Chickweed
Cup plant
Dill
Elderberry
Fennel
Feverfew
Garlic
Goldenrod
Gum plant
Hemlock
Hepatica
Hercules' club
Hops
Horsemint
Jack-in-the-pulpit
Jewelweed
Mallow
Mayapple
Milkweed
Mullein
New Jersey tea
Oak
Oregano
Ox-eye daisy
Parsley
Plantain
Poke
Pot marigold
Peppermint-Spearmint
Prickly ash
Queen Anne's lace
Red cedar
Rosemary
Rumex
Sarsaparilla
Scented mayweed
Seneca snakeroot
Smartweed
Skunk cabbage
Solomon's seal
Stoneroot
Sumac
Sunflower

Sweet ciceley
Sweet flag
Sweet violet
Tansy
Thyme
Trillium
Virginia snakeroot
Water hemlock
White pond lily
Wild coffee
Wild geranium
Wild ginger
Wild indigo
Wintergreen
Witch hazel
White pond lily
Wood sorrel
Wormwood
Yarrow

Syphilis
(See Venereal Diseases)

Thrush
(See Anti-fungal)

Thyroid
Horsenettle
Stinging nettle

Tonic
(See Alterative)

Tonsillitis
(See Gargle - Sore throat)

Toothache
Angelica
Asparagus
Balm of Gilead
Blackberry-Raspberry
Bittersweet nightshade
Blue cohosh
Butternut
Caraway
Coneflower
Coriander
Dogwood
Elderberry
Fennel
Feverfew
Garlic
Hercules' club
Hollyhock
Hops
Lavender
Mustard
New Jersey tea
Oregano
Plantain
Pennyroyal
Pot marigold
Prickly ash
Rattlesnake master
Rosemary

Scented mayweed
Slippery elm
Skunk cabbage
St. Johnswort
Sweet ciceley
Sweet flag
Tansy
Virginia snakeroot
Walnut
Wild geranium
Wild indigo
Wild strawberry
Wild yam
Yarrow

Tuberculosis
Birch
Bittersweet
Elecampane
Ginseng
Goldenrod
Hercules' club
Horehound
Jack-in-the-pulpit
Mustard
Prickly ash
St. Johnswort
Prickly ash
Red cedar
Tansy
White pond lily
Wild strawberry
Witch hazel

Tumors
(See Cancer)

Typhoid
Boneset
Lavender
Sweet flag

Ulcers - Internal
(See Demulcent)

Urinary Disorders
(Bladder, Kidney, Gravel, Stones)
Alfalfa
Amaranth
Angelica
Asparagus
Arrowhead
Balm of Gilead
Bearberry
Birch
Bittersweet
Blackberry-Raspberry
Black cohosh
Black snakeroot
Blue cohosh
Blue iris
Boneset
Borage
Burdock

Cattail
Chickweed
Chicory
Comfrey
Couchgrass
Dogwood
Dandelion
Dayflower
Devil's shoe string
Dutchman's breeches
Elderberry
Elecampane
False Solomon's seal
Fennel
Feverfew
Fleabane
Goldenrod
Goldenseal
Ground ivy
Gum plant
Hawthorn
Hepatica
Hercules' club
Honeysuckle
Hops
Horsemint
Horseradish
Horsetail
Indian hemp
Lavender
Maize
Marijuana
Mallow
Mayapple
Mugwort
Mullein
Oak
Onion
Parsley
Pennyroyal
Peppermint-Spearmint
Plantain
Poke
Prickly pear
Pumpkin
Queen Anne's lace
Rattlesnake master
Red cedar
Rose
Sarsaparilla
Sassafras
Self-heal
Shepherd's purse
Slippery elm
Smartweed
Solomon's seal
Spikenard
Stinging nettle
Stoneroot
Sumac

Sweet ciceley
Sweet violet
Tansy
Thyme
Toadflax
Virginia snakeroot
Watercress
White pond lily
White snakeroot
Wild black cherry
Wild coffee
Wild hyssop
Wild kidney bean
Wild plum
Wild strawberry
Wintergreen
Yarrow
Willow
Wormwood

Venereal diseases
(Gonorrhea, Syphilis)
Alumroot
Balm of Gilead
Birch
Bittersweet nightshade
Boneset
Burdock
Cattail
Chickweed
Coneflower
Dayflower

Devil's shoe string
Dutchman's breeches
Goldenrod
Goldenseal
Gum plant
Hemlock
Hercules' club
Hops
Horsenettle
Horsetail
Indian hemp
Indian physic
Indian tobacco
Maize
Mallow
Marijuana
Milkweed
Moonseed
Mugwort
New Jersey tea
Parsley
Peppermint-Spearmint
Plantain
Poke
Prickly ash
Rattlesnake master
Red cedar
Rumex
Sage
Sarsaparilla
Seneca snakeroot

Soapwort
Spikenard
St. Johnswort
Sweet ciceley
Sweet violet
Sumac
Twinleaf
White pond lily
Wild indigo
Wild strawberry
Wild yam
Wintergreen
Willow
Yarrow

Vermifuge
(See Anthelmintic)
Vulnerary
(See Antiseptic)
Whooping cough - Pertussis
Burdock
Catmint
Cattail
Clover
Indian hemp
Indian tobacco
Pennyroyal
Rattlesnake master
Red cedar
Skunk cabbage
Wild ginger

Appendix III: Medicinal Plants By Plant Family

(* Indicates Cultivated Plant)

Alismaceae
  Arrowhead
Amaranthaceae
  Amaranth
Anacardiaceae
  Sumac
Apiaceae
  Angelica
  Black snakeroot
  Caraway*
  Celery*
  Coriander*
  Dill*
  Fennel*
  Dogwood
  Fennel*
  Hemlock
  Parsley*
  Rattlesnake master
  Water hemlock
  Queen Anne's Lace
  Sweet ciceley
Apocynaceae
  Indian hemp
  Periwinkle
Araceae
  Jack-in-the-pulpit
  Skunk cabbage
  Sweet flag
Araliaceae
  Ginseng
  Hercules' club
  Spikenard
Aristolochiaceae
  Virginia snakeroot
  Wild ginger
Asteraceae
  Blessed thistle
  Boneset
  Burdock
  Chamomile*
  Chicory
  Compass plant
  Coneflower
  Cornflower
  Cup-plant
  Dandelion
  Elecampane
  Fleabane
  Feverfew
  Goldenrod

Gum plant
Joe-Pye weed
Milk thistle
Mugwort
Ox-eye daisy
Pot marigold*
Scented mayweed*
Sunflower*
Tansy
Tarragon*
White sage
White snakeroot
Wild lettuce
Wormwood
Yarrow
Asclepiadaceae
  Pleurisy root
Balsaminaceae
  Jewelweed
Berberidaceae
  Barberry
  Black cohosh
  Mayapple
  Twinleaf
Betulaceae
  Birch
Boraginaceae
  Borage
  Comfrey
Brassicaceae
  Horseradish
  Mustard
  Shepherd's purse
  Watercress
Cactaceae
  Prickly pear
Campanulaceae
  Indian tobacco
Cannabaceae
  Hops
  Marijuana
Caprifoliaceae
  Crampbark
  Elderberry
  Honeysuckle
  Wild coffee
Caryophyllaceae
  Chickweed
  Soapwort
Celastraceae
  Bittersweet

Chenopodiaceae
  Mexican tea
  Smartweed
Commelinaceae
  Dayflower
Cucurbitaceae
  Pumpkin*
Cupressaceae
  Red cedar
Discoroceae
  Wild yam
Ericaceae
  Bearberry
  Wintergreen
Equisetaceae
  Horsetail
Euphorbiaceae
  Castor bean*
  Indian physic
Fabaceae
  Alfalfa*
  Bush clover
  Clover
  Devil's shoe string
  Kentucky coffee tree
  Melilot
  Senna
  Wild indigo
Fagaceae
  Oak
Geraniaceae
  Wild geranium
Graminaceae
  Maize*
Hamamelidaceae
  Witch hazel
Hypericaceae
  St. Johnswort
Iridaceae
  Blue flag
  Saffron*
Juglandaceae
  Butternut
  Walnut
Laminaceae
  Basil*
  Catmint
  Ground ivy
  Horehound
  Horsemint

Lavender*
Motherwort
Oregano*
Pennyroyal
Peppermint-spearmint*
Rosemary*
Sage*
Self-heal
Stoneroot
Thyme*

Lauraceae
Sassafras
Spicebush

Liliaceae
Asparagus*
False Solomon's seal
Garlic*
Lily of the Valley
Onion*
Sarsaparilla
Solomon's seal
Trillium
Wild garlic

Malvaceae
Hollyhock
Malva

Menispermaceae
Moonseed

Menyanthaceae
Buckbean

Nyphaeceae
White pond lily

Onagraceae
Evening primrose

Oxalidaceae
Wood sorrel

Paeoniaceae
Peony*

Papaveraceae
Bloodroot
Dutchman breeches

Papilionaceae
Fenugreek*

Passifloraceae
Passion flower

Phytolaccaceae
Poke

Pinaceae
Scotch pine*

Plantaginaceae
Plantain

Poaceae
Quack grass

Polygalaceae
Seneca snakeroot

Polygonaceae
Rumex

Polypodiaceae
Bracken fern

Ranuculaceae
Black cohosh
Buttercup
Goldenseal
Hepatica

Rhamnaceae
New Jersey tea

Rosaceae
Blackberry-raspberry
Hawthorn
Rose*
Wild black cherry

Wild plum*
Wild strawberry

Rutaceae
Prickly ash

Salicaceae
Balm of Gilead
Willow

Saxifragaceae
Alumroot

Scrophulariaceae
Culver's root
Foxglove
Mullein
Toadflax
Turtlehead

Solonaceae
Bittersweet nightshade
Henbane*
Horsenettle
Jimsonweed
Pepper*

Typhaceae
Cattail

Ulmaceae
Slippery elm

Urticaceae
Stinging nettle

Valerianaceae
Valerian

Verbenaceae
Wild hyssop

Violaceae
Sweet violet
Wild pansy

Appendix IV: Botanical Terms

Achene - A small, dry, one-seeded fruit that does not split open when ripe to release the seed.

Annual - A plant that completes a cycle of development from germination of the seed through flowering and death in a single growing season.

Axil - The angle between the petiole of a leaf or branch and the stem from which it grows.

Bark - The outer covering of a woody stem or root.

Berry - A simple fleshy or pulpy fruit with one or more carpels and seeds

Biennial - A plant that requires two seasons to complete the growth cycle from germination of seed through flowering and death.

Bract - A small, modified leaf which forms either on the flower stalk or a part of the flower head. Bracts are often mistakenly referred to as flowers.

Bud - A miniature shoot, leaf or flowers; also a partially opened leaf or flower.

Bulb - An underground storage organ with fleshy leaves and a shortened stem, the whole enclosing next year's bud

Calyx - The sepals collectively; outermost flower whorl.

Capsule - A dry fruit with one or more seeds which splits open when ripe by pores or slits, but not down one side (a follicle) or down two sides (a pod).

Carpel - A part of the female organ (pistil) of a flower consisting of the stigma, style, ovary with ovules; there may be more than one carpel either joined (partitional ovary) or separate.

Catkin - A downy or scaly spike of flowers produced by certain plants. An example is the pussy on the willow.

Composite - A flower actually made of many separate flowers, complete of themselves, which are united in a single head (characteristic of the Asteraceae or daisy family).

Corm - The short, underground bulb-like base of a stem that lasts one year; the next year's growth grows at the top of the old one.

Corolla - Petals collectively; usually the conspicuous colored flower whorl.

Deciduous - A tree or shrub that produces a new set of leaves for each growing season, dropping them in the fall.

Drupe - A simple, fleshy fruit usually derived from a single carpel with one seed, in which the exocarp (outer layer of the fruit wall) is thin, the mesocarp (middle layer of the fruit wall) is fleshy, and the endocarp (inner layer of the fruit wall) is a stone.

Essential oil - A volatile oil present in aromatic plants, usually containing terpenoid substances.

Flavonoid - Any of a group of organic pigments found in plants derived from flavones and related substances, often associated with glycosides.

Follicle - A dry fruit that contains one or more seeds and splits down only one side when ripe.

Furrows - Longitudinal channels or grooves.

Glaucous - Covered with a fine, white, often waxy film that easily rubs off.

Glycoside - One of a group of plant substances containing a carbohydrate molecule that can be converted into a sugar and a non-sugar component.

Leaflet - A subdivision of a compound leaf.

Lobed - Leaves divided towards the midrib, but not into separate leaflets, with each division rounded at the apex.

Mericarp - A one-seeded part of a multi-seeded dry fruit (schizocarp).

Midrib - The central vein of a leaf, usually thickened and conspicuous.

Monoecious - Separate male and female flowers on the same plant.

Mucilage - A slimy complex gelatinous carbohydrate secreted by certain plants.

Nut - A dry, one-seeded fruit with a hard, woody outer covering that does not split open when ripe.

Node - A point on a stem where a leaf (or leaves) arises.

Obovate - A leaf that is oval, but broader toward the apex.

Palmate - Comprised of more than three leaflets or veins arising from the same point.

Panicle - A branching flower group with branches that are usually racemes: i.e., an unbranched, elongated flower grouping with the individual flowers on distinct stalks.

Pectin - One of a group of acid polysaccharides found in plants; in the right conditions they form gels with sugar.

Perennial - A plant which continues a cycle of new growth and flowering for many seasons between germination of the seed and death.

Pinnate - A compound leaf with three or more pairs of leaflets arranged in two opposite rows along a common stalk; there may be an unpaired terminal leaflet (odd-pinnate).

Pistil - The female organ of a flower, consisting of the ovary, the style and the stigma which develop into the fruit after fertilization.

Pod - A dry, many-sided, long, cylindrical fruit that splits open down both sides.

Pollen - The powdery substance produced by the anthers of a flowering plant.

Raceme - A single clustering of flowers on nearly equal length stalks along a stem with the lowest flowers blooming first and the youngest blooming at the top.

Receptacle - The cup-shaped, conical or flat uppermost part of the stem bearing the flower parts.

Rhizome - An elongated, thickened, usually horizontal, underground plant stem which sends out roots below and shoots above. It is differentiated from ordinary rootstock by the presence of nodes, buds and occasionally scale-like leaves. (From the Greek word meaning root).

Saponin - Any of a group of plant glycosides that produce a soapy foam in water.

Scale - Thin, dry structure, usually a modified leaf.

Schizocarp - A dry, many-seeded fruit that splits when ripe into one-seeded parts (mericarps).

Sepal - The outer flower leaf (usually green); the sepals collectively form the calyx.

Serration - Sawlike tooth. Many herbs have serrated leaves.

Sessile - A term referring to leaves and flowers that have no stalk.

Silicula (silique) - A pod, less than three times as long as broad, found in the Crucifer family (Cruciferae).

Spadix - A spike with a thick, fleshy stem usually enclosed in a spathe.

Spathe - A bract- or petal-like sheath enclosing one or more flowers, usually a spadix.

Stigma - The sticky or feathery tip of the pistil which receives the pollen.

Stipule - A small leaf- or scale-like appendage at the base of the leaf stalk.

Stalon - A slender, short-lived creeping stem that grows along the surface or below ground and takes root at the nodes to form new plants.

Subshrub - A plant with a stem that is mostly herbaceous, but woody at the base.

Tannin - One of a group of complex compounds found in many plants containing acids, phenols and glycosides.

Taproot - The main root which grows vertically downward and bears smaller lateral roots.

Tendril - A slender, clasping, twining organ (a modified leaf or branch) often formed from the stem, leaf or leaf stalk.

Terminal - The end of a stem or branch.

Thorn - A sharp-tipped woody structure formed from a modified branch.

Trifoliate - A leaf with three leaflets or lobes.

Tuber - An enlarged part of a root or underground stem. The potato is perhaps the most familiar tuber.

Umbel - A cluster of flowers formed by stalks of nearly equal length sprouting from a common center. The individual flowers form a flat or nearly flat surface (characteristic of the Apiaceae or carrot family).

Vein - A strand of strengthening and conducting tissue running through a leaf. The arrangement of the veins (venation) take one of several forms: i.e., the veins may form a network (net venation); be in a parallel (parallel venation); or, arise from the same point (palmate venation).

Volatile oil - An essential oil.

Appendix V: Medical Terms

Abortifacient - A substance that induces abortion.

Active constituent - A medicinally effective chemical substance, that is, a principle substance that promotes certain effects.

Acute - Rapid onset, intense severity of a disease and of brief duration.

Ague - A fever of the malarial type characterized by chills, fever and sweating at regular intervals.

Alkaloid - A large varied group of complex nitrogen-containing compounds that react with acids to form soluble salts, many of which have physiological effects on humans.

Alterative - A substance capable of favorably altering or changing unhealthy conditions of the body and tending to restore normal bodily function.

Amenorrhea - Cessation of menstruation.

Anemia - A deficiency in the number of red blood cells or in the quantity of oxygen-carrying hemoglobin in those cells: i.e., thin blood.

Analgesic - A substance that allays pain without causing loss of consciousness.

Anaphrodisiac - A substance that lessens sexual function and desire.

Anesthetic - A substance that produces loss of sensation without loss of vital function.

Anodyne - A substance that relieves pain (analgesic).

Antibiotic - A substance produced by or derived from a microorganism that kills or inhibits the growth of other microorganisms.

Anti-coagulant - A substance that prevents the formation of a clot.

Anti-convulsant - A substance that reduces or relieves convulsions or cramps.

Anti-diabetic - A substance that prevents or relieves diabetes.

Anti-diaphoretic - A substance that checks excessive perspiration.

Anti-diarrheal - A substance that combats diarrhea.

Antidote - A substance that counteracts the effects of a poison.

Anti-emetic - A substance that relieves nausea and vomiting.

Anthelmintic - A substance used to eliminate or destroy parasitic intestinal worms. Also called vermifuges.

Anti-hydrotic - An agent that checks perspiration by reducing the action of the sweat glands (the opposite of diaphoretic).

Anti-inflammatory - A substance that counteracts inflammation.

Anti-neuralgia - A substance that counteracts the stabbing pain along the course of one or more nerves.

Anti-periodic - A substance that prevents the periodic return of attacks of diseases, such as malaria.

Anti-pyretic - A substance that reduces or prevents fever. Also referred to as febrifuges.

Anti-scorbutic - A remedy for scurvy, usually a substance that supplies vitamin C.

Antiseptic - A substance that inhibits or destroys the growth of infection-causing microorganisms.

Antispasmodic - A substance used to prevent or ease muscular spasms or convulsions.

Antitussive - A substance that prevents or relieves coughs.

Aperient - Gentle laxative.

Aphrodisiac - A substance that provokes or excites sexual function and desire.

Appetizer - A substance that stimulates the appetite.

Aromatic - A plant or medicine with a fragrant, spicy smell and often a pleasant, pungent taste, used to mask less pleasant drugs.

Arrhythmia - Any deviation from the normal rhythm of the heart.

Arteriosclerosis - Hardening and constriction of the arteries.

Arthritis - Inflammation of the joints, characterized by swelling, stiffness, pain and restricted mobility.

Asthma - A condition characterized by difficulty in breathing and exhaling.

Astringent - A substance that causes contraction of the tissues and stops bleeding.

Bactericide - A substance that destroys bacteria.

Bitter tonic - A substance with an acrid, astringent or disagreeable taste which stimulates the flow of saliva and gastric juices. Such tonics are taken to increase the appetite and aid the digestive process.

Bright's Disease - Nephritis. Acute or chronic local renal dysfunction with degenerative kidney lesions, edema, hypertension and nitrogen retention.

Bronchitis - Inflammation of the air passages characterized by coughing and the production of mucus.

Bruise - 1) An injury, especially one produced by a blow or collision, that does not break the surface of the skin but by rupturing small blood vessels near the surface, causes blood to flow into the tissues, which results in discoloration; or, 2) crushing or mangling the tissues of a plant to release its properties.

Calmative - A substance that has a mild sedative action.

Cardiac - A substance that acts on the heart.

Caries - Tooth decay.

Carminative - An agent which checks the formation of gas and helps to expel whatever gas has already formed; relieves colic or flatulence.

Catarrh - An inflammation of a mucous membrane (usually of the nasal and air passages) characterized by congestion and the secretion of mucus.

Cathartic - An agent used to encourage the evacuation of the bowel (a laxative or purgative). A laxative is a gentle cathartic, while a purgative is more forceful and is used for severe constipation.

Cerebral Depressant - A substance used to depress the vital activity of the brain.

Cerebral Excitant - A substance used to stimulate the vital activity of the brain.

Chilblains - Poor circulation of the extremities caused by prolonged or repeated exposure to cold insufficient to freeze the tissue. The condition may reoccur in the same areas of the body at the onset of colder winter weather.

Cholagogue - A substance which promotes the discharge of bile from the gall bladder and bile ducts into the duodenum.

Cholecystitis - An inflammatory disease of the gallbladder and bile ducts.

Choleretic - A substance that stimulates the production of bile in the liver.

Chronic - Of long duration involving very slow changes.

Colic - Paroxysmal pain in the abdomen or bowel due to over-distention, toxemia, inflammation or obstruction.

Coma - A state of deep unconsciousness.

Compress - A wet or dry, hot or cold pad of material with or without medication applied with pressure to the affected part of the body.

Conjunctivitis - Inflammation of the mucous membrane (conjunctiva) that covers the front of the eye and lines the inside of the eyelids.

Convulsions - A violent involuntary contraction of the muscles.

Counter irritant - A substance used to produce superficial inflammation of the skin in order to relieve a deeper inflammation (rubefacient).

Cramp - A painful spasmodic contraction of the muscles.

Crohn's Disease - Regional enteritis of the intestines (ulcer, abscess and fistula formation).

Decoction - A liquid preparation made by boiling a medicinal plant with water, usually one part plant to twenty parts water, boiled in a covered nonmetal container for about fifteen minutes.

Demulcent - A medicinal liquid of a bland nature taken internally to soothe inflamed mucous surfaces and to protect them from irritation.

Deodorant - A substance used to inhibit or mask unpleasant odors.

Depressant - A substance that reduces exaggerated functional activity of the tissues.

Detergent - A substance used for cleansing.

Diabetes - A disorder of carbohydrate metabolism in which sugars in the body are not oxidized to produce energy because of the lack of the pancreatic hormone insulin.

Diaphoretic - A substance taken internally to promote sweating; it increases perspiration.

Diarrhea - An abnormal increase in the frequency of intestinal evacuations characterized by their fluid consistency.

Digestive - A substance that aids digestion.

Disinfectant - A substance used to free another substance or area of the body from infection by destroying the microorganisms that cause disease.

Diuretic - A substance that increases the volume and flow of urine, thereby cleansing the excretory system.

Dropsy - An abnormal accumulation of fluid in the body: edema.

Dysentery - An inflammation of the colon marked by intense diarrhea with the passage of small amounts of mucus and blood, usually caused by pathogenic bacteria or protozoans.

Dysmenorrhea - Painful menstruation.

Dyspepsia - A condition of disturbed digestion characterized by nausea, heartburn, pain, and gas.

Eczema - Inflammation of the skin accompanied by itching, redness and weeping from the pores.

Elixir - A sweetened aromatic preparation, about twenty-five percent alcohol, used as a vehicle for medicinal substances for its flavoring or medicinal qualities.

Emetic - A substance used to induce vomiting.

Emmenagogue - A substance that promotes or stimulates menstrual flow: once a euphemism for an abortifacient.

Emollient - A substance applied externally to soothe, soften or protect the skin.

Emulsion - A preparation composed of totally non-homogenous substances that are intimately mixed, causing one to be suspended in the other. An example is the oil and egg in mayonnaise.

Enema - A rectal injection of liquid, often used to encourage the evacuation of the bowels.

Erysipelas - Acute group A streptococcal infection of the skin (St. Anthony's Fire).

Enteritis - Internal inflammation.

Essence - A solution of an essential oil in alcohol.

Estrogenic - A substance that induces female hormonal activity.

Excretory - Concerned with the process of elimination of waste products through urine and sweat.

Expectorant - A substance that stimulate the formation and expulsion of mucus from the respiratory tract.

Extract - A concentrated preparation of the active constituents of a plant or animal drug obtained by evaporating a solution of the drug in water, alcohol or ether.

Exudate - The liquid that oozes from an inflamed area. Also the products, such as gums, resins and mucilages, formed in the metabolical processes of a number of plants.

Febrifuge - A substance that reduces or prevents fevers.

Flatulence - Gas in the stomach or bowels.

Flux - Excessive flow of any body secretion.

Galactagogue - A substance that promotes or increases the secretion of milk.

Gastritis - Inflammation of the lining of the stomach.

Gastroenteritis - Inflammation of the stomach and small intestine, usually causing vomiting and diarrhea.

Germicide - A substance that kills bacteria and other microorganisms.

Gout - A metabolic disease characterized by painful inflammation of certain joints caused by deposits of uric acid in them.

Gravel - Small stones formed in the urinary tract which are passed with the urine.

Hallucination - A false perception of something that is not present.

Hallucinogen - A substance that produces hallucinations.

Hemolysis - The destruction of red blood cells.

Hemorrhage - Profuse internal or external bleeding.

Hemorrhoids - Enlarged veins in the wall of the anus; sometimes known as piles.

Hemostatic - A substance that arrests bleeding and hemorrhages.

Hepatic - A substance which affects the liver (harmful or helpful).

Hepatitis - Inflammation of the liver.

Homeopathy - A method of medical treatment (founded by Samuel Hahnemaun in the late 1700s) where very small amounts of drugs are administered, producing in the body symptoms similar to those of the disease.

Hydrating - Having the capacity to maintain or restore the normal proportion of fluid in the body or skin. Hydrating agents are used in cosmetics to keep the skin moist, firm and young looking.

Hypnotic - A drug or other agent that produces or tends to produce sleep without disturbing alertness and receptiveness to others.

Immunostimulant - A substance that stimulates various functions or activities of the immune system.

Influenza (Flu) - A viral infection involving the respiratory tract.

Infusion - The extraction of the active properties of a substance by steeping or soaking it, usually in water.

Inhalant - A substance used to treat illnesses by inhaling medicinals rather than injecting or drinking them.

Insecticide - A substance that kills insects.

Insomnia - The chronic inability to fall asleep or to remain asleep for an adequate amount of time.

Irritant - A substance that produces irritation or inflammation of the skin or internal tissue.

Laxative - A substance that loosens the bowels and eases constipation.

Liniment - A medicinal substance, thinner than an ointment, that is gently rubbed into the skin for relief from the pain of sprains and bruises.

Liqueur - A solution of medicinal substances in water as distinguished from a tincture, which is a solution in alcohol.

Locomotor ataxia - Symptom of Tabes Dorsalis, a chronic degenerative disease involving the sensory roots of the spinal cord. It results in an impaired gait in walking.

Lotion - A medicinal solution for external application to the body.

Lozenge - A small flat candy, variously flavored and sometimes medicated.

Medicinal - Any substance used for treating disease.

Mitogenic - A substance that affects cell division.

Moxa - A dried herb that is burned on or above the skin to stimulate an acupuncture point or serve as a counter-irritant. A famous technique of traditional Chinese medicine using dried mugwort (*Artemisia vulgaris*) leaves.

Mucilaginous - Mucus-like (slimy, sticky) substance which offers a soothing quality to inflamed parts.

Mucus - A slimy protective secretion of the mucous membranes consisting chiefly of glycoproteins.

Narcotic - A drug that in moderate doses allays sensibility, relieves pain and induces sleep, but if misused, or taken in large doses, is poisonous to the system.

Nausea. A feeling of sickness in the stomach (queasy stomach).

Nephritis - Inflammation of the kidneys.

Neuralgia - A severe recurrent pain alone or on one or more nerves, usually not associated with changes in nerve structure.

Nervine - A substance that calms or soothes nervousness, tension or excitement.

Panacea - A substance that is basically a "cure-all" for any and all ailments.

Parasite - An organism that lives in or upon another organism, usually causing damage to the host organism.

Parasiticide - A substance that kills parasites.

Pectoral - A medicine for the chest.

Peritonitis - Inflammation of peritoneal (abdominal) cavity.

Plaster - A paste-like medicinal mixture which can be applied to the affected part of the body and is adhesive at body temperature.

Pleurisy - Inflammation of the covering of the lungs (pleura) resulting in pain when breathing and coughing.

Potpourri - A mixture of dried flowers and spices used for scent or perfume.

Poultice - A soft mass of fresh vegetable matter that has been crushed or soaked into a limber mass, usually heated then spread on cloth and applied to sores or inflamed area to supply warmth, relieve pain, or act as a counterirritant or antiseptic.

Purgative - A substance that causes vigorous evacuation of severely constipated bowels more quickly and forcefully than a laxative. Sometimes synonymous with cathartic.

Purge - To cleanse, rid of anything undesirable.

Purulent - Foul or puslike.

Rheumatism - An ailment characterized by stiffness, aches and pains of the joints or muscles.

Rubefacient - A substance which, when rubbed into the skin, reddens the skin by attracting blood to the area.

Sachet - A small bag of powdered flowers used in drawers and closets to scent clothes.

Salve - A healing or soothing ointment.

Saponin - A glycoside compound common in plants, which when shaken with water, has a foaming or "soapy" action.

Scrofula - A disease, once known as King's Evil, characterized by enlargement of the neck glands and eruptions that are susceptible to infections.

Scurvy - A disease resulting from impaired nutrition, especially a vitamin C deficiency.

Sedative - A substance that tends to calm, relieve anxiety and tension; it may cause drowsiness.

Spleenosis - An inflammatory disease that affects the spleen.

Stimulant - A substance which increases or quickens the various functional actions of the body, such as quickening digestion, raising body temperature, etc.

Stomachic - A medicine which gives strength and tone to the stomach or stimulates the appetite by promoting digestive secretions.

Stomatitis - Inflammation of the mucous lining (mucosa) of the mouth.

Styptic - A substance that checks hemorrhage.

Sudiforic - A substance that induces sweating. (See diaphoretic.)

Tea - An infusion prepared by pouring boiling water over an herb (one teaspoon to eight ounces water), steeping it in a covered nonmetal container and straining it. Used medicinally or as a beverage.

Tincture - An alcoholic solution of medicinal substances, usually fifty percent alcohol.

Tonic - A substance that stimulated and invigorates the body or an organ.

Toxic - Poisonous.

Tranquilizer - A substance that has a calming effect, relieving anxiety and tension; less likely to cause drowsiness than a sedative.

Urolith - A stone in the urinary tract.

Vermifuge - An agent that destroys or expels parasitic worms. Also called anthelmintic.

Vitamin - One of a group of unrelated substances that are essential in trace amounts for healthy growth and development; they cannot be synthesized in the body but occur naturally in certain plant and animal foods.

Vulnerary - A substance that counteracts inflammation and promotes the healing of wounds.

Whites - A lay term for leucorrhea, an inflammation of the uterine or vaginal mucosa characterized by a white or yellowish discharge from the vagina.

Bibliography

Balls, Edward K. 1962. *Early Uses of California Plants*. University of California Press, Berkeley Press, Los Angeles, Calif.

Biederman, Hans. 1979. *Medicina Magica: Metaphysical Healing Methods in Late-Antique and Medieval Manuscripts*. Gryphin Editions, Inc., Birmingham, Ala.

Bradford, Angier. 1978. *Field Guide to Medicinal Wild Plants*. Stackpole Books, Harrisburg, Pa.

Brill, S. and S. Dean. 1994. *Identifying and Harvesting Edible and Medicinal Plants in the Wild (and Not So Wild) Places*. Hearst Books, New York, N.Y.

Bunney, Sarah, ed. 1984. *Illustrated Encyclopedia of Herbs: Their Medicinal and Culinary Uses*. Barnes and Noble Books, New York, N.Y.

Casteneda, Carlos. 1968. *The Teaching of Don Yuan: A Yaqui Way of Knowledge*. Ballantine Books, New York, N.Y.

Cool, N. 1979. *Using Plants for Healing: An American Herbal*. Rodale Press, Emmaus, Pa.

Dispensatory of the United States of America, 23rd edition, J. B. Lippicott Company, Pennsylvania.

Duke, James A. 1992. *Handbook of Edible Weeds*. CRC Press, Boca Raton, Fla.

Duke, James A. 1985. *CRC Handbook of Medicinal Herbs*. CRC Press, Boca Raton, Fla.

Erickson-Brown, C. 1989. *Medicinal and Other Uses of North American Plants: A historical survey with special reference to the Eastern Indian Tribes*. Dover Publishing, New York, N.Y.

Fielder, M. 1975. *Plant Medicine and Folklore*. Winchester Press, New York.

Foster, S. 1984. *Herbal Botany: The Gentle Art of Herb Culture*. Peregrive Smith Books, Salt Lake City, Utah.

Foster, S. and Duke, J. A. 1990. *A Field Guide to Medicinal Plants*. Houghton Mifflin Company, Boston, Mass.

Gilmore, Melvin 1977. *Uses of Plants by Indians of the Missouri River Region*. University Press of Nebraska, Lincoln, Neb.

Grieve, M. 1974. *A Modern Herbal*: Vol 1 & 2. Dover Publication, Inc., New York, N.Y.
Grigson, G. 1975. *The Englishman's Flora*. Paladin, St. Albons, United Kingdom.

Grime, W.E. 1979. *Ethno-botany of the Black American*. Reference Publ., Algonac, Mich.

Gunther, Robert T. 1959. *The Greek Herbal of Dioscorides*. Hafner Publisher, New York, N.Y.

Haragan, P.D. 1991. *Weeds of Kentucky and Adjacent States: A Field Guide*. University Press of Kentucky, Lexington, Ky.

Hartwell, J.A. 1982. *Plants Used Against Cancer: A Survey*. Quarterman Publications, Inc., Lawrence, Mass.

Hultman, G.G. 1978. *Trees, Shrubs, and Flowers of the Midwest*. Contemporary Books, Inc., Chicago, Ill.

Hutchens, A.R. 1992. *A Handbook of Native American Herbs*. Shambhala, Boston. Mass.

Leliver, Ernest and Johanna Leliver. 1962. *Folklore and Odysseys of Food and Medicinal Plants*. Farrar Straues Giroux, New York, N.Y.

Kindscher, Kelly. 1992. *Medical Wild Plants of the Prairie*, University Press of Kansas, Kan.

Kowalchek, C. and H.W. Hylton, editors. 1987. *Rodale's Illustrated Encyclopedia of Herbs*. Rodale Press, Emmaus, Pa.

Krochmal, A., R.S. Walters and R.M. Doughty. 1971. *A Guide to Medicinal Plants of Appalachia*. Agricultural Handbook No. 400, Forest Service, U.S.D.A., Washington, D.C.

Krochmal, A. and C. Krochmal. 1973. *A Guide to the Medicinal Plants of the United States*. Quadrangle, The New York Times Book Co., New York, N.Y.

Lewis, W.H. and M.P.F Elvin-Lewis. 1977. *Medical Botany: Plants Affecting Man's Health*. John Wiley & Sons, New York, N.Y.

Mabey, R. 1988. *The New Age Herbalist*. Collier Books, MacMillan Publishing Co., New York, N.Y.

Meyer, Clarence. 1976. *The Herbalist*. Meyerbooks, Glenwood, Ill.

Mohlenbrock, R.H. 1975. *Guide to Vascular Flora of Illinois*. Southern Illinois University Press, Carbondale, Ill.

Millspaugh, C.F. 1971. *American Medicinal Plants*. Dover Publishers, Inc., New York, N.Y.

Passwater, R.A. 1981. Evening Primrose Oil: Its amazing nutrients and the health benefits they can give you. Keats Publ. Inc., New Canaan, Colo.

Peithman, I.M. 1955. *Indians of Southern Illinois*. Charles C. Thomas Pub., Springfield, Ill.

Pierce, R.V. 1885. *The People's Common Sense Medical Advisor*. World's Dispensery Medical Association, Buffalo, N.Y.

Pierce, R.V and Leo H. Smith. 1918. *The People's Common Sense Medical Advisor*. World's Dispensery Medical Association, Buffalo, N.Y.

Rafinesque, C.S. 1828. *Medical Flora or Manual of Medical Botany of the United States*, Vol. 1. Atkinson & Alexanders, Pennsylvania.

Rafinesque, C.S. 1830. *Medical Flora*, Vol. 2. Samual Atkinson, Pennsylvania.

Rose, Jeanne 1972 *Herbs and Things. Jeanne Rose's Herbal*. Grossel and Dunlop Workman Publ. Co., New York, N.Y.

Runkel, Sylvan T. and Alvin F. Bull. 1979. *Wild Flowers of Illinois Woodlands*. Wallace Homestead Book Co., Des Moines, Iowa.

Scully, Virginia. 1970. *A Treasury of American Indians Herbs*, Crown Press, New York, N.Y.

Snively, W.D. and L. Furbee. 1966. Discovery of the cause of milk sickness. J. American Medical Association 196:1055-1060.

Spellenberg, R. 1979. *The Audubon Society Field Guide to North American Wildflowers: Eastern Region*. Alfred A. Knopf, New York, N.Y.

Stary, F. 1994. *The Natural Guide to Medicinal Herbs and Plants*. Barnes & Noble Books, New York.

Tehon, Leo R. 1951. The Drug Plants of Illinois. Illinois Natural History Survey Circular 44:1-124.

Tucker, A.O., M.J. Maciarello, P.W. Burgage and G. Sturtz. 1994. Spicebush [Spicebush benzoin (L.) Blume var. benzoin, Lauraceae]: a tea, spice, and medicine. Economic Botany 48:333-336.

Vogel, Virgil. 1970. *American Indian Medicine*. University of Oklahoma Press, Norma, Okla.

Weiner, Michael A. 1972. *Earth Medicine - Earth Foods: Plant remedies, drugs and natural foods of North American Indians*. MacMillan Pub. Co., New York, N.Y.

Weiss, Gaea and Shandon Weiss. 1985. *Growing and Using Healing Herbs*. Rodale Press, Emmaus, Pa.

Werner, William, E., Jr. 1988. *Life and Lore of Illinois Wildflowers*. Illinois State Museum, Springfield, Ill.

Westland, Pamela. 1987. *The Encyclopedia of Herbs and Spices*. Marshall Cavandish Books Ltd., London.

Index of Medicinal Plants